P9-DDI-980

COSTS, RISKS, AND BENEFITS OF SURGERY

Costs, risks, and benefits of surgery

Edited by
JOHN P. BUNKER, M.D.
Professor of Anesthesia
and of Family, Community and Preventive Medicine
Stanford University School of Medicine

BENJAMIN A. BARNES, M.D.
Professor of Surgery
Tufts University School of Medicine

FREDERICK MOSTELLER, Ph.D.
Professor of Mathematical Statistics
Harvard University

New York
OXFORD UNIVERSITY PRESS
1977

Second printing, 1978

Library of Congress Catalogue Card Number 76-40739
Printed in the United States of America

Contributors

CLARK C. ABT, M.A., Ph.D.
Abt Associates, Inc., Cambridge, Massachusetts

BENJAMIN A. BARNES, M.D.
Department of Surgery, Tufts University Medical School
Interhospital Organ Bank, Boston
Board of Consultation, Massachusetts General Hospital

ERNEST M. BARSAMIAN, M.D.
Department of Surgery, Veterans Administration Hospital, West Roxbury, Massachusetts
Harvard Medical School

HENRIK H. BENDIXEN, M.D.
Department of Anesthesiology, Columbia University College of Physicians and Surgeons

JOHN P. BUNKER, M.D.
Departments of Anesthesia and of Family, Community and Preventive Medicine,
Stanford University School of Medicine

WILLIAM G. COCHRAN, M.A., LL.D. (honorary)
Department of Statistics, Harvard University

PERSI DIACONIS, M.A., Ph.D.
Department of Statistics, Stanford University

ALLAN DONNER, Ph.D.
Channing Laboratory and Department of Preventive and Social Medicine, Harvard Medical School

GARRY F. FITZPATRICK, M.D., F.R.C.S. (Canada)
Department of Surgery, University of Massachusetts Medical School

MAURICE S. FOX, Ph.D.
Department of Biology, Massachusetts Institute of Technology

JOHN P. GILBERT, S.M., Ph.D.
Office of Information Technology, Harvard University
Department of Anesthesia (Biostatistics), Massachusetts General Hospital

ALAN GITTELSOHN, Ph.D.
Department of Biostatistics, The Johns Hopkins School of Hygiene and Public Health

JERRY R. GREEN, Ph.D.
Department of Economics, Harvard University

PHILIP L. HENNEMAN, B.Sc.
Harvard Medical School

HOWARD H. HIATT, M.D.
Harvard School of Public Health

DAVID C. HOAGLIN, Ph.D.
Department of Statistics, Harvard University

BARBARA J. McNEIL, M.D., Ph.D.
Department of Radiology (Nuclear Medicine), Harvard Medical School and Peter Bent Brigham Hospital

BUCKNAM McPEEK, M.D.
Department of Anesthesia, Massachusetts General Hospital

KLIM McPHERSON, M.A., Ph.D.
Medical Statistics, Department of Social and Community Medicine, Oxford University

LILLIAN LIN MIAO, M.P.H.
Department of Statistics, Harvard University

FREDERICK MOSTELLER, Ph.D., D.Sc. (honorary)
Department of Statistics, Department of Psychology and Social Relations, and the Committee on Public Policy, John F. Kennedy School of Government, Harvard University

DUNCAN NEUHAUSER, Ph.D.
Department of Health Services, Harvard School of Public Health

RAYMOND NEUTRA, M.D., Dr. P.H.
Department of Preventive and Social Medicine, Harvard Medical School
Department of Epidemiology, Harvard School of Public Health

NICHOLAS E. O'CONNOR, M.D.
Department of Surgery, Harvard Medical School and the Peter Bent Brigham Hospital

OSLER L. PETERSON, M.D., M.P.H.
Department of Preventive and Social Medicine, Harvard Medical School

JOSEPH S. PLISKIN, Ph.D., S.M.
Faculty of Management, Leon Recanati Graduate School of Business Administration, Tel-Aviv University

NAVA PLISKIN, Ph.D., S.M.
Interdisciplinary Center for Technological Analysis and Forecasting, Tel-Aviv University

VICTOR M. ROSENOER, M.B., Ph.D., F.R.C.P., F.A.C.P.
Gastroenterological Research Unit, Lahey Clinic Foundation
Department of Medicine, Harvard Medical School

DONALD S. SHEPARD, M.P.P., Ph.D.
Center for the Analysis of Health Practices, Harvard School of Public Health
John F. Kennedy School of Government, Harvard University

WILLIAM B. STASON, M.D., S.M.
Center for the Analysis of Health Practices, Harvard School of Public Health

AMY K. TAYLOR, A.M., Ph.D.
Department of Economics, Harvard University
Center for the Analysis of Health Practices, Harvard School of Public Health

MILTON C. WEINSTEIN, M.P.P., Ph.D.
Center for the Analysis of Health Practices, Harvard School of Public Health
John F. Kennedy School of Government, Harvard University

JOHN E. WENNBERG, M.P.H., M.D.
Department of Preventive and Social Medicine, Harvard Medical School

RICHARD JAY ZECKHAUSER, Ph.D.
Committee on Public Policy, John F. Kennedy School of Government, Harvard University
Center for the Analysis of Health Practices, Harvard School of Public Health

Foreword

Almost since its beginning, the encounter between patient and surgeon has involved more than two people. With our growing capabilities, the participants have progressively increased to include not only many different specialists contributing to diagnosis and to technical aspects of the surgical procedure, but also those involved in the development and preparation of pharmaceuticals, blood products, and other essential materials, in the manufacture of highly specialized equipment, and in the construction and staffing of facilities required during treatment and recovery periods. The partnership between biology and medicine, which has helped elucidate our understanding of pathologic processes and often our approaches to them, has further widened the circle of people important to surgeon and patient.

Important deficiencies in other dimensions of surgical practice, however, have become increasingly apparent. For example, we require both better understanding of the natural history of diseases treated surgically and more accurate appraisal of the potential benefits and limitations of surgical interventions. We also need a fuller appreciation of the complexities and costs of modern surgical technology, particularly in the light of increasing demands on our resources and of a growing awareness of their limitations. What are the effects of surgical intervention on the quality of life and/or on life expectancy? How can we determine whether proposed new procedures represent improvements over present ones, or, indeed, that present procedures are more effective than doing nothing? What are the costs in lives, suffering, and money, attributable to alternative treatment plans, including doing nothing? Will the use of resources to undertake a given procedure require our giving up something else in its place, and if so, how shall we choose? What are the legal and ethical implications of what we do or propose to do?

Many fields of knowledge are required to address this panoply of questions—experts in the behavioral sciences, statistics, economics, decision analysis, law, ethics, engineering, management sciences, and others must join the surgeon in approaching a whole new range of questions. Almost always, the central figure involved must be the patient, whose appreciation of these complex matters must be sufficient so as to ensure his effective participation in the decision process. Behind the patient stands society and its increasing need to set priorities.

In the fall of 1972 Harvard's Center for the Analysis of Health Practices and its Department of Statistics, seeking to promote interactions between physicians and other professionals to improve the medical care process, joined to establish a Seminar in Health and Medicine. An immediate goal of attracting faculty and students from throughout Harvard University and its neighboring institutions was quickly achieved, thus demonstrating the widespread interest in medicine and health throughout the University community. Months elapsed, however, before the participants, more than one hundred, achieved a communality of understanding, language, and specific objectives, and before some nonphysicians came to appreciate the potential pitfalls of applying statistical, economic, legal, managerial, or other principles to the medical encounter in the absence of an understanding of the patient-doctor relationship. Many other professionals, including biologists and engineers, were stimulated to extend their interests to medical problems to meet new challenges. We, in medicine, achieved insights that had previously escaped most of us, not only in analyzing the results of experiments, but in better formulating the questions that needed asking. Further, our colleagues apprised us of previously unappreciated experimental methods and helped us to a broader understanding of questions asked, and perhaps more often, not asked by our patients. These interactions have already been extremely rewarding for the physicians and other professionals in the Seminar. It is not too soon to predict important benefits as well for society and for individual patients.

Costs, Risks, and Benefits of Surgery is the first major product to be "exported" by the Seminar. It represents the results of over two years of work by Drs. Bunker, Barnes, and Mosteller and their colleagues. Like the Seminar's several other study groups, the many authors of this volume initially met biweekly for a full evening. As enthusiasm grew, meetings were held weekly, and as the papers attest, much additional work went on between regularly scheduled sessions. The details of the operation of this Seminar group are instructive—some early participants dropped out, but the group grew in size as word spread of its activities. The participants came from many disciplines and shared a concern for assessing and improving medical care. Initially, a few papers were presented to facilitate group discussion. After the prepared papers had been repeatedly criticized and revised (and otherwise subjected to the Bunker-Barnes-Mosteller treatment), it became apparent that they would be extremely valuable to a much wider audience. Thus, the gently persuasive powers of the editors played a barely perceptible role in the group's decision to present their work in book form.

This volume is the first comprehensive treatment of surgery from the perspectives described in its title. As such, I believe it will prove of enormous value not only to the patient and his or her doctor contemplating surgical intervention for a specific problem, but to society and its decision-makers considering questions regarding resource allocation and priority setting. These latter decision-makers include the rapidly increasing numbers of managers, planners, and regulators who are charged with examining the quality and distribution of medical care, and for whom few specific and well-documented guidelines currently exist. For them, the book should prove a reference of great value. For medicine and society, it should serve as a paradigm for approaches to the several other areas of medical diagnosis and treatment where equally critical evaluation is urgently required.

Its authors hope that the volume will contribute to the realization of two long-range goals that were set for the Seminar and for the Center—to improve the care of the individual patient and to optimize benefits for society. In providing gratification for the participants involved in new partnerships, its preparation has already achieved a third.

I believe that the book will strengthen many patient-doctor relationships by facilitating decision-making on the basis of logic instead of, as is now too often the case, dogma. Of equal importance are the guidelines it offers the medical profession for exerting leadership in what has become a second critical interface—that between society and medicine. Drs. Bunker, Barnes, and Mosteller have taken a long step toward demonstrating how the physician and patient can call on others for help that will promote the benefits of all. Their efforts can serve as a model for dealing with problems that must be resolved as we struggle to ensure for all our people more equitable access to the benefits of medicine. If the medical profession responds to the challenge, the patient, society, and the practice of medicine will all, I am convinced, be the beneficiaries. If the profession turns its back on the opportunity and what I believe to be a major responsibility, the consequences will surely be government intervention and all the disadvantages that this will bring to the medical profession, the patient, and society.

Howard H. Hiatt

Preface

This book is written for physicians and surgeons, public health planners, policy analysts, faculty and students of medical schools, members of legislatures and their staffs, and others who ask, "How can we get the most from the resources we allocate to medical care?". As a start at answering this question, the authors have examined selected areas of surgical practice and research, using the methods of cost-benefit analysis and drawing heavily from decision analysis, statistics, and economic theory.

THE PROBLEM

Costs of medical care have accelerated rapidly, but the apparent improvement in the traditional indices of the health of the public in recent years has been modest. The national expenditure in the United States for health care in 1975 was $118.5 billion, an increase of 10 per cent over 1974, thus totaling 8.3 per cent of the gross national product. Per capita this amounts to an expenditure of $547 or about 10 per cent of the average personal income. For comparison, the shares of the gross national product in the federal budget allotted to national defense, education, and veterans benefits and services are, respectively, 5.6, 1.2, and 1.0 per cent.

With expenditures at this level, the public and its representatives in Congress naturally want to know what they receive in return—that is, how much do these large expenditures improve health. Unfortunately, we don't know. Life expectancy, one measure of health and certainly an important one, increased by three years between 1950 and 1973, while real per capita health expenditures* increased by a factor of two and a half during this period. This might be an acceptable return on the dollar if one could be sure that the improved life expectancy was a direct result of the investment. But we have no way of knowing how much of the effect is the result of medical care, and how much is the result of improved housing, improved nutrition, decrease in smoking, or other nonmedical factors known to have pronounced effects on how long we live. Moreover, a large proportion of medical expenditures is very properly intended to achieve goals other than increasing the length of life; these include relief of disability, discomfort, and disfigurement—that is, substantial improvement in the quality of life. Although improvement in quality of life would be a welcome benefit from this large health care expenditure, no credible data on this subject exist; we do not know whether quality of life is getting better or worse, or remaining the same.

The problem besets social programs in general, and the dearth of data for assessing social programs has been called by Elliot Richardson "a nearly fatal deficiency." Richardson believes that this deficiency can be corrected only "through rigorous evaluation; we cannot otherwise find out how well—or how poorly—a particular effort is succeeding. And only if we know this—and know also the effectiveness of an alternative approach to the same objective—can we compare the two. Only thus, moreover, can we judge the value of pursuing the objective at all versus that of devoting the same resources to some wholly different purpose."[2] It is in this spirit that the authors of this book have undertaken their assignments.

WHY SURGERY?

Modern surgery, with such techniques as cardiopulmonary bypass, organ transplantation, and total hip replacement, represents medical care at its greatest complexity and highest cost. The surgeon's successes are dramatic, but there are failures as well. This complexity of modern surgery, with the associated costs, risks, and benefits, has profound moral as well as economical implications, not only for the patients and their families, but also for the boards of trustees and hospital administrators providing the institutional environment. Additional problems arise for those responsible for the training of surgeons, anesthetists, and specialized paramedical personnel, as well as for the designers and manufacturers of appliances and instrumentation for modern medical care.

The expenses of all medical therapy, and surgical therapy in particular, put pressures on those who invent, manufacture, distribute, apply, and earn payment for providing surgical instrumentation, specialized anesthesia, expert intensive care, laboratory tests, diagnostic x-rays, and costly drugs. Inevitably, expensive therapy generates economic problems, and interests are created whose purposes may not always coincide or appear to coincide with those of the patient. Each quarter tries to justify its own particular contributions and charges.

*Increase in total expenditures corrected for price rise and population growth.[1]

But, in the end, it is the public that must pay the costs of therapy and judge the value it produces. Surgical therapy, because of its discreteness, accomplishments, and cost, appears to be particularly suited for cost-benefit analysis.

PLAN FOR THE BOOK

The book is divided into five parts. Part I, Background and General Principles, presents material to guide careful thinking, a task that frequently requires the aid of quantitative tools. Among the tools we introduce are conditional probability, decision trees, and economic analysis. These tools can contribute much to the formation of policy attitudes about the treatment of particular diseases. These attitudes in turn can help the medical profession develop standard methods of treatment from which the physician may deviate when a patient presents unusual manifestations of a disease or its complications. Thus, such analyses may help guide medical thinking without presuming to settle individual clinical decisions. The methods themselves will, for the most part, be of more permanent value than the applications or illustrations that we here draw from current experience.

In Part II, Surgical Innovation, the process of surgical innovation, in contrast to any specific innovations, is viewed in some detail. After illustrating the process of innovation through the analysis of historical and contemporary examples of surgical and anesthetic experience, we examine several instructive randomized controlled clinical trials. The examples chosen have distinctive features emphasizing both the power and the limitations of this type of validation of clinical therapy.

Part III, Assessment of Risks and Benefits by Decision Analysis: Established Procedures, scrutinizes a variety of operations. The selection of ambiguous situations is deliberate and provides instructive examples where a detailed consideration of cost-benefit analysis could be informative. For example, though many or most hysterectomies may be performed for widely accepted indications, those we consider are the troublesome minority for which the indications are marginal. Our attention to these particular situations should not be construed as opposition to the numerous operative innovations when indications are clearly defined and widely agreed upon. Indeed, cost-benefit analysis of many of these established operations would be a trivial and unnecessary application of the technique.

Part IV, Assessment of Risks and Benefits by Decision Analysis: New Procedures, directs attention to complicated and costly therapies including some of the most dramatic and brilliant extensions of medical care today. Although this Part emphasizes the mounting costs of the various treatments, it should not be inferred that all new procedures share this characteristic. Many therapeutic innovations that clearly are relatively inexpensive and highly successful would not be suitable for our analysis, because we are directing attention to the hard cases. Analysis of more costly forms of therapy is of special interest to national, state, local, and institutional policy. When the cost-benefit data seem firm and the medical process clear, these analyses help us think about each aspect of the treatment, as well as options and the cost. Society can then judge on an informed basis what resources it is willing to contribute. If the data are weak but the knowledge of the disease process firm, then special data gathering seems to be called for. If we do not understand the causes of the disease or its course, then basic medical research seems needed.

Finally in Part V, Summary Conclusions, and Recommendations, we make recommendations for further research and for education; the analyses presented herein are only a beginning, and a great deal remains to be done. We confidently anticipate that such future research will produce new and better analyses, including some that may overturn some of the findings in this book, and we look forward to such work as evidence of the book's success rather than its failure.

SOME CAVEATS FOR THE READER

Many discussions of the inefficiency and maldistribution of medical care will be familiar to the reader, for they appear frequently, even in the daily newspapers. Comfortable solutions in the past have been conspicuously infrequent; they will likely remain so in the future, partly because some of our goals are in conflict with one another, and partly because no one has shown that the "solutions" work. Only occasionally do articles suggest techniques designed to clarify our thinking about, instead of just proposing solutions for, social and medical problems.

Lest we seem to oversell the approach presented in this book, we offer a cautionary quotation from a National Academy of Sciences committee on making decisions of broad social implications in regulating the discharge of undesirable chemicals in the environment: "There is no objective scientific way of making decisions, nor is it likely that there ever will be. However, use of the techniques developed by decision theory and benefit-cost analysis can provide the decision maker with a useful framework and language for describing and discussing trade-offs, noncommensurability, and uncertainty. It can help to clarify the existence of alternatives, decision points, gaps in information, and value judgments concerning trade-offs. Furthermore, it should facilitate communication between the decision maker and his staff of analysts, and between the decision maker and the public."[3]

All told, then, the methods presented in this book are intended to create the atmosphere and provide a set of approaches that may be of continued value in reaching solutions for many surgical and medical problems. Specific chapters may be quickly outmoded, or be found to need revision. It is the thrust of the methods and the value of joining these ways of thinking to those commonly used by physicians that form a large part of what the reader should gain from this book. Other aspects, it is hoped, will contribute in concrete ways to the design of surgical research generally and to our understanding of medical issues in single diseases such as diagnosis and evaluation of therapy for the individual patient.

REFERENCES

1. Mueller MS, Gibson RM, National health expenditures, fiscal year 1975. Social Security Bulletin, 39:2 (February 1976), 12, 13

2. Richardson E, The Creative Balance: Government, Politics, and the Individual in America's Third Century. Holt, Rinehart and Winston, New York, 1976, p 138
3. Decision Making for Regulating Chemicals in the Environment. Committee on Principles of Decision Making for Regulating Chemicals in the Environment; Environmental Studies Board; Commission on Natural Resources, National Research Council-National Academy of Sciences, 1975, ISBN 0-309-02401-3.

Acknowledgments

The authors and editors acknowledge with gratitude the support of the Edna McConnell Clark Foundation through the Harvard Faculty Seminar in Health and Medicine, and of the Robert Wood Johnson Foundation through the Center for the Analysis of Health Practices at the Harvard School of Public Health. The seminars, on which this book is based, were initiated by Howard H. Hiatt and Frederick Mosteller and were sponsored jointly by the Center for the Analysis of Health Practices and by the Departments of Biostatistics and of Statistics. The chairs of the Harvard Faculty Seminar in Health and Medicine have been 1973-74: Frederick Mosteller, 1974-75: John P. Bunker, 1975-76: John Hedley-Whyte. The Seminar's Surgery Group, which is primarily responsible for this book, was chaired in 1973-75 by John P. Bunker, and in 1975-76 by Frederick Mosteller. The Seminar's Protocol Group, which contributed Chapter 11, was chaired by William G. Cochran. During the editing of the manuscript, Bunker was Guggenheim Fellow (1973-74) and Mosteller was Miller Research Professor, University of California at Berkeley (1974-75), and these posts enabled them to make substantial contributions to the development of the book. The work of Frederick Mosteller was also facilitated by National Science Foundation grants GS-32327 and SOC75-15702. The editors extend their thanks, in addition, to their respective institutions for support of their participation; to Kathleen Ittner, for her assistance in arrangements for the seminars; to Natalie Katz Fisher, Marjorie Olson, and Kyra M. Kaplan for assistance in the preparation of the manuscript; to Katherine Ford Bunker for assistance in preparation of the index; and to Charlene Levering and members of the Staff of Medical Graphics and Illustration at Stanford University for preparation of figures.

The membership of the Surgery Group over the three-year period included:

Membership of Surgery Group

Walter H. Abelmann (1974-75)
Clark C. Abt (1974-75)
Ernest M. Barsamian (1974-75)
Benjamin A. Barnes (1973-76)
David Berengut (1974-75)
John P. Bunker (1973-75)
Joan Chmiel (1975-76)
Jean Dunegan (1973-74)
Mary Ettling (1975-76)
Garry F. Fitzpatrick (1973-75)
Floyd J. Fowler, Jr. (1974-75)
Maurice S. Fox (1973-75)
Miriam Gasko-Green (1975-76)
John P. Gilbert (1973-76)
Alan Gittelsohn (1973-74)
Jerry R. Green (1974-75)
John Hedley-Whyte (1975-76)
Nan Laird (1975-76)
John J. Lamberti (1973-74)
Frederick C. Lane (1974-75)
Robert Lew (1975-76)
Willard G. Manning, Jr. (1974-75)
William V. McDermott, Jr. (1974-75)
Barbara J. McNeil (1973-76)
Bucknam McPeek (1973-76)
Klim McPherson (1973-74)
Lillian Miao (1973-75)
Alfred P. Morgan, Jr. (1973-75)
Frederick Mosteller (1973-76)
Duncan Neuhauser (1973-75)
Raymond R. Neutra (1973-75)
John Petkau (1975-76)
Joseph S. Pliskin (1974-75)
Nava Pliskin (1973-75)
John Raker (1975-76)
Mark Rogers (1973-74)
Donald Shepard (1974-75)
Richard Singer (1974-75)

Keith Soper (1975-76)
Michael Stoto (1975-76)
Judith Strenio (1975-76)
Amy K. Taylor (1973-75)
Kenneth Wachter (1974-75)
Peter Walker (1973-74)
John E. Wennberg (1973-75)
David A. Wise (1974-75)
Jane Worcester (1974-75)

Contents

I BACKGROUND AND GENERAL PRINCIPLES

II SURGICAL INNOVATION AND ITS EVALUATION

III ASSESSMENT OF COSTS, RISKS, AND BENEFITS OF ESTABLISHED PROCEDURES

IV ASSESSMENT OF COSTS, RISKS, AND BENEFITS OF NEW PROCEDURES

V SUMMARY, CONCLUSIONS, AND RECOMMENDATIONS

COSTS, RISKS, AND BENEFITS OF SURGERY

BACKGROUND AND GENERAL PRINCIPLES

The first part of the book sets forth the basic economic and statistical ideas of cost-benefit and decision analysis and illustrates them with medical and surgical examples. The reader should expect neither too little nor too much from these techniques, for many of the questions encountered are not easily answered. What costs and benefits should be included? Can they be reduced to common units? Monetary costs and survival can be measured, but how should the quality of life be valued? And who should make the value judgments implicit in every medical decision—society, the insurance company, or the individual? These, and other conceptual and methodological questions are addressed in Chapter 1 by Nava Pliskin and Amy Taylor.

In Chapter 2 Neuhauser explores in greater detail the possible conflict between the interests of society and those of the individual. In an ideal economic system, a given dollar investment in the treatment of one disease should result in an improvement equivalent to that gained by the same dollar investment in the treatment of another disease. Neuhauser suggests reasons why this is not likely to be achieved in practice and proposes a number of possible corrective measures which might be taken.

The attempt to subject surgery to cost-benefit analysis would be markedly facilitated if it were possible to measure in monetary units the psychosocial costs of illness: the pain, anxiety, grief, limitation of activities, loss of companionship, and other costs incurred by patient, family, friends, and associates. In Chapter 3 Abt proposes an approach to estimating the "shadow prices" that society or the individual might be willing to pay for the relief of these social costs.

In reducing illness and its treatment to common units, it would be convenient if we could assume, as a first approximation, that patients and thus preferences were all alike. But of course they are not, and in Chapter 4 Shepard and Zeckhauser demonstrate how the recognition of heterogeneity within a population can enhance our analyses, and how failure to recognize its presence or magnitude may lead to incorrect or incomplete conclusions.

From a purely economic point of view, there are many reasons why the prices paid for medical goods and services are not likely to reflect their true worth to society or to the individual. In Chapter 5 Green explains how and why medical care can be expected to violate the classical economic assumptions of a static economic environment, of prices unaffected by market transactions, of profit maximization, and of rationality of consumer choice.

Consideration of the efficiency and effectiveness of diagnosis is an essential first step in assessing the overall costs, risks, and benefits of surgical therapy. In Chapter 6 McNeil demonstrates the relation between diagnostic sensitivity and specificity on the one hand, and monetary costs of case-finding and life-saving on the other.

The utilization of surgical services has repeatedly been shown to vary widely among different geographic populations. In Chapter 7 Gittelsohn and Wennberg report the large variations in the rates at which adenotonsillectomy and other operations are performed in different Vermont communities. The existence of such variations strongly suggests that the allocation and utilization of surgical services are not based on a consistent or rational assessment of costs, risks, and benefits.

1

General principles: cost-benefit and decision analysis

Nava Pliskin
Amy K. Taylor

In evaluating the outcome of specific surgical operations, later chapters use the several approaches introduced and described in this chapter. Many decisions must be made when considering surgical procedures. Is it better to operate immediately or wait and see? Is a more costly procedure superior to a less expensive one? Is the difference in benefits worth the costs? Will medical treatment be more effective than surgical? Cost-benefit analysis and decision analysis are two techniques that help answer such questions.

Part I of this chapter presents economic principles involved in cost-benefit analysis. This method is often used to compare programs with the intent of maximizing the difference between properly measured benefits and costs. Economists usually value benefits in terms of dollars, and in a beginning analysis assume that the values are known with certainty. Medical problems involve benefits and costs not easily measured in monetary terms, and thus they require an appropriate adaption of cost-benefit analysis.

Surgical decision-making is often plagued by uncertainty, complicating a straightforward cost-benefit analysis. Decision theory deals with this difficulty. The basic notions are presented in part II, "Decision Analysis and Surgical Applications."

The multidimensional aspect of surgical outcomes creates another complica-

The first part of this chapter (Economic Issues in Cost-Benefit Analysis) was written by Dr. Taylor, the second part (Decision Analysis and Surgical Applications) by Dr. Pliskin, and the third part (Discussion) by both authors.

tion both formal approaches must treat. Multiattributed preference and utility functions offer one way of looking at this problem. Another section of this chapter, "On Measuring Health Outcomes," will discuss these functions briefly with respect to quality of life and other aspects of health outcomes. The measurement of quality of life is illustrated through the examples of coronary-bypass surgery and kidney transplant.

Finally, in part III we preview some of the specific studies to follow and relate them to the theoretical approaches described.

I. ECONOMIC ISSUES IN COST-BENEFIT ANALYSIS

The techniques of cost-benefit analysis were first developed to ensure the efficient allocation of resources to government investment projects. In several analyses, this technique has been applied to public health projects (Acton, 1970; Weisbrod, 1961, 1971), and it can be expected to have increased use if national health insurance is implemented. Since resources available to the health sector (as well as to the rest of the economy) are scarce, society cannot undertake all seemingly worthy projects. Choices must be made among health programs and beyond this, between health programs and other social goals. Economic analysis cannot make value judgments for society, but it can frequently clarify the issues by identifying advantages and disadvantages, quantifying effects, and measuring the resources involved.

General Principles

Cost-benefit analysis compares the advantages and disadvantages of a project. More formally, cost-benefit analysis is a systematic method of setting out the relevant factors for choosing among investments in public projects including, for example, medical care which consists of both investment and consumption aspects. The basic rule is that a project should be done if benefits exceed costs; this is straightforward enough in theory, but the calculation of these values can be difficult in practice. When considering several projects, those with the largest difference between benefits and costs are done first. This process is continued until the available funds are exhausted. The benefits and costs must be enumerated correctly and evaluated considering effects both now and in the future, and accruing to society as a whole as well as to individuals.

The general approach to cost-benefit analysis can be summarized essentially by a series of questions (Prest and Turvey, 1965; Layard, 1972):

1. What costs and benefits should be included?
2. How should these costs and benefits be valued?
3. What is the appropriate discount rate?
4. What are the relevant constraints?

All possible advantages and disadvantages of the project must be included in the initial stage of cost-benefit analysis. The analyst sets forth the effects on both individuals and society, those occurring in this and subsequent years, the direct and indirect costs and benefits, and intangible benefits as well as those more readily quantifiable.

After identifying costs and benefits, we measure and evaluate them. To compare the costs and benefits, it is convenient to express them in common units. The economist's usual approach is to measure the benefits as well as the costs in monetary terms. Monetary units pose no problems in evaluation of items bought and sold in the marketplace. Market prices provide a convenient measure of the value of a good or service. Furthermore, market prices reflect individuals' preferences, given the distribution of income, provided that certain other conditions are met. An example of the use of a market price to value a given service is the widespread use of the wage rate as a measure of the cost of labor. However, imperfections in the market require market prices to be modified for use in cost-benefit analysis where prices have been distorted by taxes, monopoly power, price controls, and so on. Modifications must also be made when markets are not in equilibrium, as when unemployment exists. Another example of under-utilized resources is the availability of unoccupied hospital beds. When an empty bed becomes occupied by a surgical patient, no other patient has been denied the use of that bed; in other words, the opportunity cost of using the hospital bed is less than if the hospital had been full before the surgical patient had been admitted. For nonmarket items, other difficulties arise in evaluating social costs and benefits. It is important not to ignore items difficult to measure, since this could lead us to under- or overestimate the benefits or costs of certain government projects (particularly in the health field). An example is a project producing benefits not accruing to specific individuals, and thus hard to value as seen in what economists call public goods, such as defense, and externalities, such as air pollution.

"An externality exists when the actions taken by an individual household or firm will impose costs or confer benefits on other households or firms, and where no feasible way exists of arranging direct compensation for these costs or benefits. . . . A classic example of an externality is the costs of air pollution imposed on others by the smoke emanating from a factory. Another classic example is the benefit to society that results when an individual decides to be vaccinated or treated for a communicable disease." [Fuchs, 1972]

Public goods cannot be provided through the market system because they may possess the following characteristics:

1. Nonrivalness in consumption–my partaking of benefits does not reduce the benefit to others.
2. Nonexclusion–it is inefficient and often impossible to exclude some individuals from partaking of the benefits.

An example in the health field would be the draining of a swamp and ridding an area of malaria-carrying mosquitoes. Once done, everyone in the area benefits. Intangible benefits, such as reduction of pain and suffering, recreational facilities, scenery, and leisure time are a further problem, since they are not only impossible to measure, but difficult to quantify, and almost impossible to value in monetary terms. Many attempts have been made to put dollar values on these intangibles, some more successful than others. For example, Klarman (1965b) attempts to value the stigma associated with having syphilis.

Another approach when the benefits cannot be valued is that of cost-effectiveness. This technique compares the costs of providing the same benefit (e.g., lives saved) in different ways. However, few projects produce exactly the same benefit, and so we are thrown back to the problem of comparing different types of benefits. For example, is saving one year of life the same for a young person as an old one, or for the rich as for the poor? Further, many health projects produce more than one type of benefit at the same time, such as reducing pain as well as increasing life expectancy. Thus, cost-effectiveness must compare several different types of benefits.

In investment decisions, all benefits and costs are not immediate but are spread out over future years. When the net benefits in each future year are known, some way of aggregating them is necessary. Economists generally agree that one dollar today is worth more than one dollar next year, even in the absence of inflation, because individuals prefer consumption today to the same amount of consumption in the future. The reluctance of consumers to postpone current for future consumption is known as time preference, and the social rate of time preference is used to measure the value of next year's consumption relative to this year's. Another reason that a dollar today is worth more than a dollar in the future is that investments in the private (and often public) sector generally yield a positive rate of return over time. Thus, we must take into account the opportunity cost of alternative uses of the funds to be spent on a given government project. The rate used to express future benefits in terms of their present value is known as the discount rate. If the rate per year is r, then \$1 today is worth \$1 + r next year; or, \$1 next year is worth \$1/(1+r) this year. That is, one dollar spent today is really equivalent to (1+r) dollars next year since the same dollar in the bank could have earned interest worth $r \times \$1$. This formula can be extended to deal with benefits which accrue over many years. One dollar two years from now is worth $1/(1+r)^2$ dollars, three years from now it is worth $1/(1+r)^3$ dollars, etc. Thus, we say that the present value of a benefit stream $B_0, B_1, B_2, B_3 \ldots B_T$, where the subscript represents years in the future, is equal to

$$B_0 + \frac{B_1}{1+r} + \frac{B_2}{(1+r)^2} + \ldots + \frac{B_T}{(1+r)^T} = \sum_{t=0}^{T} \frac{B_t}{(1+r)^t}.$$

Given a corresponding stream of costs $C_0, C_1, C_2, \ldots, C_T$, net present value is defined as

$$\sum_{t=0}^{T} \frac{B_t - C_t}{(1+r)^t}.$$

The preceding discussion has assumed that the discount rate, r, is known and is unique. However, many different interest rates exist in the economy, and economists disagree over the correct rate to be used in making public investment decisions (Feldstein, 1964b, 1974; Harberger, 1968, 1972; Marglin, 1963; and Prest and Turvey, 1965). Although this issue is beyond the scope of the present discussion, the basic question is whether the proper discount rate for public projects is the opportunity cost of capital in the private sector, or the social rate of time preference. Economists often use the rate of interest on a savings account as a measure of the social rate of time preference; similarly, the pretax rate of return in the corporate sector is considered the private opportunity cost of capital. Generally, the social rate of time preference is thought to be lower than the interest rate in the private capital market. This suggests that society is willing to accept a lower interest rate for money lent out to create future social goods than individuals are willing to accept for private goods (Feldstein, 1964a; Klarman, 1965a; and Weisbrod, 1961).

In the absence of a universal discount rate, cost-benefit studies may present results based on several different rates. Then the government decision-maker, guided by society's preferences, decides which rate is appropriate. The choices of a high or low discount rate can affect choices among projects with different patterns of benefits and costs over time. More specifically, the use of a lower rate gives greater weight to benefits (or costs) occurring in the future, while a high rate weighs the present more heavily. This is particularly important for health projects because they often entail large costs initially, and have benefits spread out over many years.

The previous paragraphs have described the process of identifying, valuing, and discounting the costs and benefits of a public project. The next step requires the results to be reviewed in the light of the criteria used to decide whether a given project should be undertaken. The basic decision rule is: Do the project if the net present value

$$\Sigma (B_t - C_t)/(1 + r)^t$$

is greater than zero; or, a project should be done if its discounted benefits exceed its discounted costs. When choosing among several mutually exclusive projects, the rule becomes that of maximizing the net present value of the alternative programs. (See Appendix.) This rule has to be modified somewhat in cases when there are budget constraints and different size projects being considered, and special techniques have been developed to deal with these problems. (Feldstein, 1964c; Weinstein, 1972; Marglin, 1963).

Application to Health Projects

The utilization of health services is viewed as a joint process of investment and consumption. It has investment aspects because it may increase income and productivity in the future and consumption aspects because it brings direct satisfaction. Both of these benefits must be taken into account in the cost-benefit calculations. The usual approach to measuring the benefits of a health project is to equate them with the total costs (both monetary and in terms of morbidity, lost productivity, and mortality) of the illness prevented or alleviated by the project. Clearly, if a certain disease is avoided or cured, society no longer incurs the costs associated with that disease; these avoided costs are then considered the benefits of the health-care project. There are few conceptual problems in determining the costs of the project itself; they basically consist of personnel and materials valued at their market prices.*

The benefits of a health project can be classified into three types: direct, indirect, and intangible. Direct benefits are measured by current expenditures for health services; that is, those medical expenses attributable to poor health which will be prevented by the project. These represent tangible savings in the use of health resources. This is the simplest part of the benefit calculations, and it is often assumed that direct benefits or costs can be measured accurately. If the costs have been incurred over several years, the present value of medical expenses associated with a given disease should be used.

Indirect costs are those due to loss of productivity; thus, indirect benefits are measured by the earnings lost because of premature death, morbidity, or disability.** This benefit calculation is complicated by such issues as the proper treatment (valuation) of transfer payments, taxes, consumption, and housewives' services. Some agreement on these issues has been reached. First, we are concerned only with earnings, and not unearned income which would continue even after death. Next, should earnings be measured after subtracting consumption? Klarman argues convincingly that since everyone is a member of society from a prospective viewpoint, consumption should not be subtracted from gross earnings (Klarman, 1973). Finally, the positive value of housewives' services is recognized, even though these are not included in the calculation of GNP. One approach values a housewife's services at the wage rate of a domestic servant; another uses the opportunity cost of a woman's forgone earnings by summing the wages she would have earned if she had been a regular member of the labor force. Of course, both measures are approximations and, although many consider them unsatisfactory, no better measures have been devised. A similar problem is the value to be assigned to lost productivity in the total valuation of a human life. That is, what is the relationship between the value of a person's life and the amount he (or she) could earn and produce over his (her) lifetime? The problems of using discounted future earnings as a benefit measure have been discussed by Fein (1971). He points out many inequities that might occur if the criterion of maximizing future production is used. For example, the Medicare and Medicaid programs might never have been enacted if the decision were based solely on increasing productivity in the economy. As Prest and Turvey (1965) point out,

"Other things being equal, these calculations are worth undertaking only if we believe that more resources should be devoted to saving a more 'productive' life than a less 'productive' life—e.g., the average man in preference to the aver-

*This may be complicated somewhat by the use of indivisible capital equipment, and the presence of joint products or multiple diseases.

**Rice (1968) calculated the present value of earnings lost due to mortality for a number of diagnostic categories. She also estimated 1-year earnings lost due to disability and morbidity.

age woman of the same age, a white Protestant American in preference to a colored one, the average Englishman rather than the average Scot, a young worker rather than a baby. To put the question this way outrages many people's feelings who do not see that the 'other things' which are here assumed 'equal' include one's estimate of the moral worth and human value of the different people and of the sorrow caused by their death."

Finally, intangible benefits include such items as reducing pain, discomfort, grief, and death. Even though these items are not traded in the market place, it is important to take them into account, and economists would like to know what individuals would be willing to pay to avoid them. (See Chapter 3 by Abt.) More generally, what amount is society willing to sacrifice (in economic terms) to save a life? At present, all that can be said is that the amount is greater than zero (since money is spent to save lives) and that it is less than infinity (because there are avoidable deaths) (Prest and Turvey, 1965). Still, there have been many attempts to estimate more exactly the value of a human life per se (versus livelihood). (See Zeckhauser, 1975.) Other intangible benefits such as relief from pain and suffering, are even harder to measure (Pliskin, Shepard and Weinstein, 1975). Estimates of these benefits may be implicit in values inferred from observable behavior regarding life and death matters. Life insurance holdings and court verdicts have been analyzed (Weisbrod, 1961; Acton, 1970). But life insurance cannot be used for the whole population (such as bachelors) and court decisions are often inconsistent. Further, the problem of inferring values from existing programs is more fundamental than these examples illustrate. If it were true that decisions have been good and consistent in the past, why should we try to change the decision-making process now? Or, if they have not been consistent previously, why should we pretend that they were? A different approach to the problem has been developed by Schelling (1968), who suggested that a life be valued by the amount people are willing to spend to reduce the statistical probability of death.

This section has raised many difficult questions concerning the evaluation of the benefits of health projects. Cost-benefit analysis will be more useful if all the possible benefits can be included, and should be adapted to deal with projects in the field of medical care. Studies in later parts of this book illustrate the ways cost-benefit analysis can be used in the health field and some of the difficulties arising in its application.

II. DECISION ANALYSIS AND SURGICAL APPLICATIONS

Decision theory offers a mathematical tool for handling the logic of surgical care once it is viewed as decision-making under uncertainty. Basic notions of this methodology are introduced through a simple surgical example—appendectomy. Benjamin A. Barnes has provided the following statement of the problem:

"The symptoms and signs of patients considered for appendectomy—the location and degree of abdominal pain, nausea, vomiting, fever, leucocytosis, rectal tenderness, to mention a few—range widely. Patients are seen when the aggregated symptoms and signs merely raise suspicions of appendicitis or when the symptoms and signs are severe enough to warrant immediate abdominal exploration for appendectomy. Thus, prompt surgery is indicated for obviously advanced cases, but if symptoms and signs are mild, observation of the patient is usually the choice. The management of a patient suspected of having appendicitis between the extremes is a matter of controversy. Some surgeons choose to operate early, while others prefer to wait and see, allowing the evolution of the illness to clarify the diagnosis. A decision analysis for such controversial patients is worthwhile."

Figure 1-1 captures the decisions and the main uncertainties underlying the appendectomy problem for the patient with "not so severe" symptoms (we now

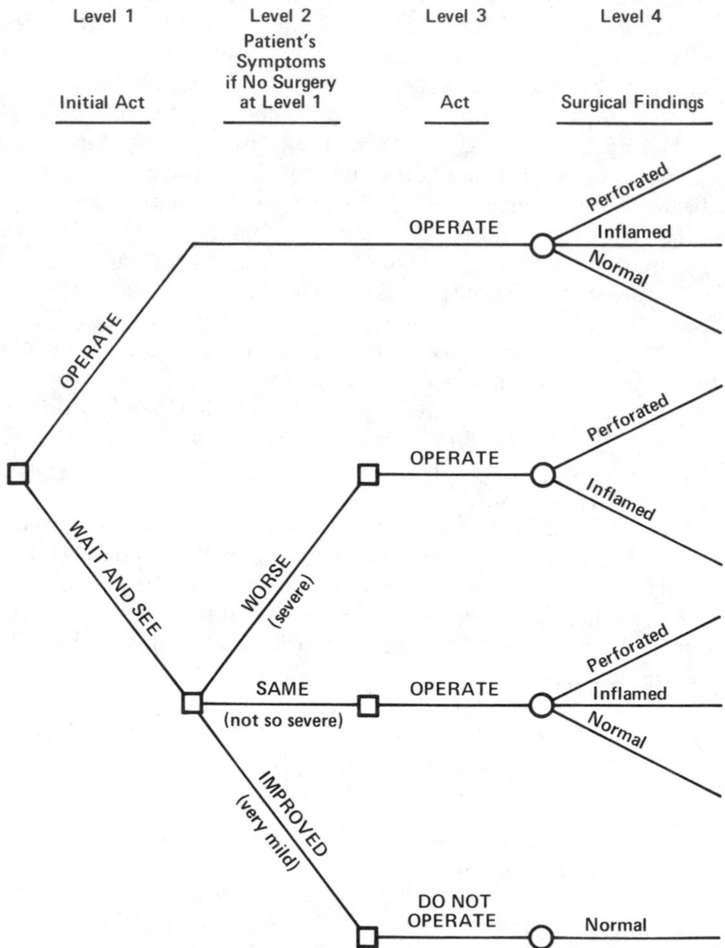

Figure 1-1. Appendectomy decision tree for patients under suspicion for appendicitis.
See text for description.

use "symptoms" to represent the aggregate of the symptoms and signs). The surgeon may either operate or choose to wait several hours and see how the patient progresses. This is indicated by a square decision node on the left of the figure. Surgery (upper branching) may uncover an inflamed or a perforated appendix, but there is also a chance that the appendix will be found to be perfectly normal. The branches, depicting the three possible events, emanate from a round node, a chance node indicating the uncertainty from the surgeon's viewpoint. If surgery is postponed and the patient is observed for several hours (lower branching), the symptoms may get worse, remain the same, or improve. Unless symptoms subside, most surgeons tend to opt for surgery at this point, as depicted by level 2 of the decision diagram. A normal appendix is considered unlikely, in this example, if symptoms become severe. The second branching of level 4 of the tree is pruned to reflect this assumption. If the patient's condition improves, the appendix is assumed normal. To illustrate by an application in the clinical situation we have assigned probabilities for the branches emanating from chance nodes which appear in Figure 1-2. These illustrative numbers are informed guesses suggested by Benjamin A. Barnes, M.D., and are compatible with those used in Chapter 18 by Neutra. For example, if surgery is postponed and the symptoms remain unchanged, the figure gives a .05 chance that a perforated appendix will be uncovered in surgery, and a .55 probability that the appendix will be inflamed. Otherwise, it will be found to be normal.

Avoiding death is the main concern of the surgeon. The probability of death following surgery on a perforated appendix was set at .05, on an inflamed appendix at .002, and on a normal appendix at .001. Obviously, if a healthy patient is not operated on, the risk of appendicitis-related-death is zero. A surgeon, when considering an appendectomy for a patient suspected of having appendicitis, wishes to minimize the risk of death. To do so, one has to proceed from right to left along the tree (Fig. 1-2) towards the origin. First, the combined probability of death is calculated at the right-most chance nodes. For example, following immediate surgery, there is a .0066 risk of death

$$.0066 = (.10)(.05) + (.70)(.002) + (.20)(.001).$$

Likewise, if surgery is postponed there is a .0092 risk of death if symptoms become severe, and a .004 mortality if there is no change. Based on the last two figures and the zero mortality if no action is taken when symptoms subside, one can calculate the mortality rate if the surgeon opts to wait and see. The probabilities of the three possible symptom states are multiplied by the respective risks of death: (.70) (.0092) + (.10) (.004) + (.20) (0) to yield a .0068 risk of death. Thus, a wait and see approach, on the average, results in an estimated mortality practically the same as for immediate surgery, considering the uncertainty of our numbers. Barnes says that this similarity in mortality is in accord with current surgical practice, since immediate or delayed operations are considered by experienced surgeons as appropriate care in individual cases of suspected appendicitis.

The probabilities of death associated with the two options are extremely close, but the subjectivity of the different probability assessments along the tree leads

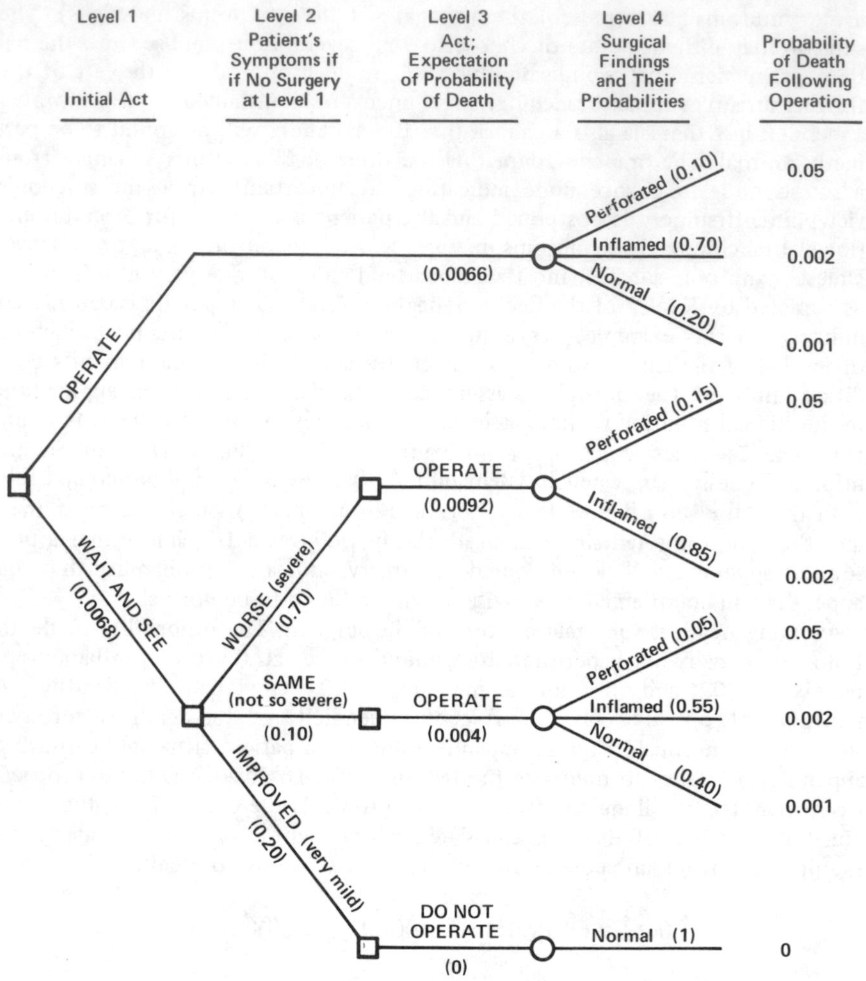

Figure 1-2. Appendectomy decision tree for patients under suspicion for appendicitis with mortality data.

The numbers along the tree are judgmental estimates of Benjamin A. Barnes, M.D. The analysis based on these numbers shows a slight preference for operating on this type of patient as the risk of death .0066 is less than .0068 associated with "wait and see." Considering the uncertainty in the numbers, the results are nearly identical and we examine them further in the text.

one to question the conclusion of the analysis. Is it possible to base practical decisions on these values (.0068 versus .0066)? One must first undertake a sensitivity analysis to see whether a small shift in the probabilities (especially those that are considered "soft") leads to a reversal of the favored decision at level 1. Sensitivity analysis is the process of testing how variations in the assessments along the decision tree affect decisions. Sensitivity analysis may also be worthwhile when the values associated with the different alternatives are not as close as in Figure 1-2. For example, a probability assessor may be confident about specifying a range for a certain probability rather than pinpointing a specific value. Clinicians often put risks within a range instead of committing themselves to a figure. The decision analyst may do well to accept such assessment and to test whether, over the specified range, decisions vary. If the decision is consistent over all possible or likely values, the analyst need look no further. If the decisions are reversed within that range it will be necessary to obtain more reliable data or to make the decision on the basis of the most likely data. When the outcomes are very close sometimes considerations not included in the tree may sway the choice. Sensitivity analysis is one of the attractions of decision theory because it allows us to consider alternative numbers when they are uncertain, and through the variation in outcomes provides valuable insight into the decision-making process. (See Chapter 15 for a fuller presentation of sensitivity analysis.)

The appendectomy decision tree presented here is simple. Some might argue that it fails to reflect the complications in the problem. Such a simple tree helps introduce the methodology. For most medical problems, the decision tree is more complicated. There are more decision points and additional uncertainty levels. Sometimes, the tree becomes so complicated that pruning is a necessity prior to analysis. Pruning involves the elimination of clearly inferior acts at decision nodes, very unlikely branches at chance nodes, and so forth. The appendectomy decision tree, for example, was pruned at level 4.

Assignment of probabilities in practice is often difficult. The interested reader may consult Raiffa (1969a), Schlaifer (1969), and Forst (1971a). In the medical setting, the determination of probabilities is further complicated if the risks vary among patients. In such cases, probabilities have to be assessed for different, sometimes many, types of patients. In the appendectomy context, the mortality figures depend on age and possible associated disease such as heart disease, diabetes, etc. Also, the probability of appendicitis, inflamed or perforated, is an increasing function of the progressive symptoms and signs of appendicitis in our example, which varies even within the intermediate range of values considered.

Expectation over probabilities of death at end points of the decision tree yields the risk of death which the surgeon wishes to minimize. For many medical problems, mortality is not the most important variable. Lost days of work, cost of treatment, quality of life, etc. might be given greater weight where mortality risks are negligible. Sometimes expected values of the quantities at end points of the decision tree are not a guide for decision-making under uncertainty. Using two criteria other than expectation, identically handicapped patients may make different choices about having a major operation intended to cure them.

The concept of a utility function is designed to handle cases for which averages over end consequences are not acceptable as guides for decision-making. Function values (utilities) are assigned to end consequences such that not only preferences are reflected, but, under risk, the expected utility (the sum of utilities multiplied by the respective probabilities) is a guide for rational decision-making. Utility theory is beyond the scope of this review, and the interested reader is referred to Raiffa (1969a).

The applicability of decision analysis to the evaluation of surgical procedures has been illustrated. Structuring the decision tree is, by itself, a worthwhile informative process. The need to assign numerical values for further analysis should be regarded as an appropriate challenge, not a disadvantage. In the absence of objective data for probability assessments, the analysis must rely on subjective estimates. Implicitly, these subjective estimates are being used by surgeons all the time! The capability to undertake a sensitivity analysis with regard to subjective assessments offers an advantage over the normal subjective evaluation of surgical procedure.

On Measuring Health Outcomes

The application of decision analysis to surgical problems is further complicated by the multidimensional nature of the outcomes. Usually it is difficult to quantify medical end consequences in terms of one attribute only, as sickness affects several aspects of a person's life and death. The next section presents a short theoretical discussion of multidimensional preferences and the reader may choose to skip on to a review of medical preference functions.

Preference Structure—Theoretical Notes

A decision-maker is often faced with a multidimensional outcome space. (Cost-benefit analysis is a two-dimensional problem. Cost, x, is one dimension, and benefit, y, is another.) In quantitative analysis of decision-making one wishes to reflect the implicit preferences of the decision-maker over possible outcomes.

A *preference function* (or *value* function or *index*) assigns a value to each point in a multidimensional space such that, the more the point is preferred, the higher the value. (In cost-benefit analysis $v(x, y) = y - x$ is the value function, since the objective is to maximize benefits (y) minus costs (x).) Preference functions are representable in terms of indifference curves. All points in the multidimensional space that are equally preferred compose an indifference curve. The curves in cost-benefit analysis are as shown in Figure 1-3. The equation characterizing these lines is $y - x = c$, where c is the intercept on the y axis, and both axes are measured using the same scale. Line B, for example, represents all combinations of cost and benefits with

$$c = \text{benefits} - \text{costs} = 0.$$

More generally, the net value at every point along a 45° line is the same.

The definition of a preference function is straightforward, but the assessment in practice is not. Mathematicians have developed methods of simplifying the assessments. Specifically, properties of the preference structure which yield an additive index have been identified. When a decision-maker considers his rank ordering to have these properties, the value function can be formalized additively as a weighted sum of unidimensional value functions (Raiffa, 1969b). When

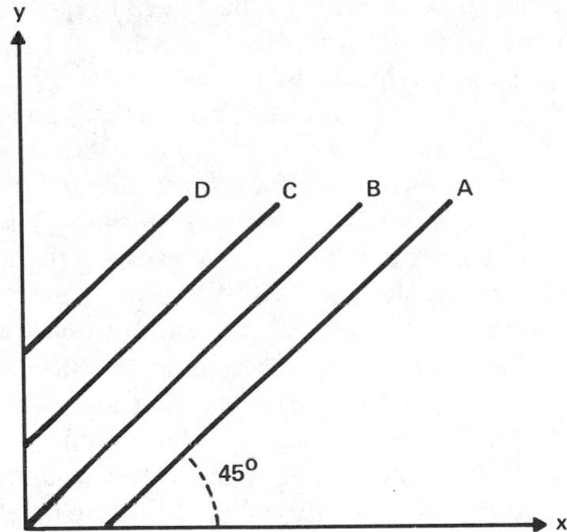

Figure 1–3. Indifference curves in cost-benefit analysis.

each attribute is quantifiable (e.g., dollars, years, etc.), the variable itself may serve as a unidimensional preference function. Under such circumstances the assessment task reduces to determining the scaling constants which represent the trade-offs between attributes.

A Review of Medical Preference Functions

Several attempts at designing value functions over health outcomes have been reported in the literature. Grogono and Woodgate (1971) proposed an index based on ten attributes: work, recreation, physical suffering, mental suffering, communication, sleep, dependency on others, feeding, exertion, and sexual activity. Each attribute can take three values: normal, impaired, and incapacitated. The index is additive with equal weights (1/10) to each dimension. Each unidimensional value function takes three values: 0, 1/2, and 1 for incapacitated, impaired, and normal, respectively. Although no rational basis is provided for these figures, Grogono and Woodgate are satisfied with the consequent ordering. Moreover, they believe that weighting the index over years evaluates health over time and they propose its use in the evaluating of outcomes of surgery. In other words, a fraction of a year in full health (index 1) is treated as equivalent to one year with health index equal to the same fraction. We note that rough and ready methods like these often prove reasonably satisfactory because modest changes in weights usually matter little to the overall assessment. Large changes can, of course, create large disagreements.

The Visick scale was proposed (1948) to classify patients into categories according to the symptoms following surgery for peptic ulcer. (See Chapter 11 on duodenal ulcer and Chapter 10 on quality of life). This index has been modified and repeatedly cited in the literature (Goligher et al., 1968, 1970) but does not lend itself to numerical analysis. Cay et al. (1975) report results of a more quantitative scale for the same condition but fail to report the functional form.

Katz et al. (1963) in studying illness of the aged have looked at attributes of disability (such as bathing, dressing, toilette, continence, and feeding) and have categorized patients. Garrad and Bennett (1971) discuss measures of disability. Rather than sum the various component scores, they chose to present four scores, one for each area of essential activity (mobility, self-care, domestic duties, and occupation) as a profile. Thus, they avoided the loss of information associated with having only one score, but unless a preference function is assigned over the four-dimensional profile, we cannot order the patients. Larson (1963) developed a rating scale for hip disabilities. Essentially, it is an additive function over freedom from pain, function, gait, freedom from deformity, and motion. The weights, as well as the individual value functions, are set so that the consequent ordering conforms to the experience of the evaluator.

A more formal approach to quantifying medical benefits was proposed by Williams (1974). He described indifference curves over painfulness and over degree of restriction of activity, each attribute taking several possible values. An indifference curve is associated with a value reflecting society's judgments concerning the relative importance of seeking one state of health rather than another.

Multidimensional Preferences Under Uncertainty

Utility functions have been briefly mentioned in the section on decision analysis. These functions have been designed as tools, to account for preferences as well as for attitudes towards risk, by making expected utilities a guide for rational decision-making. Following the introduction of utility functions for one dimension, decision analysts recognized the need to extend the theory to several dimensions. However, the assessment procedures in the unidimensional setting are rarely feasible in the multiattribute case. Thus, investigation of simple functional forms was initiated. Certain properties of preferences under risk have been identified, such that if acceptable to the decision-maker, the utility function is either additive or multiplicative. That is, in n dimensions $x_1, x_2, \ldots, x_n$ the utility function is representable as a weighted sum,

$$\sum_{i=1}^{n} k_i u_i (x_i)$$

or product,

$$\prod_{i=1}^{n} k_i u_i (x_i)$$

of the unidimensional utility functions u_i (Keeney, 1972, 1974).

Assessments of utilities in the medical area have already been attempted. They are associated with specific medical problems and do not provide a framework for utility assessments over health, in general, and on quality of life, in particular. Still, awareness of available applications may help in the development of more general health quantifiers.

Ginsberg (1971) sets up a three-dimensional space which translates medical outcomes into equivalent dollar amounts. The "translation" method involves certain restricting assumptions which to many are not acceptable for medical problems. Forst (1971b, 1972) tried to avoid the resulting additive utility by proposing simple, yet less restrictive functional forms. As an example, he developed a utility function over the following three attributes: the probability of death to the individual within a year, the duration of incapacity incurred in years, and the market value of treatment.

Using more recent developments in multiattributed utility theory, Giauque (1972) addressed the prevention and treatment of streptococcal sore throat and rheumatic fever in children. In addition to dollar costs, he took into account health-related consequences such as: immunity developed, days ill, method of receiving medication, and antibiotic reaction. The multiattributed utility function was structured as weighted sums and products of unidimensional utilities. Krischer (1974) examined the problem of treating cleft palate and cleft lip in children. The utility over the four crucial attributes—amount of speech impediment, amount of hearing loss, cosmetic appearance, and amount of money spent—was brought to a manageable format by employing several simplifying assumptions.

Some Thoughts on the Evaluation of Medical Outcomes

The evaluation of medical outcomes depends upon the evaluator. The surgeon, the patient, the insurance company, or any other body in a decision-making capacity, has an individual order of priorities. Due to the multiattributed nature of medical outcomes, the difference in preferences between evaluators probably results from different trade-offs among the attributes. Therefore, no matter who the decision-maker is, identification of relevant factors is essential.

A checklist of variables for surgical decision-making would provide a source of attributes for specific analyses. Some suggestions towards the development of such a list will be offered here and in the next section.

Variables related to medical decisions fall into three categories: monetary aspects, survival measures, and quality of life (including morbidity). The first two categories have been widely discussed by the economic and medical literature. Within monetary aspects one may include direct expenses (or income) to the patient, to the surgeon, to the hospital, and others. Further discussion of economic considerations can be found in Chapter 2. Possible measures of survival are: age at death, lost years of life (see Neuhauser's herniorrhaphy example), and the probability of death or survival within a certain period. The choice of monetary and survival measures depends on the evaluated procedure as well as on the level of detail, accuracy, and reality of the analysis.

Quality of Life

The difficulty encountered in quantification of quality of life should not deter one from considering this important aspect in evaluation of a surgical procedure. Quality of life is a general term that covers may interrelated aspects. When a surgical procedure is considered, suffering of the patient is one of the decision-making factors. But, suffering is difficult to measure. Instead, one may wish to reflect suffering through other, more quantifiable, elements: duration of pain, severity of pain as suggested by potency of drug needed for relief (aspirin or morphine, etc.), cost in time (to measure inconvenience), and time of immobility (in predefined levels). Interpretation of the "suffering" variables is difficult since these will vary depending on the motivation the patient has to ignore or amplify complaints of pain and on the emotional qualities of the patient's personality. Other aspects of quality of life such as recurrences of the original disease or specific complications may be measured in probabilistic terms or by the expected time of the event. The list of factors affecting useful and happy longevity is still not exhausted. Earning capacity, ability to pursue normal activities (sex, sports, hobbies), dependency on others, feelings of well-being, and worrying are a few such factors. Some of these are not easily measured and much methodological work is still needed for the necessary quantification.

Is there a way of handling nonquantifiable aspects in a formal analysis? It is possible to base the analysis on the quantifiable variables. Then, if the optimal strategy is not clearly superior, other variables, not considered because of methodological obstacles, may be introduced to break the tie. For example, analysis of the herniorrhaphy problem may be based on longevity only. But, if truss and surgery are found to be of equal value, patients' worries about strangulation or the discomfort of wearing a truss may lead to surgery. This approach will not be useful for those patients for whom the unquantifiable secondary considerations are more significant than the few aspects that can be readily measured.

The checklist idea is a very general approach to the evaluation of medical outcomes, in particular, the quality of life. Other approaches may also produce acceptable results, and sometimes a simple quality of life measure may serve the analysis. To illustrate this point, two examples will be presented.

In a study of hemodialysis versus kidney transplantation in the treatment of end-stage renal disease, five quality of life levels were considered (Pliskin, 1974):

A = The patient is carrying a functioning transplant, working full time, and has returned to preuremic level of activity.

B = The patient is on dialysis, working full time, and has returned to preuremic level of activity.

C = The patient is carrying a transplant, has multiple physical and/or emotional problems, and there are limitations on activity.

D = The patient is on dialysis, has multiple physical and/or emotional problems, and there are limitations on activity.

E = The patient is chronically ill and almost totally disabled (on dialysis or carrying a transplant).

The expert assessor involved in the analysis graded the quality states as listed and the following utility function over quality of life was determined:*

$$U(A) = 1 \qquad U(B) = .88 \qquad U(C) = .7 \qquad U(D) = .55 \qquad U(E) = 0.$$

The utility for quality of life was incorporated into a more general utility function that also included life years having the form:

$$U(Y, Q) = .71\, f(Y) + .29\, g(Q)$$

as a general utility for the kidney problem for a specific patient, where f and g are utility functions for survival (Y) and quality (Q), respectively.

In the analysis of coronary artery bypass surgery (see Chapter 21) quality of life was also considered. Symptomatic relief of anginal pain in relation to desired level of activity served as the indicator. Three quality levels were considered:

A_0–no pain
A_1–pain with strenuous activity only (mild to moderate)
A_2–pain with minimal activity or pain at rest.

These value trade-offs are patient-dependent. We have $g(A_0) = 1$, $g(A_1) = .8$, and $g(A_2) = 0$ for an active patient, and $g(A_0) = 1$, $g(A_1) = .95$, and $g(A_2) = 0$ for a sedentary patient. Not surprisingly, a sedentary patient puts a higher value on A_1 because of his limited activity. Here again a more general utility function, including life years, was employed: $U(Y,Q) = (1 - P)Y + PYg(Q)$ where P is the fraction of remaining length of life the patient would sacrifice for a pain-free existence.

The two examples illustrate the dilemma of the decision analyst: how to balance generality and practicality. For the kidney and heart applications, a workable scheme was developed. It is generalizable to other problems where quality of life can be graded in terms of a few levels.

III. DISCUSSION

Cost-benefit analysis and decision theory are useful tools for decision-making. Although theoretically attractive, currently several obstacles and unanswered questions impede practical implementation. We shall consider five that are pertinent to medical application.

Identification of the decision-maker

Several authors (Forst, 1971b; Giauque, 1972; Ginsberg, 1971; Krischer, 1974) have considered this problem and most have advocated the involvement of the patient, if possible, but for practical considerations have used physicians' atti-

*It should be pointed out that in both examples the utility function has been scaled to range from 0 to 1. The choice of these numbers is arbitrary, 0 does not mean worthless, nor 1, 100%

tudes only. Some have investigated possible differences among utilities assessed by patients, physicians, public-health personnel, etc., and, it is important to note, found little disagreement or none. The optimal strategy was insensitive to the identity of the assessor. Proponents of having the doctor responsible for utility assessment argue that, as a primary decision-maker with a better understanding of the treatment process and end consequences, the physician should assess the preferences for the patient. The physician's role is especially important if the patient is unfit to assume the task. Still, some people do not wish to have someone else represent their preferences. Consultation among physicians and family members offers substantial help.

Level of detail of analysis

Many studies were based simply on expected mortality as the criterion for evaluation. Other studies have considered additional factors and have asked whether averages are sufficient for an analysis in the multidimensional case. Unless certain very restricting assumptions about the preferences of the decision-maker hold, averages would probably not suffice. For example, it might be meaningless to know that a surgical procedure involves, on the average, 5 days of severe pain and 1.5 complications. Where averages are inappropriate, a more extensive analysis is required. We may need to resort to utility functions and distributions rather than averages.

The time horizon, or how far into the future the analysis must extend, and the complexities introduced by sequential decision making are additional examples of analytic detail requiring careful definition for each study.

Generalization options

Here we consider two separate issues: (a) Is there a general utility function for health? and (b) How are utility functions adapted to a specific patient? One may wish to view these two questions differently—how to generalize from utilities of specific problems to a universal health-utility function, and how to make a utility function (general or for one problem) specific to a patient.

A general health-utility function could be practical if it were attainable from patients through a simple questionnaire. But even prior to this is the issue of what variables should be included. They must be general, yet specific. A list of these variables is a prerequisite to a practical utility assessment procedure. The attributes proposed by Forst (1971b, 1972)—risk of death, duration of disability, and monetary costs—seem general enough. Yet, for the cleft-palate (Krischer, 1974) these would not suffice because appearance, for example, is not included. Some ideas for an attribute list for surgical procedures have been presented in a previous section. Even if a complete list were available, constructing a general utility function would face another obstacle. Assessment of a general utility function must take place prior to the occurrence of medical problems. Yet, the ability of a healthy person to quantify attitudes toward sickness and health, in the abstract, is questionable. Healthy and remote from suffering, the potential patient cannot conceive and fully understand the complete meaning of health outcomes.

If a general utility function is proved impractical, a partition of medical problems into categories, such that for each a specific utility function applies, is indicated. This would save reassessment for every new problem and seems more practical. For example, chronic diseases where quality of life is a major issue could be separated from acute emergency situations where survival is the issue.

Another practical aspect of utility assessments is patient specificity. While this must be ignored in a general evaluation of a medical treatment, the individual physician should take into account patients' preferences. How to do it formally within the tight schedule of the physician is an unresolved question. Developing utility functions for different types of patients (optimist, pessimist, etc.) or else attempting to reach easily assessed utility structures are two possibilities of approaches to patient specificity.

Comparison of medical benefits by means of monetary costs

When it is not possible to express all the benefits and costs in commensurate terms, another approach is to measure in dollars all those benefits which can be valued plausibly, and then simply list the remaining benefits. Thus, the final product of such an analysis would include the net social value of the measured and valued part of the project, along with an itemization of the expected physical benefits and other intangible effects. In this manner, cost-benefit analysis remains useful in evaluating projects in the health area even when benefits are difficult to value. The analysis can rarely be summarized in a single number, but the systematic approach of identifying the various types of benefits and comparing them with the associated costs is critical in decision-making. Many studies in this book include such worked out examples. (See Fitzpatrick's study of cholecystectomy, Chapter 16, Bunker's analysis of elective hysterectomy, Chapter 17, and Neuhauser's study of inguinal herniorrhaphy, Chapter 14.)

Discounting procedures

The difference between the social rate of time preference and the rate of return to capital in the private sector is one aspect of this problem. Since different interest rates occur at the same time in the capital markets of this country, economists may use different rates in the analysis to test the sensitivity of the results to this variable. Often, the conclusions are unchanged because the choice of rate is not crucial to the analysis.

The role of time in medical decision-making is important for several reasons. Different procedures use medical resources in ways which differ greatly over time. For example, a kidney transplant has immediate costs in terms of a surgeon's time, nursing care, and hospitalization for the patient. On the other hand, hemodialysis is an ongoing procedure, with costs spread out over a longer period of time. The timing of the costs and benefits to the patient is also a consideration. The case of an elective hysterectomy in a 40-year-old woman, discussed in

Chapter 17 of this book is illustrative. The immediate risks of this operation, in part due to surgical mortality, can be compared with the benefits of eliminating the possibility of cancer of the uterus or cervix many years in the future.

Thus we have seen that many of the studies of surgical procedures in this book can be viewed within the analytic framework of cost-benefit analysis. The data and analyses presented make up a significant part of a cost-benefit procedure. And, although the studies included here may not definitively answer the question of whether or not to perform certain operations, they do provide much information that can be helpful to rational decision-making.

Acknowledgments

The authors would like to thank all members of the surgical group in the Faculty Seminar on the Analysis of Health Practices, especially Professor Fred Mosteller for help at the initial stages of the manuscript and Drs. R. Neutra and J. Pliskin for providing medical examples. The authors would also like to thank the Editors and other members of the Faculty Seminar for helpful comments on an earlier draft.

APPENDIX

Maximizing the net present value is the theoretically correct rule in choosing among mutually exclusive projects because it leads to equal benefits and costs at the margin. There are, however, several other decision rules which appear frequently in the cost-benefit literature. Besides being theoretically incorrect, there are practical problems associated with them also. More specifically, one rule often used involves the internal rate of return. The internal rate of return (*irr*) is defined as that interest rate for which net present value would be equal to zero; the decision rule then used is: do the project if the *irr* is greater than the discount rate, and choose the project with the highest *irr*. However, several problems may arise when trying to follow this rule. First, if the discount rate changes over time, there is more than one value to which the *irr* must be compared. Next, when comparing projects of different sizes or lengths, this rule may lead to incorrect rankings. For example, a \$10,000 investment with an *irr* of 10% will yield a lower net benefit than a \$100,000 project with an *irr* of 8%. Finally, if the cost and benefit streams are not well behaved, solving the equation

$$\sum \frac{(B_t - C_t)}{(1 + irr)^t} = 0$$

may not yield a unique value for *irr*.

Another decision rule commonly used is based on the benefit-cost ratio, defined as

$$\sum \frac{B_t}{(1+r)^t} \Big/ \sum \frac{C_t}{(1+r)^t}.$$

A project should be undertaken if the benefit-cost ratio is greater than one. This condition holds if and only if the net present value is greater than 0. Problems can arise, however, in the actual calculations of the benefit-cost ratio. That is, it is not always easy to tell whether something is a negative benefit or a positive cost. Although this distinction makes no difference in the net present value calculation, it is important in calculating both the numerator and denominator of the benefit-cost ratio.

References

Acton JP: Evaluation of a Life Saving Program: The Case of Heart Attacks. Ph.D. Dissertation, Harvard University, Cambridge, Massachusetts, 1970

Cay EL, Philip AE, Small WP, et al: Patient's assessment of the result of surgery for peptic ulcer. Lancet 1:29, 1975

Fein R: On measuring economic benefits of health programs, Medical History and Medical Care. Edited by G McLachlan, T McKeown. London, Oxford University Press, 1971

Feldstein MS: The social time preference discount rate in cost-benefit analysis. Econ J 74:360, 1964a

Feldstein MS: Opportunity cost calculations in cost-benefit analysis. Public Finance 19:2, 1964b

Feldstein MS: Cost-benefit analysis and investment in the public sector. Public Administration, Winter 1964c

Feldstein, MS: Financing in the evaluation of public expenditure. Public Finance and Stabilization Policy: Essays in Honor of Richard E. Musgrave. Edited by W Smith, et al, Amsterdam, North Holland Publishing, 1974

Forst BE: A Doctor's Introduction to Decision Analysis. Professional Paper No. 82, Center for Naval Analyses, Arlington, Virginia, 1971a

Forst BE: The Grisly Analytics of Death, Disability and Disbursements. Paper presented at the 40th National Meeting of the Operations Research Society of American, Anaheim, California, October 1971b

Forst BE: Quantifying the Patient's Preferences, Health Status Indexes. Proceeding of Health Services Research Conference, Tucson, Arizona, October 1972

Fuchs V: Health care and the United States economic system: an essay in abnormal physiology. Milbank Mem Fund Q, 50:211, 1972

Garrad J, Bennett AE: A validated interview schedule for use in population surveys of chronic disease and disability. Br J Prev Soc Med 25.97, 1971

Giauque WG: Prevention and Treatment of Streptococcal Sore Throat and Rheumatic Fever—A Decision Theoretic Approach. Unpublished Ph.D. Dissertation, Harvard University Graduate School of Business Administration, 1972

Ginsberg AS: Decision Analysis in Clinical Patient Management with an Application to the Pleural Effusion Syndrome. Santa Monica, California, Rand Corporation R-751-RC/NLM, July 1971

Goligher JC, Pulvertaft CN, de Dombal FT, et al: Five- to eight-year results of Leeds/York controlled trial of elective surgery for duodenal ulcer. Br Med J 2:781, 1968

Goligher JC: The comparative results of different operations in the elective treatment of duodenal ulcer. Br J Surg 57:780, 1970

Grogono AW, Woodgate DJ: Index for measuring health. Lancet 2:1024, 1971

Harberger A: The Social Opportunity Cost of Capital: A New Approach. Paper presented at the Annual Meeting of the Water Resources Research Committee, December 1968

Harberger A: The Opportunity Costs of Public Investment Financed by Borrowing: Cost-Benefit Analysis. Edited by R Layard. England, Penguin Books, 1972

Katz S, Ford AB, Moskowitz RW, et al: Studies of illness in the aged. The index ADL: a standardized measure of biological and psychological function. JAMA 185:914, 1963

Keeney RL: An illustrated procedure for assessing multiattributed utility functions. Sloan Management Review 14:37, 1972

Keeney RL: Multiplicative utility functions. Operations Research 22:22, 1974

Klarman HE: The Economics of Health. New York, Columbia University Press, 1965a

Klarman HE: Syphilis control programs, Measuring the Benefits of Government Investments. Edited by R Dorfman. Washington DC, The Brookings Institution, 1965b, p 367

Klarman HE: Application of cost-benefit systems technology, Technology and Health Care Systems in the 1980's. Edited by MF Collen. (DHEW Publication (HSM) 73–301b), 1973

Krischer JP: An Analysis of Patient Management Decisions Applied to Cleft Palate. Unpublished Ph.D. Dissertation, Harvard University, 1974

Larson CB: Rating scale for hip disabilities. Clin Orthop 31:85, 1963

Layard R: Cost-Benefit Analysis. England, Penguin Books, 1972

Marglin SA: The social rate of discount and the optimal rate of investment. Quart J Econ 77:274, 1963

Pliskin JS, Shepard DS, Weinstein MC: Utility Functions for Life Years and Health Status. Discussion Paper, CAHP, 1975

Pliskin JS: The Management of Patients with End-Stage Renal Failure: A Decision Theoretic Approach. Ph.D. Dissertation, Harvard University, 1974

Prest AR, Turvey R: Cost-benefit analysis: a survey. Econ J 75:685, 1965

Raiffa H: Decision analysis, Introductory Lectures on Choices Under Uncertainty. Reading, Massachusetts, Addison-Wesley, 1969a

Raiffa H: Preferences for Multiattributed Alternatives. The Rand Corporation, RM-5868-DOT/RC, 1969b

Rice DP: The direct and indirect cost of illness. Federal Program for the Development of Human Resources, A Compendium of Papers, Vol. 2 Part IV, Health Care and Improvement, Washington, DC, 1968

Schelling TC: The life you save may be your own, Problems in Public Expenditure Analysis. Edited by SB Chase Jr, Washington, DC, The Brookings Institution, 1968, p 127

Schlaifer R: Analysis of Decisions Under Uncertainty. New York, McGraw-Hill Book Company, 1969

Visick AH: A study of the failures after gasterectomy. Ann R Coll Surg Engl 3:266, 1948

Weinstein M: An introduction to project evaluation, Teaching and Research Materials, Public Policy Program, Kennedy School of Government, Harvard University, Vol. 1, 1972

Weisbrod BA: Economics of Public Health. Philadelphia, University of Pennsylvania Press, 1961

Weisbrod BA: Costs and benefits of medical research: a case study of poliomyelitis. J Polit Econ, 79:527, 1971

Williams A: Measuring the effectiveness of health care systems. Brit J Prev Soc Med 28:196, 1974

Zeckhauser RJ: Procedures for valuing lives. Public Policy 23:45, 1975

Additional Readings

Fein R: Economics of Mental Illness. New York, Basic Books, 1958

Glass NJ: Cost-benefit analysis and health services. Health Trends, Vol. 5, 1973

Grosse RN: Analysis in health planning, Analysis of Public Systems. Edited by AW Drake, RL Keeney, and E Mase, Cambridge, MIT Press, 1972

Musgrave RA: Cost-benefit analysis and the theory of public finance. J Econ Lit 7:787, 1969

Musgrave R and P: Public Finance in Theory and Practice. New York, 1973

Mushkin S: Health as an investment. J Polit Econ 70:129, 1962

2

Cost-effective clinical decision-making: implications for the delivery of health services

Duncan Neuhauser

The use of health services has created an inherent conflict. On the one hand, the compassionate physician and the sick patient desire that everything be done and no expense spared to help the sick and the suffering. On the other hand, the socially responsive health-care manager or planner and the well public who pay the bills through insurance premiums desire that costs be contained. This creates a conflict we have to live with. At best we can only define acceptable rules to contain the conflict.

The traditional basis for medical practice is that the doctor do his utmost for his patient. Each patient, one at a time, should get the doctor's full attention. The idea of scarcity of time and resources has no explicit role in this logic. Scarcity implies that when one patient is treated, others go untreated. The doctor cares for those who seek his help. He has no obligation to inquire after those who did not appear at his clinic. If I am a patient in pain, this is exactly the way I would wish my doctor to approach me. Of course, this traditional plan cannot always be implemented. The doctor in time of plague or on the battlefield has to choose among many who need his help.

From an historical perspective, the introduction of health insurance has served to reinforce the traditional philosophy. Now the doctor does not have to take into account the insured patient's ability to pay when deciding what might be done on behalf of this patient. This smoothed the path of rapidly rising health-care costs.

*Supported in part by a Grant from the Robert Wood Johnson Foundation and the Commonwealth Fund, and a USPHS Grant (GM-1-8674).

THE HEALTH-CARE MANAGER AND THE PAYING PUBLIC

Independent of the evolution of health services, there has grown up a managerial philosophy that owes a substantial debt to economic theory. It assumes that resources are scarce, and efforts spent here cannot be spent there. It provides a calculus for relating benefits to costs and distributing costly resources in a way that will produce the most benefit. The assumptions of this approach are different and at odds with those of the traditional doctor-patient approach described above. Cost-effective clinical decision-making is simply the application of the managerial-economic approach to how doctors make decisions.

There is nothing new in this approach applied to health care. Sir William Petty (1623-87) understood the essential idea in his *Political Arithmetick* (1690). Petty studied medicine at Leyden, Paris, and Oxford. He was Professor of Anatomy at Oxford, a founding member of the Royal Society, a member of Parliament, and a pioneer in "political arithmetic," which he defined as "the art of reasoning by figures upon things relating to government" (Hull, 1899; Fein, 1971; Glass, 1973; Roberts, 1974). He considered the value of human life based on the person's productive contribution to society.

Fein (1971) has described some of Petty's analyses as follows.

"In his plan 7 October 1667, 'Of lessening ye Plagues of London,' Petty estimated that 'given the value of an individual and the cost of transporting people outside of London and caring for them for three months, thus increasing the probability of survival, every pound expended would yield a return of £84.'

"In 1676 in a lecture on anatomy, Petty noted that the value of better medicine was that it could save some 200,000 lives. Even valued at only £20, the lowest price of slaves, this was a large sum and better medicine therefore represented a sensible expenditure 'wherefore it is not in the interests of the state to leave physicians and patients to their own shifts.'"

Here we have, three hundred years ago, the evaluation of human life in terms of productivity, numbers of lives saved, estimates of program costs and benefit to cost ratios; in short, the core concepts of cost-benefit analysis. Also unchanged are the use of almost outrageously approximate numbers for the analysis, and bold leaps to major public policy pronouncements.

Cost-benefit analysis was used by Lemuel Shattuck to justify his proposals for sanitary reforms in Boston in 1850 (Shattuck, 1850), and George Bernard Shaw's play *The Doctor's Dilemma* (1906) was constructed on the question of whose life is more valuable and therefore merits scarce medical attention. But except for the few recent efforts summarized in the preceding chapter, cost-benefit analysis has been applied to health care infrequently and sporadically.

That the systematic consideration of costs and benefits has not been more widely adopted in clinical medicine is understandable given the traditional doctor-patient decision-making framework. A framework that led one compassionate physician to say:

"Throughout my medical school education and training, I was taught to base my decisions primarily on the effectiveness and benefit of performing a particular action and rarely was it ever emphasized that the costs of a particular procedure or action was of significant importance. Implied throughout the cost-benefit analytical techniques is the constant placement of a value on each individual action, procedure, and resource that goes into the problem-solving plan. Such subjective and formally unquantifiable items as the value of a life and the cost of dying are met head on. Life is assigned a price tag in the same fashion that a stock clerk places a price tag on his merchandise. For one who has not been brought up to put price tags on one's actions and outcomes, I find this quite distressing and unethical—unethical because physicians take an oath to do all they can for their patients."

There is a great value in this traditional approach that should not be lost sight of. One can imagine as a patient being told by one's doctor that one's life is not worth the effort involved in trying to save it. There is one chance in twenty that one's life can be prolonged by 5 years and the cost of treatment is $20,000. However, those odds are not good enough so we must go home to die, even though we have paid a lifetime's worth of health insurance premiums. To live in such a callous world would seem more than one would wish explicitly to tolerate (Schelling, 1968).

Albert Jonsen (1975) states:

"Soon there may be need to make an explicit choice . . . when healing is contraindicated by cost benefit analysis. This constitutes a very real if most repugnant limitation on therapeutic freedom of choice."

If there is something to be gained by both approaches, can we obtain the benefits of both? What kind of institutional arrangements would allow this? A variety of approaches suggest themselves. Before turning to these approaches, let us summarize the cost-effective approach to clinical decision-making.

PUTTING IT ALL TOGETHER

One could, at least in theory, develop production curves for each of the major treatment categories that would plot benefits against cost. Such a production curve would look like the one shown in Figure 2-1. For each treatment category, the most cost-effective interventions are shown on the left of the curve and the least cost-effective are shown on the right (Leftwich, 1962, Neuhauser, 1974, Douglas, 1948). Benefit would be a combined index of quantity and quality of life.

Figure 2-1 can be viewed as a guide to rational resource allocation. It implies that decision makers can rank those patients who will benefit most per dollar spent. Secondly, it implies that for a given amount of money, the decision makers will then work down this ranking, starting with the patient who benefits most, then second most, then third, and so on, until they have run out of money.

To be specific, consider inguinal herniorrhaphy. The younger the patient, other things being equal, the greater the benefit from the procedure. Assuming this to be true, then the youngest patients should be cared for first. As additional dollars become available, older and older patients are cared for. As this happens, the benefits per dollar expended decline.

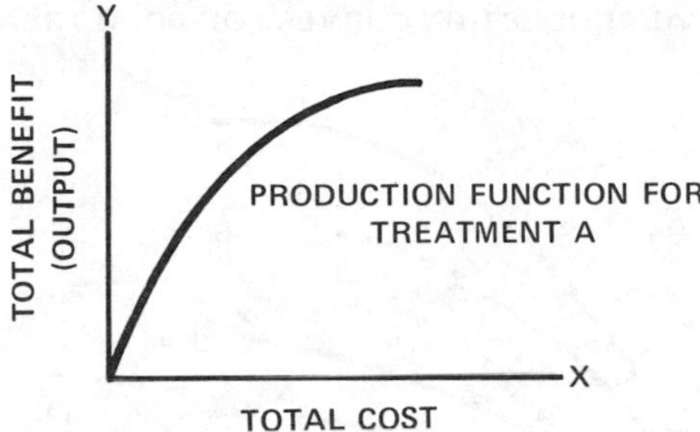

Figure 2-1. Production function for treatment A.

For example, say, the cost per patient is $10,000. Patient 1 will benefit by 10 years' additional life. The first point on this curve would be X = $10,000, $Y = 10$. Patient 2 will benefit by 9 years' additional life, so the second point on the curve is X = $20,000, $Y = 19$. If patient 10 receives no benefit, the curve would be horizontal at that point. If patient 11 would lose a year of life, then the curve would slope downward.

If there are massive economies of scale for the first few patients, the curve would start flat, rise steeply, and then level off.

By rank ordering the interventions and creating a smooth curve, we have created a production function curve with a slope:

$$\frac{Y_2 - Y_1}{X_2 - X_1} \quad \text{or} \quad \frac{\Delta Y}{\Delta X}$$

that declines from left to right.* This slope at the point which defines the amount we now spend for treatment A defines the marginal return for this treatment.** As more money is spent, the marginal benefit per dollar declines, perhaps even to a point where more money spent lowers the benefit.

*More precisely, $(Y_2 - Y_1)/(X_2 - X_1)$ is the slope of the chord (straight line between two points on a curve) from point number 1 to point number 2, both of which must lie on the curve. The slope of the curve at a point (dY/dX) is the limit of the slope of this chord as the abscissa of the second point approaches the first. That is, the slope of the function at the point is the derivative (found by use of differential calculus) rather than the slope of the chord.

***Marginal Costs and Average Costs: Marginal cost* is an abbreviation for marginal cost per unit produced where the unit might be a year of life saved, a patient day in the hospital, a case of cancer detected or such. The *marginal cost* of the 101st unit is defined algebraically as (the total cost of producing 101 units) minus (the total cost of producing 100 units). This should not be confused with the average cost of producing 101 units, which is defined as (the total cost of producing 101 units) divided by 101. Defined in terms of Figure 2-1, the marginal cost for the nth unit of benefit would be the reciprocal of the slope.

$$\text{Marginal Cost of the } n^{th} \text{ Unit of Benefit} \qquad \frac{X_n - X_{n-1}}{Y_n - Y_{n-1}}$$

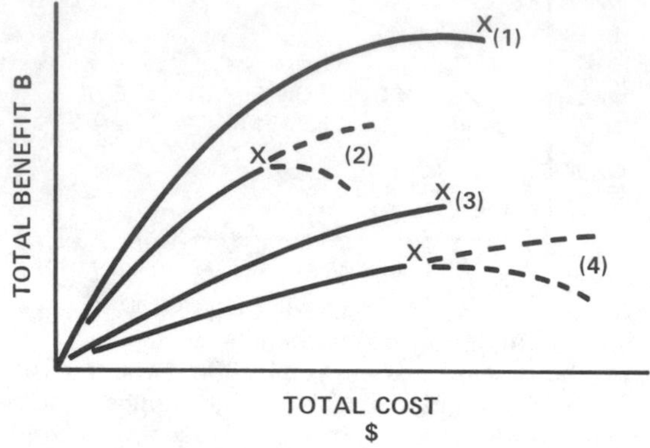

Figure 2-2. Hypothetical production curves for four treatments.
The vertical axis measures total benefit for each treatment and total costs are measured on the horizontal axis. The *X* marks indicate the current cost and benefit position for each treatment. The dotted lines indicate uncertainty about benefit or the lack of benefit for large expenditure on these treatments. (1) is a hypothetical curve for hypertension; (2) for hernia; (3) for appendectomy; and (4) for coronary artery bypass graft.

If we were able to construct such curves for a variety of treatment forms, the result might look like Figure 2-2.* The *X*'s indicate our current position on these production curves. This assumes that the benefits for each treatment are measured in the same way on the same scale.

Suppose Curve (1) is for Hypertension. If we can generalize from the V.A. trials (Veterans Administration, 1967, 1970) to the population at large, it appears that we have the potential of prolonging life significantly at little cost, but perhaps as much as 50% of the population goes untreated.

Curve (2) is for Herniorrhaphy. It is possible that we do too many such operations, as discussed in Chapter 14. If we are on a part of the curve where the slope is negative, we could increase benefit if we spent less money here.

Curve (3) is for Appendectomy. The analysis presented in Chapter 18 indicates that we could do more operations and continue to save lives but only at great cost per year of life saved.

---

where $Y_n - Y_{n-1}$ is one unit of benefit, and therefore, the marginal cost of the nth unit of benefit is $X_n - X_{n-1}$.

Marginal return is the slope in Figure 2-1 and defines how many more units of benefit we will get for an additional expenditure of dollars. If we are willing to assume that providers will spend limited money on the cases that will benefit most, then we can consider a curve as in Figure 2-1, where the marginal return is always declining. Whether this is now true is debatable. However, it might be the national basis for resource allocation for a defined population.

*These curves are only approximations for the sake of demonstrating this approach. The reader with different information or different evaluations may wish to redraw these curves and assign the *X*'s to different locations.

Curve (4) is for Coronary Bypass Surgery, which may be vastly expensive and yield relatively little benefit at the margin.

If we are willing to accept these curves and current marginal costs per unit of benefit as indicated by the *X*'s in Figure 2-2, then we spend too much on some treatments and too little on others. The point that maximizes benefit can be defined mathematically as:

$$\frac{\Delta B_1}{\Delta \$_1} = \frac{\Delta B_2}{\Delta \$_2} = \ldots = \frac{\Delta B_n}{\Delta \$_n}$$

That is to say, we have maximized benefits (*B*) for a given level of money spent ($) when the *X* marks are at the points where the slopes are equal; in other words, when the marginal return is the same for all treatment forms. In terms of Figure 2-2, we should spend more on treating hypertension and less on herniorrhaphies. Since the above equation is satisfied for an infinite number of slopes, there is a second piece of information required for a single solution. Two approaches are possible. The first is to define a budget constraint *Z* so that,

$$\sum_{i=1}^{k} \$_i = Z$$

where k is the number of treatments and $\$_i$ is the cost for treatment i.

An example of this approach would be to say we will spend 8% of our gross national product on health care. If this amounts to $120 billion, then this is the value of *Z*. For any value of *Z*, the constraint on total cost, we can imagine an assignment of expenditures $\$_1, \$_2, \ldots, \$_k$, and a corresponding set of *X*'s on the curves as in Figure 2-2. For that *Z* we can sum the benefits. As *Z* increases, the allocation of dollars changes, generally increasing. But each one need not increase as there may be some tradable therapies involved (for some disease, hospital care expenditures could go up while home expenditures went down or vice versa). For each *Z*, we make the cost allocation and add up the benefits and get a total benefit *B*.

The second approach is to define a marginal rate of return that we will match but not exceed. For example, we will spend up to the marginal point of $10,000 per year of life saved (of constant quality), but no more, regardless of how much or how little money it will cost in total. Although one can conceptually separate out these two approaches, in the real world they are likely to be used in a poorly defined combination.

In theory this seems easy. In practice it is not. Comparison across treatment forms is difficult because of poor data. For example, there may be only two-year follow-up data for bypass surgery, fifteen-year follow-up for colon cancer surgery, and lifetime estimates for hysterectomies—and treatments keep changing. But perhaps most important of all, there is disagreement as to the value of life, and the weighing of your benefit against mine, to say nothing of the empirical measurement of quality of life. There is hope for some resolution of the methodological problems, but not for the underlying value judgments.

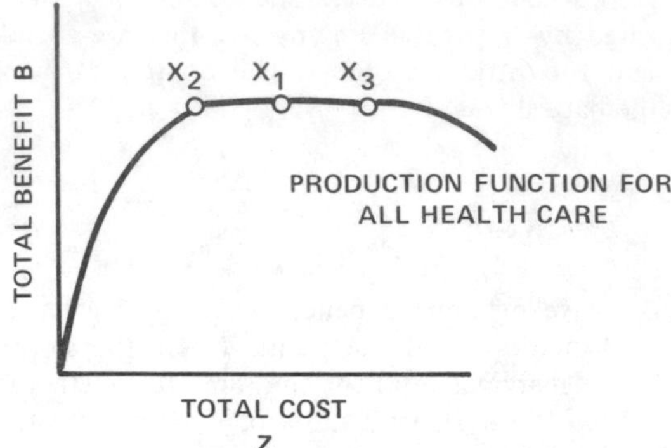

Figure 2-3. The sum of the production function curves for health services
The effect of adding up total benefits and total costs for all treatments X, might reflect current U.S. expenditure and benefits. If we are at point X_1, "total benefits," which we equate with overall public health, will be indifferent to a large increase or decrease in expenditures on health care.

In practice, we do not have to value a year of a person's life within the context of health services. We can still consider life to be priceless,* assign it an index number 1.0 for each year. We could deflate that index for a future year against a present year, a low quality year against a high quality year, a year at age 75 versus a year at age 25. We could then use our limited resources to maximize the number of units of life saved. It is only at the level of deciding how much to spend on education or defense, versus medical care, where one might be compelled to value a life.**

National Health Insurance comes at a price. It will, in an approximate way, give us all a single level of health care, a single marginal rate of return, whether we wish more or less.

This will lead to an aggregate curve like that shown in Figure 2-3. Different strategies of allocation would lead to different curves. The best possible strategy would produce the highest curve. In principle, we can always prevent the curves from turning down by stopping spending in a category when we reach the maximum for it as shown in Figure 2-2. Though we do need to know that the maximum has been reached. Formally then we introduce a k+1st category "invest elsewhere" and any excess money in Z would form $\$_{k+1}$.

*Perhaps it would be more accurate to say "unpriceable."

**To assume that we can measure benefits of different treatments for different people with different diseases on a single scale assumes more than our technology and social agreements on values can deliver today. (Gilbert, McPeek, and Mosteller in Chapter 9 use two scales, survival and frequency of complications, in discussing surgical innovations and these do not cover outcomes for all operations. Furthermore Chapter 10 points out that we are not far along in measuring quality of life.) To assume further that we can add the social benefits so computed may not trouble the reader as much as the first assumption. (For an attempt to carry out such evaluations in dollar values see Chapter 3.)

IS THE TOTAL THE SUM OF THE PARTS?

If we were to sum all the production functions as those in Figure 2-2, the aggregate curve might be as shown in Figure 2-3.

The effects of all doctors, hospitals, drugs, nursing homes, and such on health at the margin may well be zero (Neuhauser, 1974). This point is indicated by X_1. In the United States, about 8% of our GNP is spent on health. In England, it is about 5½%, and reportedly Kuwait spends about 10% of its GNP on health care. These points might be equivalent to X_1, X_2, and X_3, respectively in Figure 2-3. To spend a million dollars more or less at point X_1 (at the margin) would have no noticeable impact on the quantity and quality of life. This might suggest we should spend less, but this is not likely to occur in health care, where the cry is usually for more, not less. This phenomenon can be equated with the pessimism that now seems to pervade health services (Cochrane, 1972; Illich, 1974). In the last decade we have been spending vastly more without any obvious benefit reflected in national life expectancy. Apparently, 1974 is an exception. The reduced speed limit and gas shortage sharply reduced automobile fatalities and one result was a notable increase in U.S. life expectancy.

However, this may be an inappropriate way to consider the input-output relationship in health care. Consider the following hypothetical patients:

1. *65-year old hernia patient undergoing elective herniorrhaphy:*
On the average, we may shorten his life slightly, but we will improve its quality.
2. *kidney dialysis patient:*
We prolong his life at great expense by using a technique that results in a low quality of life.
3. *patient with myocardial infarct:*
The study by Mather et al., (1971) showed no difference in survival between home care and hospital treatment for some patients suffering myocardial infarction.
4. *noncompliant hypertensive:*
His life can be prolonged, but he fails to take his medication.
5. *coronary bypass surgery patient:*
His quality of life has probably been improved but the effect on length of life is not yet clear.
6. *patient with radical mastectomy:*
The evidence that radical surgery for breast cancer is more beneficial than other treatment forms is questionable. Yet, it would probably be considered unethical to do the randomized clinical trial of surgery versus no surgery to determine net benefits. So, we may be indefinitely committed to a procedure the value of which we may never know. (There are signs that this procedure is being questioned. See Chapter 19.)
7. *patient undergoing psychoanalysis:*
Let us suppose that for this patient the treatment is ineffectual. Since that patient pays out of his own pocket and of his own free will, it may be no concern of ours in a society that believes in the free market.

For the above patients, if we were to sum up the changes resulting from treatment in quantity of life and the change in the quality of life, they might both sum to zero. We may have prolonged life as much as shortened it. We may have decreased the quality as much as increased it. The sum is perhaps zero on the benefit side, although the costs are clear and large. But each individual patient has possibly asked to be changed, and those who live to tell us about it may come away pleased with the result. If life is too uncomfortable, perhaps making it a few days shorter and more comfortable is an agreeable bargain. If life is too short, perhaps the discomfort associated with prolonging it is also an acceptable exchange. The total is not the sum of its parts.*

Our current pessimism is concerned with the marginal relationship between health care and health. Medicine has been singularly effective in largely eradicating smallpox, puerperal fever, and poliomyelitis. It has been so effective that an insignificant fraction of the medical effort is now spent on these diseases. Our efforts are now directed to the diseases that we can scarcely cope with—notably, cancer, heart disease, and stroke. It may be inherent in medicine that the greater effort is spent on the areas where least can be done.

COST-EFFECTIVE CLINICAL DECISION-MAKING AND THE PRESENT SYSTEM OF HEALTH CARE

This cost-effective approach to resource allocation is quite different from the usual logic inherent in health insurance. The insurance approach undertakes to distinguish "necessary" from "unnecessary" care. As the above analysis suggests, this is a false dichotomy. It is a matter of providing more or less that will vary with patient preferences and resources available. The insurance approach is concerned with deductibles, co-insurance, upper limits, and exclusions. All this may have very little relation to the benefits of the treatment being insured. Health insurance may make a useless operation "free" to the patient, but exclude from coverage potentially beneficial treatments such as screening for colon cancer, or measuring blood pressure in the doctor's office. The actuaries who define health insurance coverage and therefore define the type of health care provided are interested directly in the solvency of the insurance plan and only indirectly in the benefit to the patient.

The cost-effective approach suggests a number of avenues for restructuring the delivery of health services. Here are a few examples:

(1) It is not simply a matter of the cost-effective approach being "unethical" because patients are denied treatment. The traditional approach of one patient at a time may also be viewed as being "unethical" because other patients are denied treatment: those who do not or cannot demand care. The problem is that the former are visible to the health-care providers and the latter are not

*This can only be true because we use "objective" measures of quality of life, like ability to perform activities of daily living or days lost from work. If accurate "subjective" measures were used, this dilemma would be resolved. However, such subjective measures are not likely to be used as the basis of health planning and evaluation, if for no reason other than that the patient may not tell the truth. If the criterion for receipt of free care is demonstrated subjective benefit, there is good reason for the patient to conceal his true feelings.

patients and therefore invisible. The cost-effective approach may be most relevant to Health Maintenance Organizations. In fact, this way of allocating resources could be the HMO's major distinction. Allowing as large a proportion of the population as possible a choice between these two alternatives seems reasonable. Letting both alternatives compete with each other may allow a wider understanding of the differences in these two approaches.

(2) Linking the size of a worker's payment with the benefit he achieves is surely older than history. If we wish to gain the most benefit from health care, and we assume that the size of the doctor's fee influences his behavior, we might wish to link the size of physicians' fees with the marginal benefit for the procedure. At the extreme, this would mean not paying anything for some treatments considered useless. If we wish to encourage herniorrhaphy in the young, the surgeon's fee for a herniorrhaphy might be an inverse function of age. Or it might be, for example, five times higher for an emergency strangulation than for an elective operation, if one wished to encourage the use of trusses (see Chapter 14). On the other hand, George Crile, Jr., the surgeon, would have surgeons paid by salary because, in his judgment, fee-for-service provides an incentive for excessive surgery (Crile, 1975).

(3) If patient preferences vary and are essential in evaluating the benefits from surgery, then patients with similar preferences might be grouped together into experience-rated insured groups, where each member is charged the actuarial cost of the benefit package.* Now such groups are usually based on place of employment. This has been expedient, but seems a poor way of grouping people by their preferences for quantity and range of health services desired. A preferred mechanism would be one analogous to the computerized blind date or roommate-matching programs. Each person would indicate his or her preference as to health care, such as desire to prolong life, yearly expenditure, discount rate, preferred way to die, desire for psychoanalysis, and such. Then, the computer would group people with similar preferences. A random sampling of these people could form a committee to design their insurance coverage, contract with providers, and monitor member usage.** Consistent with A.L. Cochrane's slogan that "all effective health care should be free," the government would pay for the first X hundred dollars of premiums, age-adjusted for basic care, and the experience-rated group would pay more if they want more costly benefits or get a rebate if they want less (Cochrane, 1972).

(4) Another resolution of the provider-patient and manager-taxpayer dilemma is somewhat like the approach of the British National Health Service. The government provides a uniform number of hospital beds, physician posts, personnel, and supplies, that on a per capita basis is low by American, Soviet, Swedish, or Canadian standards. Then they allow the physicians to use these

*To be more precise, there are two components to expected use of services. First, some people have a higher probability of needing care because of age, sex, or pre-existing conditions. Secondly, there is variation according to patient preferences. One may wish to make transfer payments to cope with the former (the young pay for the old), and experience rate the latter (those who want more psychoanalysis pay for it themselves).

**One possible example would be to have people enroll for care in a neighborhood health center, paying a fixed amount per year to the center. The center would purchase hospital care in volume from the hospital which sells them the best package.

facilities as they see fit. The Consultant-Surgeon has, say 20 beds, and he or she chooses the patients who are to fill them. Presumably, such a physician chooses the urgent cases who will benefit most and lets the elective cases wait. As a first approximation, this probably works rather well. Some observers disagree, suggesting that the interesting cases come first and the uninteresting ones wait. However, much of the great variation in lengths of stay and volume of diagnostic tests from one hospital and one surgeon to another appears to depend on local custom rather than on patient condition (Simpson et al., 1968; Heasman, 1964; Smedby, 1967).

Controlling total beds, personnel, and resources, however, sets a limit on the surgeon's capacity to make choices. A doctor's commitment to the compassionate view that he should do everything for his patient results in his giving up some freedom to make choices. That is the price the physician may have to pay for his compassion.

(5) The introduction of new surgical procedures may in the future be centrally controlled in a manner analogous to the Food and Drug Administration's control over new drugs. New surgical procedures may have to be proved safe and efficacious based on randomized clinical trials before they can be paid for (Cochrane, 1972). One can easily foresee the problems associated with trade-off between the control of costly new procedures and some stifling of innovation.*

Some combination of the approaches above is likely to evolve in the coming decades. Based on my belief that history is a random walk, I have no ability to predict the outcome, but I would expect that the process will be one of incremental change consistent with our country's values and traditions.

SUMMARY

Although the basic ideas behind cost-effective clinical decision-making have been in existence for almost three centuries, it provides a distinctive approach to deciding what medical care to deliver to whom, based on the assumption of scarcity and a goal of obtaining as much benefit as possible from limited resources.

Applying this point of view to a national health service, health insurance, payment of physicians, and grouping of insured patients, leads to some interesting ways of thinking about these problems.

I think the most interesting issue raised by this approach is the explicit trading of dollars for lives. If this trade-off is not considered, then health services may be inefficient in that we do not save as many lives as we could. If we do consider this trade-off, we may be in danger of losing a compassionate concern for human suffering. Is to be compassionate and humanitarian to be inefficient? To be efficient must we be inhumane?

Perhaps true compassion must be efficient. How can we develop a health service where this is true?

*The analogy between surgery and drugs is an oversimplification. Surgery may evolve slowly so that a long series of small changes spread out over the decades may result in major differences (see Chapter 9). If so, then regulation analogous to drug regulation would be difficult to carry out.

References

Cochrane AL: Efficiency and Effectiveness. London, Nuffield Provincial Hospitals Trust, 1972

Crile G Jr: Kicking the fee-for-service habit. Hospital Physician 11:34, 1975

Douglas PH: Are there laws of production? The American Economic Review 38:1, 1948

Fein R: On measuring economic benefits of health programs, Medical History and Medical Care. Edited by G McLachlan, T McKeown. London, Oxford University Press, 1971, p 179

Glass NJ: Cost benefit analysis and health services. Health Trends 5:51, 1973

Heasman MA: How long in hospital? Lancet 2:539, 1964

Hull CH, ed: The Economic Writings of Sir William Petty, together with the observations upon the bills of mortality, more probably by Captain John Graunt. Cambridge, The University Press, 1899

Illich I: Medical Nemesis. London, Calder and Boyars, 1974

Jonsen AR: Scientific medicine and therapeutic choice. N Engl J Med 292:1126, 1975

Leftwich R: The Price System and Resource Allocation. Revised edition. New York, Holt, Rinehart and Winston, 1962, chapter 7

Mather HG, Pearson NG, Read KLQ: Acute myocardial infarction: home and hospital treatment. Br Med J 3:334, 1971

Neuhauser D: The future of proprietary hospitals in American health, Regulating Health Facilities Construction. Edited by C. Havighurst. Washington, DC, American Enterprise Institute, 1974, p 233

Roberts JA: Economic evaluation of health care: a survey. Br J Prev Soc Med 28:210, 1974

Schelling TC: The life you save may be your own, Problems in Public Expenditure Analysis. Edited by SB Chase Jr, Washington, DC, The Brookings Institution, 1968, p 127

Shattuck L: Report of a General Plan for the Promotion of Public and Personal Health. Boston, Dutton and Wentworth, April 25, 1850

Simpson J, Mair A, Thomas RG: Custom and Practice in Medical Care. London, Oxford University Press, 1968

Smedby B: Vortiden for Brackoperation vid olika sjukhus. Lakartidning 64: 3525, 1967

Veterans Administration Cooperative Study Group on Anti-Hypertensive Agents: Effects of treatment on morbidity in hypertension: results in patients with diastolic blood pressures averaging 115 through 129 mm Hg. JAMA 202:1028, 1967; Effects of treatment on morbidity in hypertension. II. Results in patients with diastolic blood pressure averaging 90 through 114 mm Hg. JAMA 213:1143, 1970

3

The issue of social costs in cost-benefit analysis of surgery

Clark C. Abt

In surgery cost-benefit analyses we must not avoid the measurement problems of economic, social, and psychological effects inherent in expressing payoffs of alternative surgical decisions in expected *quantity* of life terms just because important *quality* of life factors are invariably involved.

The crucial issue in methodology is that of translating quality of life data into quality of life costs and benefits consequent to a particular operation. Without some method of translating data on the duration and severity of pain, on inconvenience, and on anxiety, to mention only a few qualities, into costs commensurable with the known dollar costs of operating or not operating, quality of life factors cannot rationally be weighed against quantity of life (longevity) factors in reaching decisions about individual operations and overall surgical policy.

A major motivation in attempting to place a dollar "price" on pain is to provide it with a tangible and quantitative attribute for surgeons and other medical decision-makers. *Ceteris paribus,* when weighing tangible benefits, such as life extension, against previously intangible benefits, such as reduced pain, many humane physicians, like most rational individuals, would tend to give more weight to the tangible side of the balance. Since this tendency is reinforced by the statistics of medical effectiveness being frequently expressed in concrete terms of reduced mortality or extended survival, rather than in measures of reduced pain, it is all the more important to find ways to give weight to quality of life factors such as relief from pain and suffering.

THE SHADOW PRICE

How can such quality of life factors be "shadow priced" into respectable tangibility? Shadow pricing developed by welfare and public finance economists provides prices for alternative "free" public goods not traded in any market. Without such relative prices, cost-benefit comparisons could not be made among such "free" goods as alternative parks, roads, dams, etc. These shadow prices are determined by the worth imputed to the particular items by the costs of the actions devoted to obtaining them. These are opportunity costs.

The shadow prices of quality of life factors such as pain, restriction of freedom, inconvenience, and anxiety can be estimated insofar as we can determine what people are willing to pay to be rid of them. Sometimes market data are available—e.g., the price paid for drugs to reduce the pain of a headache. In other problems, such as anxiety, market prices exist for a variety of responses ranging from psychotherapy to compensatory behaviors like overdrinking and overeating. For qualities of life that are difficult to evaluate, such as companionship, it is necessary to determine the typical opportunity costs expended to achieve such usually nonmonetized qualities. Dues for social organizations and expenses of traditional family reunions are examples.

Our approach identifies as far as possible the major psychological and social variables likely to affect the quality of life of individuals directly or indirectly involved with a disease, and then uses shadow pricing to determine their impact. This approach has been used to estimate total annual national social costs of cancer (Abt, 1975). For each therapy and person, we quantify major "psychosocial" costs and benefits of the decision, and then balance them against the other aspects. Psychosocial costs and benefits refer to the quality of life impacts on all individuals affected, exclusive of direct economic costs such as medical treatment or the patient's forgone earnings. Techniques for estimating these are already well developed (Weisbrod, 1961; Rice, 1967; Fuchs, 1972). For each individual case, the total quality of life or social costs of a given disease and its alternative treatments are then obtained by summing all the specific social costs and benefits over the specific people involved. This is made possible by quantifying costs and benefits in common money terms. Had the various impacts been left in qualitative terms, they could not have been added to obtain a total net social cost or benefit for comparison with other alternatives.

In our approach we ask:

1. *Who* is likely to be significantly affected by the disease process in the patient?
2. *In what respects, and to what degree* are these involved individuals affected?
3. *What are the equivalent social costs of these effects* for the individuals affected, in terms of market or shadow prices for what is lost or must be compensated.

The first question can be answered by interviews and surveys of patients, physicians, and close relatives of patients. Substantial social research has already been done and is available in the social, psychological, and psychiatric literature (George and Wilding, 1972; Krant and Sheldon, 1971; Parkes et al., 1969; Stein and Susser, 1969; Reiss, 1969; Maddison and Viola, 1968; Rees and Lutkins,

1967; Parkes, 1964; Shoor and Speed, 1963; Brown, 1961; Feifel, 1959; Dyk and Sutherland, 1956; Feifel, 1956; Wahl, 1954; and Anderson, 1949). These reports document the psychological and social costs of disease and death for the immediate family of the patient–particularly children and spouses. Although few analyses assess the quality of life impact of disease on individuals involved with the patient other than children and spouses–parents, siblings, close friends, colleagues, coworkers, and health personnel–often are significantly involved.

ESTIMATES OF THE PRICE OF LIFE

For a comparison of the total benefits (net quantity *and* quality of life) of each treatment alternative, the net benefit of the quantity of life has to be expressed in common units as well. Otherwise we would be attempting to compare such measures as survival probabilities and monetized quality of life aspects–a not impossible but confusing task. One way of expressing the value of a given quantity of life suggested by Schelling (1968) is the price imputable to it from the amount people are willing to spend to reduce the probability of death.

The collective "price of life," in the sense of what this society appears willing to pay to keep people alive in nursing homes, is about $10,000 per year.* Since a patient's family is probably willing to pay for somewhat higher quality care in a private nursing home (if it has the resources or the insurance), this annual "price of life" may be closer to $20,000. The results of a comparative analysis of different treatment benefits may be sensitive to the number assumed, when the total monetized worth of the net quality of life benefits are close to the same amount. Different assumptions of $10,000, $20,000, or $40,000 per year as the average imputed "price of life" may change the rational choice of treatment in some cases.

AN EXAMPLE WITH BREAST CANCER

For purposes of a simple illustration (and not for advocating one method of treatment or another), let us apply the method of analysis to decisions concerning treatment of breast cancer in a 40-year-old female with a normal life expectancy of 35 years. We "price" each year of life at $20,000 and assume a life expectancy of 2 years if no treatment is obtained, or of 5 years if some form of mastectomy is obtained without additional radiotherapy, chemotherapy, or immunotherapy. (See Chapter 19 for discussion of evidence of effectiveness of various treatments.) The patient is aware of these conditions, and we endeavor to evaluate some of the complex realities she is intensely concerned about. Table 3-1 lists some quality of life factors for "no mastectomy" and "mastectomy":

The longer list of psychosocial costs associated with mastectomy should not

*Court judgments awarding damages for loss of life of middle-aged individuals have ranged from $200,000 to $300,000 for 10 to 30 years' reduction of life from the duration normally expected. This $10,000 to $30,000 annual price seems roughly consistent with the otherwise derived figure used here.

Table 3-1. Psychosocial costs for the patient.

No Mastectomy versus	*Mastectomy*
Grief at impending death (expected in two years)	Grief at loss of body part
Pain and suffering of terminal cancer	Pain from the operation
Family conflict (over choice of no treatment)	Inconvenience of hospitalization and limited arm use
Worry over impending death, and disruption of child development (motherhood expected to be limited to two more years)	Possible limitation of sex life
	Possible limitation of physically active work
	Possible limitation of physically active sports
	Worry over disfigurement and disease recurrence
	Reduced aesthetic qualify of life

Table 3-2. Psychosocial benefits for the patient.

No Mastectomy	versus	*Mastectomy*
For Patient: Avoidance of pain, discomfort, grief, and inconvenience of operation, loss of body part		Reduced worry over proximate death*
For Husband: Reduced worry over wife's disfigurement and its impact on her.		Reduced worry over proximate death
For Children: Disrupted child development		Increased time for child development

*It might be argued that an expectation of death in 5 years yields a total amount of grief *greater* than an expectation of death in 2 years. However, the psychiatric literature suggests that intensity declines rapidly with reduced proximity, and more rapidly than time increases to the event, so that my assumption is that the total amount of grief at an impending death declines with increases in time to it, at a very high discount rate.

be interpreted to indicate this as the less desirable choice. In addition to the postulated increased length of life, there are offsetting psychosocial benefits.

To determine whether "no mastectomy" or "mastectomy" yields the greater *quality* of life for all concerned, and to weigh the difference against the value of greater *quantity* of life expected from mastectomy, we quantify these impacts and aggregate them by market and shadow pricing techniques illustrated for a few factors below. We start with the psychosocial costs of "no mastectomy."

Grief and worry can be shadow priced through the diverse, compensatory actions of individuals coping with such grief and worry, ranging from such low social cost activities as prayer and reflection, through medium- cost compensations of pleasure seeking, to higher cost behaviors of self-destruction and destructive acts.

Indicators of the price of grief and worry include suicide and mental illness.

Rees and Lutkins (1967) found the incidence of suicide in surviving close relatives to be ten times higher than age-matched controls, yielding an expected cost of $20 per patient or $40 per 2-person family.

Stein and Susser (1969) found the average annual rate of patients requiring psychiatric care to be over twice as high for widows as for married individuals. Assuming a general incidence of mental illness requiring hospitalization of 1% being doubled for surviving spouses of cancer deaths, the expected additional cost is 1% of the annual average mental hospitalization cost of $20,000, for a shadow price of grief and worry of $200—hardly adequate.

While psychiatric care is not a specific for this disease, it may be used as one proxy measure for the price people are willing to pay to reduce the unusual emotional stress encountered before the patient dies. Another estimate for the price of grief might then be the average cost of psychotherapy, at $50 per hour, once a week, or about $2,500 per year.* Since these three risks are not mutually exclusive and may in large part be independent, we add their costs for a total of $2,740. The additional cost of a few more drugs, sleeping pills, drinks, and incidental anodynes might bring the annual average shadow price of grief and worry to about $3,000. This may seem a conservative estimate indeed, until one considers that, as an *average,* this represents more than one-quarter of the after-tax income of the median wage earner.

Pain and suffering may be shadow priced by the amount people are willing to spend for its elimination or relief. This may be the cost of drugs administered to reduce it, plus the cost of side effects such as reduced mental awareness. Assume the cost of drugs is $500 per year and administration costs another $500 per year, which would cover visits to a physician's office or clinic, visiting nurse expenses, etc. Add to this an assumed 300 hours of reduced mental awareness at a cost of the patient's average hourly wage of $6 for $1,800 more. The total annual shadow price of pain and suffering is thus $2,800.

Family conflict is more likely to occur as patients fear losing their independence and make demands on healthy members that are not easily satisfied, resulting in conflict and guilt. Case histories reveal effects on marital relationships caused by resentment on the part of healthy spouses as they assume the added burdens occasioned by the patient's illness, by resentment on the part of the patient to insufficient attention, by reduced sexual interest and satisfaction on both sides, and by anxiety and poor self-esteem, resulting in reduced tolerance to the increased tensions and surfacing emotional conflicts (Reiss, 1969). If psychotherapy is the minimal cost of family conflict, then an annual average shadow price of $1,000 is assumed on the basis of a weekly session at $50 over 20 weeks.

Disrupted child development may result if children deprived of a parent by cancer express the emotional conflicts of a progressive lack of attention and bereavement in reduced school achievement and delinquency. George and Wilding (1972) found that 32% of the children with widowed fathers suffered

*It is not complete faith in the efficacy of psychotherapy that causes us to use it for shadow pricing, but rather its conventional application in dealing with grief. The frequent residual grief after psychotherapy requires analysis beyond the scope of this discussion.

deterioration of school progress. Assuming completion of college is reduced by 10% in those affected, college graduation will be reduced 3%. Translated into a cash equivalent, the 3% is multiplied by the discounted present value of the difference (currently about $100,000) between the average lifetime earnings for college and noncollege graduates (Rice and Cooper, 1967), or $3,000. From the case study evidence of increased delinquency rates (Shoor and Speed, 1963), we estimate an expected cost of $100. The $3,000 and $100 are cumulative, not annual costs.

Since it was assumed that death would come in an average of two years in the "no mastectomy" alternative, its total quality of life cost is (2)(3000+2800+1000) + 3000 + 100 = $16,700. If the life expectancy benefit of mastectomies is assumed to yield an average of 5 years' life expectancy, or 3 years more than the "no mastectomy" alternative,* the additional *quantity* of life benefit of mastectomies is 3 years × $20,000 per year, or $60,000. This suggests that unless the quality of life costs of mastectomy are equal to or greater than the $60,000 life expectancy benefit plus $16,700 quality of life cost of the alternative, or $76,700, the mastectomy is the rationally preferable choice. Let us see if it is.

Since current research (see Chapter 19) indicates no significant difference in survival benefit between simple and radical mastectomies, we should rationally choose the simple mastectomy to compare to "no mastectomy" for quality of life costs. A display of the net psychosocial quality of life costs of the simple mastectomy may tabulate the psychosocial costs *minus* the benefits as follows:

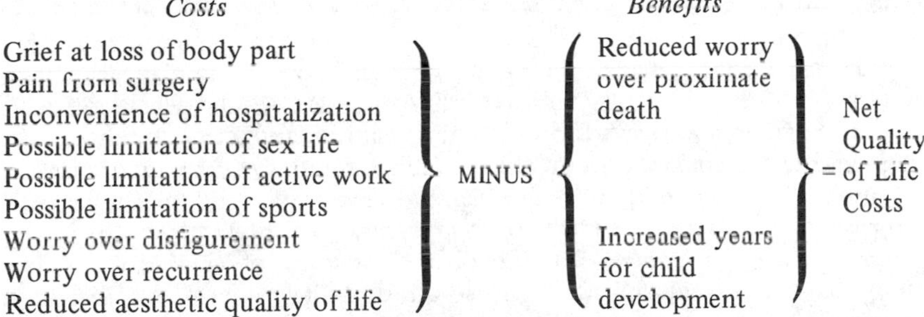

Figure 3-1. Simple mastectomy.

This net cost, subtracted from the survival or quantity benefit, yields the overall net benefit or cost to be compared with that of the alternative choice of "no mastectomy."

Grief at loss of a body part is a distressing reality for many women and is very difficult to shadow price. An indirect approximation might be based on empirical evidence of the average years of life women are willing to sacrifice rather than suffer this loss. Given the shadow price of a year of life at $20,000, we could convert the years of life women are willing to lose to retain a breast into the

*These values are chosen to illustrate the methodology, and each reader may substitute values more relevant to his or her experience.

equivalent shadow price of life cost. Although we have no survey data on actual preferences, for illustration we assume that women would sacrifice a year of life to avoid the loss of a breast, suggesting a shadow price of $20,000.

Pain from surgery involved in the mastectomy is readily estimated on the basis of market prices for the anesthesia and related medical services prescribed to minimize it. In the aggregate this might amount to about $500.

Inconvenience of hospitalization is also easily computed on the basis of the average opportunity cost of one week of time corresponding to an average hospital stay for the operation. This is a combination of the loss of a week's earnings of about $250 plus an equivalent leisure-time loss worth a similar amount for a total of about $500.

Possible limitations of sex life is complicated by the need to estimate the *probability* (rather than certainty) of some limitation of sex life, since many women would have only a temporarily interrupted sex life as a result of a mastectomy. We resort to assumptions for illustration until surveys give us empirical data.

If we assume the shadow price of a sexual experience is roughly $40,* and if we assume an average frequency of 50 per year, the annual shadow price is $2,000, or a total of $4,000 for the 2 years of life during which the sex life the "no mastectomy" alternative affords is unaffected by mastectomy. This "cost" must be discounted by the probability of a satisfactory sexual adjustment. Assuming this probability is 50% (we need surveys to develop reasonable estimates), the shadow price of a possible limitation of sex life would be some $2,000.

Limitation of active work is relatively unlikely unless the patient has a physically demanding job. Assuming that the probability of this is 20%, and that a limitation is 50%, the cumulative probability of an active job being sacrificed is 10%. Assuming this job pays $15,000 and a year is required to find substituting employment, the shadow price of this possible limitation is $1,500. Limitation of sports such as swimming or tennis can be shadow priced by the annual costs of the activities forgone, or some $500, for 5 years for a total of $2,500.

Worry over disfigurement may be compensated by psychiatric counseling during the time of adjustment. It is also a probability rather than a certainty. Assuming an expectation of a 20-week emotional adjustment period, with 2 counseling sessions per week at $25 each, the total shadow price is $1,000. *Worry over recurrence* can probably be included in this. Reduced *aesthetic quality of life* can be substantially compensated by specially tailored clothing and/or other cosmetic means at an estimated annual cost of $500 or $2,500 for the total 5 years. In summary: Tables 3-3 and 3-4 give the results.

The worry over proximate death that is now reduced by roughly (5-2)/5 years or 60%, and thus as a reduced worry constitutes a gain, was previously shadow priced at $6,000. It is now only $2,400 worth of worry. The disruption of child development from proximate death priced at $3,100 is now removed or greatly

*We emphatically do not suggest that patients are likely to, or advised to, "buy sex," at these or any other shadow prices. The reader it is hoped will not be repelled by what is merely a theoretical device for estimating an equivalent cost for an important quality of life.

Table 3–3.

Grief at loss of a body part	$20,000
Pain from surgery	500
Inconvenience of hospitalization	500
Possible limitation of sex life	2,000
Possible limitation of active work	1,500
Possible limitation of active sports	2,500
Worry over disfigurement and recurrence	1,000
Reduced aesthetic qualify of life	2,500
	$30,500

Table 3–4.

	Quantity of Life Benefit	+	*Quality of Life Benefit (Cost)*	=	*Net Benefit (Cost)*
No Mastectomy:					
2 years' life expectancy	0	-	$16,700	=	- $16,700
Mastectomy:					
5 years' life expectancy	$60,000*	-	$32,900	=	$27,100
Difference:	$60,000	-	$16,200	=	$43,800

*5–2 = 3 years' added life at $20,000 per year = $60,000. Perhaps this should be discounted to present value @ 5% to about $50,000, but we have avoided discounting the other quantity of life benefits also for the sake of simplicity of illustration.

reduced. Thus the net psychosocial quality of life cost of mastectomy is: $30,500 + 2,400 + 0 = $32,900.

Clearly, on the basis of the assumptions made, simple mastectomy with 5 years' life expectancy is preferable to the "no mastectomy" treatment with 2 years' life expectancy, because the greater quality of life costs of mastectomy are not sufficient to cancel out its greater *quantity* of life benefit over "no mastectomy." Since the quality of life costs are about the same for the mastectomy, no operation would be preferable if the mastectomy yielded no additional life expectancy. Although any experienced physician would reach intuitively the same conclusion in this example, the techniques employed could be of considerable help in reaching decisions in less obvious cases. These techniques are in their infancy, and the current stage of their development should not obscure possible applications as shadow costs are evaluated with increasing sophistication.

The above conclusions may be sensitive to the assumptions, such as the estimated price of 1 year of life or $20,000 being the shadow price of grief at the loss of a body part. If survey data could show that this was actually 2 years or $40,000, then the difference in quality of life costs would be $36,200 in place of $16,200 and for an operation to provide a compensating benefit, it would have to yield at least an additional year of life expectancy. In the example we have assumed 3 years' added life expectancy from mastectomy. Thus, for a woman whose grief at the loss of a breast is equivalent to 3 or more years of life, the operation costs her more in quality of life than it benefits her in quantity of life. The occasional patient completely demoralized and depressed following mastectomy may be such an individual.

This is a crude analysis for integrating quality of life factors with survival probabilities in the comparison of treatment alternatives. It neglects the heterogeneity of breast cancer and the many variations in the shadow pricing of specific quality of life benefits and costs. These variations arise from individual preferences and from different medical and other circumstances. In any event we have here a start for a rational framework to help patient, physician, and health policymaker alike, in their common efforts to achieve a medical decision of maximum satisfaction to the patient in the light of the best scientific knowledge of both the medical and the quality of life outcomes of alternative treatments.

AN EXAMPLE WITH END-STAGE RENAL DISEASE

A second example of integrating shadow-priced qualities of life into medical decisions is the treatment of end-stage renal disease (ESRD). Four treatment alternatives are considered: home dialysis, hospital-based dialysis, transplantation from a living donor, and transplantation from a cadaveric donor. We assume for simplicity that once started on chronic hemodialysis a patient is not considered for transplantation and that failure of an initial transplant is not followed by a secondary transplant but only by chronic hemodialysis. Such constraints would not alter the disposition of over 80% of patients under current treatment patterns for ESRD.

It may be estimated from the data in Chapter 20 that the median survival times of patients on home dialysis, hospital dialysis, or receiving a transplant from a living donor or cadaveric donor are respectively: 11.2 years, 6.1 years, 12.5 years, and 4.5 years. Since the follow-up data are not of sufficient duration to permit calculation of the life expectancy of these four treatments, we shall use these values in lieu of life expectancy for the purpose of illustration.

In the following tabulation of treatments and their quality of life attributes note that the benefits to the kidney donor are included in the living donor transplant treatment, and corresponding benefits accrue to the family of a cadaveric donor. The quality of life impact of the usual three to six months' preliminary hospital dialysis in preparation for the transplant treatment must also be considered.

Comparing quality of life costs for dialysis and transplants, we see significant discomfort, inconvenience, isolation, immobility, dependency, and loneliness for dialysis patients, with only relatively minor inconveniences from preparation and follow-up care for transplant patients. For the dialysis patients, home dialysis has somewhat lower psychosocial costs than hospital dialysis. For the transplant patients, living transplants have higher quality of life costs than cadaveric transplants, because a living donor suffers some temporary quality of life costs. Let us quantify these relative quality of life costs of the four ESRD treatment alternatives and then incorporate them with their respective quantity

Table 3–5. End-stage renal disease.

Treatment	*Quality of Life Benefits*	*Psychosocial Costs*
Home Dialysis *Estimated median survival = 11.2 yrs.		Discomfort Disrupted professional and work relations Loss of community contributions and participation Segregation Isolation and discrimination Infantilization Loss of leisure time Reduced aesthetic quality of life Inconvenience Immobility Dependency Limitation of normal activity: work, social life, sex, recreation Family conflict Loneliness Loss of self-esteem Anxiety Worry and depression
Hospital Dialysis (average 3/week, 6–8 hrs. each) Estimated median survival = 6.1 yrs.	Less medical worry Immediate medical supervision	All of the above, *plus:* *More* loneliness *More* limitation *More* inconvenience, reduced use of home environment
Hospital Dialysis and Transplant from Living Donor Estimated median survival = 12.5 yrs.	*Patient:* Restored fertility Convenience Mobility Independence Restored normal activities Reduced cost of medical care *Donor:* Family harmony Companionship Self-esteem	*Patient:* *During Hospital Stay:* Same as hospital dialysis, above *After Discharge from Hospital:* Some worry; inconvenience of follow-up checks, dependence on living donor may cause resentment *Donor:* *During Hospital Stay:* Same as above *After Discharge from Hospital:* Same as above
Hospital Dialysis and Transplant from Cadaver Estimated median survival = 4.5 yrs.	*Patient:* Same as for patient with living donor transplant *Donor's Family:* Consolation to donor's family from their generous act of consenting	*During Hospital Stay:* Same as above *After Discharge from Hospital:* Same as above

*Median survival rates are used because life expectancies are not available.

of life benefits, to determine if inclusion of quality of life factors makes any difference in preference.

Quality of life costs of discomforts for home dialysis, including inconvenience and immobility, can be shadow priced by what United States government programs or patients ineligible for them have been willing to pay for a transplant to end their dependency on home *or* hospital dialysis. The mid-range cost of transplantation including donor costs is $15,000 in the first year plus about $1,500 for each subsequent year for follow-up therapy. Over an 11.2 year period this would amount to about $30,000.

This is obviously a minimum shadow price, based on actual costs, since presumably most patients with ESRD would pay even more if they could, were it necessary to do so to obtain a transplant. We must also add the cost of inconvenience, temporary loss of gainful employment, risk, and pain to the living donor—perhaps $15,000 for that, based on a few days of life expectancy lost due to the minimal operative mortality, plus the pain and inconvenience of the nephrectomy.

We should probably add to this the quality of life costs of infertility for the dialysis patient, since successful transplants do usually restore this lost capacity. For the roughly 50% of the patients of fertile age, assume that half want children or more children. Given an estimated average cost of adoption and adjustment to it of $2,000, plus another $2,000 psychic cost at not having a natural child, we have an added quality of life cost of $.5 \times .5 \times (2{,}000 + 2{,}000) =$ $1,000.

Thus the total minimum shadow price of the quality of life costs of home dialysis is $30,000 + 15,000 + 1,000, or $46,000 for 11.2 years.

Quality of life costs of the loss of the home environment for hospital dialysis can be shadow priced at a minimum by estimating the costs of all the activities required to make the hospital environment as homelike as possible. These activities include frequent and lengthy visits by close relatives and provision of various home conveniences (desk, library, appliances). Privacy and aesthetic qualities of the home must also be added.

Costs of visiting include transportation out-of-pocket costs and the opportunity cost of the time spent in commuting between home and hospital for close relatives living in the home. Assuming one spouse, possibly accompanied by one or more children, and only one daily commute, estimated costs are $2 for transportation (20 miles round trip at 10¢ per mile) plus an hour of lost time at an average of $5, for an average daily visit cost of $7 three times a week, or about $1,000 per year. Diverse home conveniences might cost another $500 a year to rent.

The loss of home privacy and aesthetics in the hospital can be estimated from what is paid on the average to achieve it beyond a similar level of purely physical convenience attainable in rented rooms. Assuming one can rent a standard room with shared use of a bathroom and kitchen for about $1,000 a year and that the average private apartment or home rental (including utilities) is about $3,000 a year, the annual loss of privacy and aesthetic choice is estimated conservatively at the difference or $2,000 per year. For the three 8-hour days a week of home environment lost to hospital dialysis this amount must be multiplied by $3/7 \times 8/24$ or .14, to give $280 per year. Limitation of the geographic location of dial-

Table 3-6.

Treatment	*Quantity of Life Benefit*	–	*Quality of Life Cost*	=	*Net Benefit*
Home Dialysis 11.2 years' median survival	11.2 × $20,000		45,000 kidney shadow price 1,000 infertility		
	= 224,000	–	46,000	=	178,000
Hospital Dialysis 6.1 years	6.1 × 20,000		46,000 17,000		
	= 122,000	–	63,000	=	59,000
Living Donor Transplant 12.5 years	12.5 × 20,000		13,000 15,000		
	= 250,000	–	28,000	=	222,000
Cadaver Transplant 4.5 years	4.5 × 20,000		4½ × 1000 ½ × 5000		
	= 90,000	–	7,000	=	83,000

ysis patients to urban areas having hospitals with hemodialysis equipment imposes an additional estimated opportunity cost of $1,000 per year. Over the expected 6.1-year period of hospital dialysis, a total of (1000 + 500 + 280 + 1000) (6.1) or $16,958–roughly $17,000–is the quality of life cost of hospital dialysis beyond that of home dialysis.

The hospital dialysis has all the quality of life costs associated with the inconveniences of any kind of dialysis, represented by the kidney transplant shadow price of $46,000, plus the loss of the home environment cost of $17,000, for a total of $63,000.

In both transplant treatments, the quality of life *cost* is composed of the hospital stay, plus the inconvenience and time for follow-up check-ups estimated at $1,000 per year, and costs to the living donor of $15,000. The hospital stay quality of life cost was estimated at $5,000 per year or $1,250 for the three-month average wait for a living donor transplant, and twice that for the cadaveric transplant (rounding to $1,000's).

The patient's descending order of preference, on the basis of these assumptions, would thus be:

Table 3-7.

		Net Benefit
Living Donor Transplant	(best)	$222,000
Home Dialysis		178,000
Cadaver Transplant		83,000
Hospital Dialysis	(worst)	59,000

These magnitudes of difference significantly alter the rational preferences that would have been based on purely medical, quantity of life maximizing considerations:

Table 3–8.

Medical *Life Quantity Maximizing*		*Medical and Social* *Life Quantity and Quality Maximizing*
Living Donor Transplant (12.5 years' life expectancy)	BEST	Living Donor Transplant (12.5 years' life expectancy)
Home Dialysis (11.2 years' life expectancy)		Home Dialysis (11.2 years' life expectancy)
Hospital Dialysis (6.1 years' life expectancy)		Cadaver Transplant (4.5 years' life expectancy)
Cadaver Transplant (4.5 years's life expectancy)	WORST	Hospital Dialysis (6.1 years' life expectancy)

Note that the reversal of preference order in the third and fourth choices, based on an analysis recognizing quality of life factors, is *not* trivial because the first and second choices remain unchanged. Both the first and second choices are severely constrained by scarce resources of living donor kidneys and training programs for home dialysis, respectively. Thus, the reversal of the third and fourth choices by this kind of quality of life quantification and integration with life expectancy factors may offer a significantly improved quality of life for many kidney patients with end-stage renal disease.

The worth of the switch to an individual patient is the difference between the worth of the choice not including quality of life, and the worth of the choice including quality of life.

Table 3–9.

		"Worth"
Pre-QOL:	3rd choice (Hospital Dialysis) (6.1 years @ $20,000) =	$122,000
	4th choice (Cadaver Transplant) (4½ years @ $20,000) =	90,000
		32,000
Post-QOL:	3rd choice (Cadaver Transplant)	83,000
	4th choice (Hospital Dialysis)	59,000
		24,000

Thus, before QOL analysis, a patient might feel a mild preference (12 to 9) for hospital dialysis over cadaver transplant. After QOL analysis, he should prefer cadaveric transplant more than hospital dialysis. Assuming the second (QOL-including) analysis is the most correct one, a decision based on the least correct

(QOL-excluding) analysis would have cost him the difference between the total worth of the "best" third choice (cadaveric transplant, at \$83,000) and the "worst" third choice (hospital dialysis, at \$59,000), or \$83,000-\$59,000 or \$24,000. This is a significant difference in quantity and quality of life benefits, even in shadow pricing. The current queuing of ESRD patients by the thousands for a cadaveric transplant is evidence of their intuitive judgments confirming this analysis.

Considering that a full 70% of all kidney patients are given either hospital dialysis (50%) or cadaveric transplants (20%), the social significance of such a modified preference sequence is substantial. Assuming an annual cohort of 8,400 patients (see Chapter 20), the annual social cost of the error committed by not including the quality of life analysis is .70 X 8,400 X 24,000 or \$141,000,000 over five years, or over \$28 million per year. This computation of the social cost of the error assumes, for the purposes of illustration, that both forms of treatment are available to a patient. In reality there are medical indications for each of these treatments so that far less than 70% of the treated population has a choice, and the social cost of the error is correspondingly reduced.

SOME CAVEATS

This entire approach to quality of life cost-benefit analysis as applied to decisions in surgery does not take into account the variance in preferences for qualities of life among consumers and the cost of the information needed for this kind of analysis. Assumptions are made about the shadow price of life, and the nonuniform application of the discounted present value of benefit or cost streams.

There is a wide dispersion of preferences concerning life expectancy, quality of life factors, and their trade-offs for which we have assumed average values based on market or shadow prices. To provide more appropriate mean values for the quantity and quality of life preferences for subgroups, stratified sample surveys of consumer preferences might be helpful.

For the decision analysis to use empirical data rather than informed guesses for information, surveys are needed to increase precision, credibility, and confidence. If standardized quantity and quality of life preferences survey questionnaires were administered to patients routinely at the start of medical care, the monetary cost of obtaining such information would be reduced to only a few dollars per patient. This is a small cost, compared to the expected gain in the consonance of patient quantity and quality of life preferences with medical decisions, likely to amount to thousands of dollars per patient. However, the human cost of obtaining such information from patients must also be added, in terms of such quality of life costs as increased anxiety. As patients would experience psychological trauma in dwelling on the various trade-offs between treatments and results in lethal diseases, such trauma will be part of the cost of the information needed for this kind of analysis.

The price of life assumption used in the above analysis is a simplification of what should be an entire study. The use of nursing home annual patient costs as a shadow price for life is open to question, since for many individuals an added year of life is worth either much more, perhaps, at age 30, or less, perhaps, after age 90. The price used here is only for illustrative purposes. To obtain more precise and believable data, surveys should be considered to determine actual consumer valuations of life under conditions of varying quality. Yet it will be exceedingly difficult to obtain from health consumers quantitative evaluations of both quality and quantity of life factors. The concepts are unfamiliar, laden with emotional connotations, and concerned with possible states of illness never experienced or witnessed. Clearly investigation is indicated.

The application of quality of life factors and their shadow pricing to cost-benefit analysis of medical decisions has been illustrated by some crude estimates. Next in developing this approach is research to prepare for possible consumer surveys, and if sound data could be obtained, the analyses presented in this chapter could be completed with more confidence and with more ultimate utility.

SUMMARY

Quality of life factors associated with surgery are identified, quantified in terms of their equivalent social costs by shadow pricing, and balanced against *quantity* of life as also expressed in commensurate shadow price terms. The average "market" price of life is estimated. Examples of the surgical treatment of breast cancer and end-stage kidney disease are developed, with the collateral social costs and benefits of treatment alternatives. Preferred treatment alternatives, in terms of maximizing patients' utility, are compared for quantity of life, and quantity plus quality of life cases, demonstrating that the integration of quality of life factors with survival probabilities may significantly alter the treatment preference.

References

Abt CC: The social costs of cancer. Social Indicators Research 2:175, 1975

Anderson C: Aspects of pathological grief and mourning. Int J Psychoanal 30:48, 1949

Brown F: Depression and childhood bereavement. J Ment Sci 107:754, 1961

Dyk RB, Sutherland AM: Adaption of the spouse and other family members to the colostomy patient. Cancer 9: 123, 1956

Feifel H: Attitudes toward death in some normal and mentally ill populations, The Meaning of Death. Edited by H Feifel. New York, McGraw-Hill, 1959

Feifel H: Older persons look at death. Geriatrics 11:127–130, 1956

Fuchs VR: Health care and the United States economic system. Milbank Mem Fund Q 50:211, 1972

George V, Wilding P: Motherless Families. London, Routledge and Kegan, 1972

Krant MJ, Sheldon A: The dying patient–medicine's responsibility. J Thanatology 1:1, 1971

Maddison D, Viola A: The health of widows in year following bereavement. J Psychosom Res 12:297, 1968

Parkes CM, Benjamin B, Fitzgerald RG: Broken heart: a statistical study of increased mortality among widowers, Br Med J 1:740, 1969

Parkes CM: Recent bereavement as a cause of mental illness. Br J Psychiatry 110:198, 1964

Rees WD, Lutkins SG: Mortality of bereavement. Br Med J 4:13, 1967

Reiss PJ: Bereavement and the American family. Arch Found Thanatology 1:102, 1969

Rice DP: Estimating the cost of illness. Am J Public Health 57:424, 1967

Rice DP, Cooper BS: The economic value of human life. Am J Public Health 57:1954, 1967

Schelling TC: The life you save may be your own, Problems in public expenditure Analysis. Edited by SB Chase Jr. Washington DC, The Brookings Institution, 1968

Shoor M, Speed MH: Delinquency as a manifestation of the mourning process. Psychiat Q 37:540, 1963

Stein Z, Susser M: Widowhood and mental illness. Br J Prev Soc Med 23, 106, 1969

Wahl CW: Some antecedent factors in the family history of 392 schizophrenics. Am J Psychiatry 110:668, 1954

Weisbrod BA: Economics of Public Health. Philadelphia, University of Pennsylvania Press, 1961

4

Heterogeneity among patients as a factor in surgical decision-making

Donald S. Shepard
Richard Jay Zeckhauser

The effective physician is an intuitive statistician. He collects data about many variables on each patient. On the basis of these observations, he predicts the likelihood of various outcomes depending upon the treatment that is administered. Moreover, when extrapolating from his experience or past studies, the physician recognizes patient-to-patient variability, what we refer to here as heterogeneity, as a key predictor of differential response to treatment.

This paper formalizes the concept of heterogeneity and demonstrates that it can serve as a useful tool to help organize information in a variety of contexts that an analyst, a policymaker, or a physician may confront. First we show that explicit recognition of heterogeneity can aid the physician dealing with an individual patient in (a) formulating diagnoses, (b) predicting response to treatment, and (c) selecting the therapy that best meets the patient's preferences. In the following section we employ the heterogeneity concept as a tool for refining the analysis of populations from which there are dropouts due, for example, to deaths. In the final section we address the implications of heterogeneity for the formulation of policy, a context in which the use of medical resources must be included as a consideration. Our analysis proceeds by examples. Because our objective is to demonstrate a methodology and not to generate clinical insights, we sometimes oversimplify to enhance clarity. For the reader's convenience, we rely heavily on studies reported elsewhere in this volume.

This research was supported in part by grants from the Robert Wood Johnson Foundation and the Commonwealth Fund through the Center for the Analysis of Health Practices of the Harvard School of Public Health.

CHOICE OF APPROPRIATE THERAPY

Heterogeneity and the Meaning of Diagnostic Signs and Symptoms

Neutra's systematic analysis (Chapter 18) of the decision to operate on a patient with abdominal pain of acute onset provides a concrete example of how the interpretation of symptoms varies according to the characteristics of a patient. For simplicity, Neutra assumes that the diagnosis has been narrowed to a choice between two conditions: appendicitis (APP), for which surgery is best, or non-specific abdominal pain (NSAP), for which medical management is appropriate. Neutra showed that a diagnostician could obtain relatively good discrimination between APP and NSAP cases based on four signs and symptoms: location of pain, severity of pain, rebound tenderness, and rectal tenderness. Neutra made the simplifying assumption that among patients with one of these two conditions, these four signs and symptoms are probabilistically independent.

Suppose that patients presenting to a surgeon for this differential diagnosis are heterogeneous, i.e., that they are drawn from at least two distinct subpopulations. Each subpopulation differs in its likelihood of having APP or NSAP, and of presenting various signs and symptoms given each underlying condition. We will show that if the characteristics that distinguish the subpopulations are observed, then diagnostic accuracy will be improved; if these characteristics are not observed, then diagnostic accuracy will be diminished. In either case, failure to recognize heterogeneity, if it is present, may produce misleading assessments.

Consider first an observed characteristic, sex, and its influence on the differential diagnosis of APP versus NSAP. Using the data of de Dombal et al. (1972), Neutra estimated that 64% of patients presenting with undiagnosed acute abdomen had NSAP, and the remaining 36% had APP. Another report from the same data source (Staniland et al., 1972) showed that 60% of the APP cases were in males, compared to only 42% of the NSAP cases, a pattern consistent with the wider variety of causes of intra-abdominal pain in women. Thus 48.5% of the patients are male. Applying Bayes Theorem, we find that the probability of NSAP in males is 55.4%, and in females it is 72.0%. Thus we have a quantitative indication that sex conveys information for differential diagnosis.

When used in conjunction with information on signs and symptoms, consideration of sex can help to refine the type of calculation conducted by Neutra. Working with both sexes combined, Neutra examined the 24 possible combinations of the 4 signs and symptoms. He ranked these combinations in order of increasing likelihood of APP. He then considered alternative cutoff levels, above which all patients would be operated on. Assuming that 30% of APP cases would perforate in the absence of an operation, and that the objective was to minimize deaths regardless of resource costs, Neutra found that the optimal cutoff level for both sexes combined was a rank score of 8.

If we disaggregate by sex and perform an analogous computation, we may possibly find a different cutoff level for male and female patients, and thereby be able to prescribe therapies with greater precision. In carrying out these sex-disaggregated calculations, we assume that the four signs and symptoms continue

Table 4-1. Expected deaths and operations under alternative treatments at rank risk scores 7 and 8, by sex.[a]

Rank Score of Risk	*Patient Classification*	*Number Receiving Score in U.S. in a Year*	*Deaths Under Alternative Treatments*	
			If Operate	*If Do Not Operate*
7	General Population	5087	3.43	2.99*
	Male	2198	1.50*	1.80
	Female	2889	1.93	1.20*
8	General Population	4255	2.91*	3.53
	Male	1859	1.30*	2.12
	Female	2396	1.62	1.41*

*Preferred treatment for that patient classification.

Expected outcomes under optimal treatment

Rank Score of Risk	*Patients Eventually Operated*[b]		*Deaths*		*Deaths Averted Through Ability to Classify by Sex*
	If Classify by Sex	*If Do Not Classify by Sex*	*If Classify by Sex*	*If Do Not Classify by Sex*	
7	2334	340	2.70	2.99	.29
8	2019	4255	2.71	2.91	.20
Total for Two Ranks	4353	4595	5.41	5.90	.49

[a]Deaths may not add exactly in categories due to rounding. Note the differences for the *general population* between *deaths if operate* and *deaths if do not operate,* 0.44 = 3.43 - 2.99 and –0.62 = 2.91 –3.53, are identified as marginal deaths in Neutra's Table 18–6.

[b]These categories include: (1) all patients for whom surgery is initially preferred, and (2) patients for whom surgery is not initially preferred who are subsequently discovered to have true appendicitis and then operated upon (with higher mortality).

to be probabilistically independent within categories, with the categories now defined both by condition and by sex. For example, among males with APP, we assume that the probability of rebound tenderness is independent of the presence of rectal tenderness.

As shown in Table 4-1, the optimal cutoff level is lowered to 7 in males and raised to 9 in females if sex is monitored.* Using these cutoffs would reduce the expected numbers of deaths among the patients at ranks 7 and 8 from 2.99 and 2.91 per year (derived from Neutra's data) to 2.70 and 2.71, respectively. Thus, .49 deaths are saved per year at these ranks. There is also a reduction of 242 appendectomies, a consideration that could be important if savings in medical

*Following Neutra's assumption, 6.4% of the APP cases of each sex have been removed from the grouping by rank scores because they represent unavoidable perforations prior to hospitalization.

resources were considered as well. This example estimates the gains offered by distinguishing populations on an observable characteristic—sex in this instance. In this example the gain from the additional information is modest.

Age of the patient is another commonly considered factor that potentially might alter the interpretation of physical signs and symptoms used in the diagnosis of APP and NSAP. It turns out, however, that in Neutra's data source (Staniland et al., 1972) the relative incidence of APP and NSAP is virtually identical for each decade of age. Thus, unlike sex, age is of little value in distinguishing these two conditions. On the other hand, although the costs of mistakes—operate with NSAP or delay with APP—both increase with age, they increase at different rates. Thus, according to Neutra's calculation of the cost ratio, it turns out that surgeons should be slightly more interventionist with older patients than with younger patients presenting the identical signs and symptoms, despite the fact that their probabilities of APP are the same.

Consider now heterogeneity on an unobserved characteristic, tolerance to pain. To be specific, let us assume that patients presenting with acute abdomen belong to one of two subpopulations. The "pain-prone" population is more likely to report at least two of the symptoms considered, severe pain and rectal tenderness. Given either underlying condition, the probability that a member of the "pain-resistant" population will report these symptoms is below average. Again, we assume that the four signs and symptoms are independent within each condition and patient-type combination. It can be shown, however, that some of these symptoms are no longer independent within condition groups once the pain-resistant and pain-prone subpopulations are combined, as they would be if we could not distinguish between these two subpopulations. In fact, the symptoms would be positively correlated. Regardless of whether the underlying condition is APP or NSAP, a patient reporting one symptom is more likely to be pain prone, and therefore more likely to report the other symptom. Ignorance as to which patients are pain prone, in effect, introduces noise into the system; we cannot interpret the diagnostic information as accurately as we could if everyone were uniformly prone to pain, or if we could and did monitor such proneness.

Clinicians are sensitive to the possible variations in meaning of diagnostic signs and symptoms in different groups of patients, and prescribe therapies accordingly. Still, as we showed with our examples of classification by sex and pain sensitivity for suspected appendicitis, explicit consideration of the implications of heterogeneity may at times provide useful information for diagnosis; at other times it may suggest the important negative conclusion that diagnostic capabilities are limited.

Heterogeneity of Effect of Treatments and Preferences

Clinicians know from experience that individuals suffering the same disease can be expected to react differently to a given treatment, and that therapeutic decisions should therefore be individualized. Weinstein et al. (Chapter 21) formalize this notion in their comparison of coronary artery bypass graft and medical management for five hypothetical male patients suffering coronary artery

Table 4-2. Quality-adjusted life expectancy for two sets of preferences.

	Active Preferences	*Sedentary Preferences*
Surgical Treatment	12.62 yrs.	12.90 yrs.
Medical Management	12.22 yrs.	13.00 yrs.

(Data drawn from Weinstein *et al.*, Table 21-4.)

disease. The patients differ in age and medical characteristics. Weinstein et al. value outcomes in terms of "quality-adjusted life expectancy," an index that is computed as life expectancy minus a penalty for each year at reduced quality due to angina. They specifically recognize heterogeneity by scaling the magnitude of the penalty to reflect the hypothetical patient's preferences and lifestyle.

Economic considerations aside, if surgery offers a greater quality-adjusted life expectancy than the alternative of medical management, then surgery is indicated. (This decision rule may prove contrary to the sometimes-heard casual dictum that surgery is contraindicated in very sick patients who would have high surgical mortality.*) The salience of variations in medical condition is revealed in the analyses of Weinstein et al. when they assign the five hypothetical patients identical sedentary preferences. For three, surgery is preferred; medical management is superior for the other two. An extreme example of a very sick patient for whom surgery is preferred is the third patient. He is a 50-year-old male with severe congestive heart failure for whom surgical mortality is estimated at 50%. His resulting quality-adjusted life expectancy under surgery is only 1.17 years. Yet his adjusted life expectancy under medical management is estimated to be still lower, only 0.89 years. (See Weinstein et al. Table 21-4).

The patients of Weinstein et al., with "active" preferences would sacrifice greater shares of their life expectancies than would those with "sedentary" preferences, in order to conduct their normal activities free from angina. The choice of optimal therapy for a particular patient, therefore, may depend on his preferences, as is seen with the second hypothetical patient, a 60-year-old male. Here active preferences favor surgical treatment. Table 4-2 provides the numerical comparison.

IMPLICATIONS OF HETEROGENEITY IN THE ANALYSIS OF LONGITUDINAL DATA

An understanding of heterogeneity should make us more sensitive to problems of drawing inferences from longitudinal studies in which there is a changing composition of population at risk. The analysis which follows considers two such populations: patients free of recurrence of hernias after herniorrhaphy, and surviving patients after a kidney transplant. These examples are designed to il-

*See Moses (1969) and other chapters in the National Halothane Study for data on surgical mortality by patient characteristics.

Table 4–3. First recurrence after herniorrhaphy.

Interval After Surgery (Years)	*Proportion of Survivors Free of Recurrence at End of Interval*[a]	*Annual Rate of First Recurrence During Interval*[b]
0– 1	1 – .1 × .30 = .970	30.0
1– 5	1 – .1 × .65 = .935	9.1
5–10	1 – .1 × .81 = .919	3.4

[a]This value is computed in the table as 1 – (proportion of patients eventually suffering recurrences) × (cumulative proportion of recurrences up to the end of this interval). Data derived from Neuhauser (Chapter 14).
[b]Per 1,000 free of recurrence at beginning of interval.

lustrate a more general phenomenon: The early dropouts from a heterogeneous population are high-risk individuals; therefore through a selective process such a population becomes stronger over time.

An Example: Recurrences of Hernias

Using data on hernia recurrences summarized by Neuhauser (Chapter 14), we will show that heterogeneity of patients with respect to their risk of first recurrence offers a simple and consistent explanation for the pattern of first recurrences. If an individual suffers a recurrence, he is removed from the population under study, which consists of all individuals still free of recurrence. This is a simple first-failure analysis, with hernia recurrence playing the role that death does in other more familiar analyses.

Combining the results of several studies, Neuhauser estimated that 10% of the patients who undergo herniorrhaphies eventually suffer one or more recurrences. In Table 4–3 we restate these results in terms of the proportions of surviving patients who are still free of recurrences at various periods after surgery. From the ratio of proportions at the beginning and end of each interval, we estimate the annual first recurrence rate in that interval.* These rates decline with increasing length of time after surgery. Heterogeneity of patient characteristics and, conceivably, of surgical technique offer a possible explanation for this pattern.

What alternative explanations might there be? First, we might think that the true probabilities of recurrence are constant each year, and that the variations observed above are therefore a result of chance. This hypothesis doesn't seem likely because, given constant probabilities, there is less than 1 chance in 1,000 that such a large departure as that reported by Neuhauser would be observed. Second, we might think that the probability of recurrence for each patient falls over time as the tissues heal and strengthen after surgery. Our surgical colleagues suggest that this explanation is unlikely after the initial weeks of healing. There is a brief initial period when sutures provide protection against recurrence; scar

*For the 4-year interval years 1–5, for example, the calculation is
Annual Rate = $1 - (.935/.970)^{1/4}$.

Table 4-4. Demonstration of declining recurrence rates in a heterogeneous population.

Interval After Surgery (years)	*Number of Patients Free of Recurrences at End of Interval*			*Annual Rate of First Recurrence, During Interval*[a]
	Low Rate Group (.01 per year)	*High Rate Group (.25 per year)*	*Total*	
0– 1	99	75	174	130
1– 5	95	24	119	91
5–10	90	6	96	42

[a]Per 1,000 free of recurrence at beginning of interval.

tissue then forms and the wound gains maximum strength within a few weeks, not a few years.

To develop our preferred explanation that the pattern is due to heterogeneity of patients who have completed surgery, we begin with a simple model that generates the qualitative characteristics of the observed pattern. Subsequently, we refine the type of heterogeneity considered to reproduce the quantitative characteristics of the observed pattern as well.

In our simplified model, the patients receiving herniorrhaphy are of two types distinguished by their probability of a first recurrence in any given year. Initially there are 100 patients of each type. Patients in the low-rate group have a chance of .01 of having a recurrence in any given year, that is, a chance of .99 of not having a recurrence. Patients in the high-rate group have a chance of .25 of having a recurrence in any year. For this analysis we will ignore the possibility of death; it could be incorporated using models of competing risk.* After one year the numbers of patients in each group still free of recurrences are $100 \times .99 = 99$ and $100 \times .75 = 75$, respectively. Since the total number of patients free of recurrence is $99 + 75 = 174$, the recurrence rate during the initial year is $1 - 174/200 = 130/1000$. For the 4-year-period 1 to 5 years after surgery, the comparable rate is $1 - (119/174)^{1/4} = 91/1000$. Table 4-4 presents the data and rates. Qualitatively, we have shown that in a heterogeneous population where the risks of some event like recurrence for each individual remain fixed over time, the overall rates of the event decline over time. Thus by assuming heterogeneity, we can reproduce the general pattern of declining recurrence rates calculated in Table 4-3.

Once we recognize that patients differ with respect to their risk of recurrence, there is no reason to restrict our analysis to two categories. We have extended our analysis of hernia recurrences using a continuous spectrum of annual recurrence rates across the population. To keep the analysis tractable, we employed a distribution belonging to the gamma family.** Distributions in that family, which

*See Chiang (1968).

**This is an example of a mixed exponential model of selective survival. For a mathematical discussion of such models, see Mann et al. (1974).

includes the exponential and the chi-square as special cases, are flexible and computationally straightforward. Moreover, unlike the well-known normal distribution, gamma distributions take only positive values, a necessary property because recurrence rates cannot be negative.

The best-fitting gamma distribution reproduces the data in Table 4-3 exactly to three decimal places. The individuals in the population at time 0, right after the completed herniorrhaphy, have a mean recurrence rate of .0552 per year; the standard deviation among their rates is .3296.* The distribution of recurrence rates is highly skewed to the right; that is, the bulk of the patients have low rates, but a few have quite high rates. To be more precise, individuals at the 10th (high risk), 50th (median), and 90th (low risk) percentiles have probabilities of at least one recurrence within 5 years of .408, .009, and .004.** The risk at the 90th percentile is 100 times as great as at the 10th percentile.

This analysis suggests that the variability in risks of recurrence is substantial and of potential clinical importance. Weak abdominal tissue, imperfect surgical repair, chronic cough, susceptibility to septic complications in the surgical incision, and malnutrition have been mentioned as possible factors contributing to the recurrence of hernias. Our analysis of heterogeneity underscores the importance of the current clinical practice of studying these and other conceivable correlates of risk. Investigations may suggest interventions to lower these risks. Even in the absence of such interventions, merely identifying patients at elevated risk of recurrence may be of value, since their ultimate responses to treatment are so distinctive. For these patients, alternative or supplementary treatments might deserve special consideration.

The primary purpose of this recurrence example was to show the potential magnitude of heterogeneity within a population, and to show the way its existence could be inferred and estimated. Thinking of the model more broadly, as one in which individuals have varying risks of dropping out of the population, it offers a qualitative result that has widespread application.*** Any such population will "improve" itself as it differentially eliminates individuals at high risk.

Consider now a situation where risk rates for specific individuals increase regularly with age, a situation that would seem to correspond to many medical phenomena. The heterogeneous-risk model suggests that observed changes in risk rates for the cohort as a whole will underestimate the increase in risk rates for particular individuals. Particular individuals, after all, do not benefit from the elimination of the high-risk members of the population; the cohort does.

*The distributions must be written in terms of instantaneous recurrence rates, what are sometimes called "hazard rates." The observed annual rate of recurrences, q, will be related to the hazard rate, μ, by $q = 1 - e^{-\mu}$. The more familiar term "force of mortality" is the corresponding instantaneous mortality rate.

**These calculations were made by fitting a lognormal distribution to the first two moments of the hazard rate distribution.

***We have demonstrated (1975) its relevance to such diverse problems as interpreting time trends in age-specific mortality rates and assessing the benefits from automobile safety programs.

Changes in Average Quality of Life in a Heterogeneous Cohort

Parallel implications apply for longitudinal patterns of quality of life. We next present a hypothetical example motivated by Barnes's projections of survival for recipients of kidney transplants (Chapter 20, Table 20-1). This example demonstrates that the average quality of life of the members of a cohort will reflect the changing composition of the cohort due to selective survival.

Suppose that a patient surviving kidney transplantation belongs to one of two subcohorts with different prognoses. Let us assign the living donor subcohort a mortality rate of 5% per year, and the cadaveric donor group a rate of 9%. To exclude complications of the operation and immunosuppresive therapy immediately following surgery, we base our analysis on survivors one year after surgery. We consider a total cohort of 500 survivors, of whom 200 received living kidneys and 300 cadaveric kidneys. As a readily measured, concrete proxy for quality of life, we shall use restoration of ability to pursue employment. Following the suggestions of Dr. Benjamin Barnes, we assume that 80% of the surviving recipients of living kidneys are employed at any point in time in a job as demanding as the one they held prior to renal failure. The comparable rate for cadaveric kidney recipients is 40%. To calculate the overall employment rate, we compute the number of survivors from each subcohort at any time, and multiply these numbers by the appropriate employment rates. Table 4-5 displays these calculations.

Table 4-5. Hypothetical example of survival and employability following transplant surgery.

	Living Donor		*Cadaveric Donor*		*Total Cohort*		
Years Postsurgery	*Survivors*	*Employed*	*Survivors*	*Employed*	*Survivors*	*Employed*	*Emp. Rate*
1	200	160	300	120	500	280	.56
5	163	130	206	82	369	212	.57
10	126	101	128	51	254	152	.60

As would be expected, the overall employment rate in the cohort increases over time, though no single individual has an expected gain in employment probability.

Reporting the employment rates of the two subcohorts separately could control for this heterogeneity, thereby increasing our predictive ability. Moreover, such a classification could be readily accomplished in this instance.* There may be equally significant heterogeneity, however, in cohorts or subcohorts within

*This classification by subcohorts is analogous to the cross classification used to reduce confounding in observational studies (See, for example, Cochran, 1965.) In observational studies the confounding arises because the populations receiving different treatments differ on important characteristics. In our analyses of longitudinal studies of heterogeneous populations, we assume that the groups are initially similar. Due to selective removal from the populations, however, the groups do not remain the same and confounding enters.

which further classifications are not made. In such instances, if quality of life and survival probability are positively correlated, we will observe that the average quality of life for the undifferentiated cohort decreases less rapidly or increases more rapidly than it does for the individuals who comprise the cohort. Thus, the selection effect may mask the rate of deterioration in quality for each individual member.

A closely related problem arises in the interpretation of cross-sectional data on persons of different ages or at specified lengths of elapsed time after receipt of particular treatments. It is well known, for example, that the average levels of such cardiovascular risk factors as blood pressure and cholesterol are higher in samples of older patients. Because individuals with the highest levels of these risk factors die faster, cross-sectional studies, if naively extrapolated, would understate the average rate of increase in these risk factors for an individual.

Changing Mortality Rates Over Time

Medical treatments and interventions, as we have stressed, produce varying responses within a population. Surgical procedures often provide an extreme example. In a very short period of time, say a year, these procedures will result in death for some individuals, yet will permit survival for others. Changes in short-run mortality rates, however, can hardly serve as a summary measure of the benefits from surgery. They indicate nothing about quality of life; neither do they provide information about expected future mortality rates. It is widely understood that the individuals who are "saved" through surgical intervention ordinarily do not take on the average mortality characteristics of their age cohort.

An understanding of the possible relationships between short- and long-run mortality may aid the patient and his physician in the choice of appropriate therapy, and may assist the researcher who wishes to plan longitudinal studies and derive inferences from the results that they generate. We illustrate with another hypothetical example based on kidney transplantation. Suppose that we wished to choose between a new form of immunosuppressive therapy and the existing therapy. The new therapy is expected to be more effective in protecting the transplanted kidney, but might render some patients excessively prone to infection. Azathioprine is an immunosuppressive drug that might be thought of as the new therapy. It sometimes causes severe leukopenia (an extremely low white blood cell count), followed by septic death. Surgical mortality will not be affected by the choice of therapy. Patients surviving surgery under the old treatment are expected to face a constant force of mortality of .10 per year. For patients surviving surgery and receiving the new therapy, the force of mortality is expected to be constant over time, but the rates will differ within the population treated by the new therapy according to the individual responses of the patients.

We assume that a gamma probability distribution, the same distribution used in the analysis of hernia recurrences, can represent the variability in individual mortality rates resulting from application of the new therapy. Suppose that the force of mortality is distributed with a mean of .25 per year, and a standard

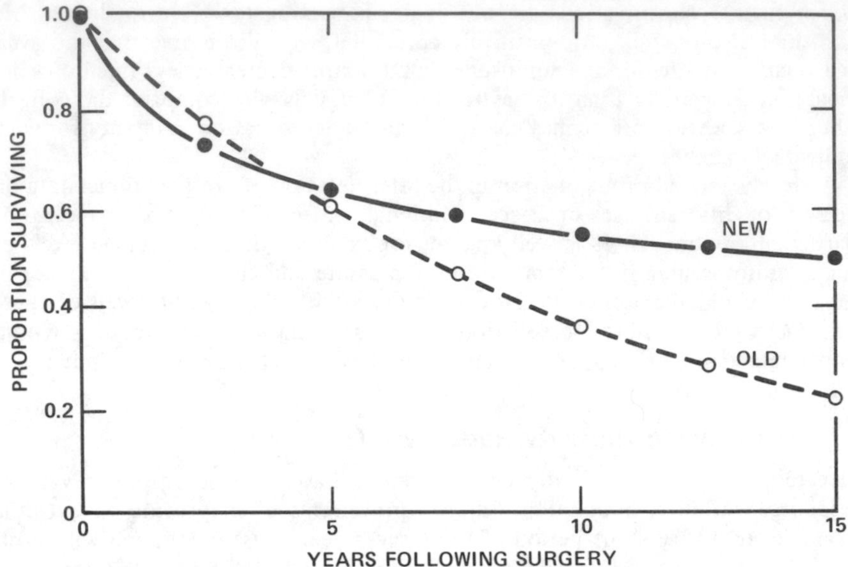

Figure 4–1. Projected survival under new and old therapies.

deviation of .50.* Due to the changing composition of the population, the force of mortality under the new therapy will then fall from .25 per year initially to .01 per year after 15 years. Since the mortality under the old treatment remains constant at .10 per year, the new treatment is inferior initially, but subsequently surpasses the old treatment. Figure 4-1 shows the proportion of patients surviving surgery who are still alive varying numbers of years later. Notice that if our criterion for choice of policy were short-run survival (1 or even 3 years) we would favor the older treatment. Yet the new therapy offers greater long-term survival and life expectancy. The explanation is similar to that in our earlier discussions of heterogeneity: initial death (or morbidity) rates are high as the high risk members of the population succumb. Thus the remaining population at subsequent times has been selected in favor of low-risk persons and has a lower force of mortality.**

*For simplicity, the present example ignores deaths unrelated to transplantation and its complications. Thus mortality and survival cannot meaningfully be calculated beyond 15 years under the present model. The curves in Figure 4–1 would be steeper in the more realistic, and more complicated, situation where force of mortality increases over time. See Shepard and Zeckhauser (1975) for a discussion of heterogeneity in populations with an increasing force of mortality.

**For a hypothetical individual patient whose reaction to the immunosuppressive drug is unknown beforehand, the best estimates of his survival under the alternative treatments are provided by the graphs in Fig. 4–1. If he counts short-term survival very heavily relative to long-term, the old therapy may be preferable; otherwise, the new one should be selected. Similar consideration of personal preferences may apply when a patient may choose to risk surgical mortality to increase expected long-term benefit.

As the example with immunosuppressive therapy illustrates, if we know that a population is likely to respond in a more variable fashion to a new treatment than to its predecessor, then we can expect mortality (or morbidity) rates to decline more sharply or rise less swiftly for the new treatment as opposed to the old. Surgery provides another illustration on a shorter time scale. If a surgical operation entails a substantial risk of death, then it will also induce a highly variable response among patients who receive it. The initial mortality rate with surgery will generally be higher than it would have been under medical treatment. The more strongly this mortality operates selectively against individuals who would have been at highest future risk, the lower will be the future mortality rates of those surviving surgery.

This observation suggests that when trying a new intervention, even if it yields inferior survival rates in the short run, we may wish to continue its use. We should extrapolate its expected future mortality rates using a model that pays explicit attention to the increased heterogeneity of the response it produces within the population.* That extrapolation may show that the poorer results to date with the new intervention lie within the bounds that suggest that the long-run cumulative performance of the intervention will be superior.**

Treatments that cut short-run mortality at the expense of introducing long-run risks will produce quite the opposite pattern. If, for example, multiple examinations by mammography with surgical follow-up for the detection and treatment of breast cancer could be shown to yield only a modest short-run reduction in mortality, we might want to discontinue the use of that procedure. In this instance, it has been suggested that the heterogeneous patient response would produce mortality results that were inferior in the future, assuming that the radiation from the multiple mammographies induced some future malignancies.***

The general inference that can be drawn from these examples is that if the population of potential patients is heterogeneous and/or if treatment will be applied differently, then we must expect varying short- and long-run responses to treatment. Modeling with explicit attention to the heterogeneity concept may help to extrapolate from a limited data base. To derive conclusive results, the

*The authors have looked elsewhere (1975) at the unfavorable implications for future mortality of the lives "saved" from an intervention such as air bags for automobiles or mobile cardiac units. Those who benefit most from these interventions, high-risk drivers and cardiac-prone individuals, will be at higher future risk as well. This same phenomenon, a positive association between the degree of reduction in short-term mortality and future mortality, could even apply if, as might be the case with certain preventive measures such as vaccinations, we cannot identify the actual beneficiaries from the intervention.

**This eliminates an ethical issue frequently encountered in clinical experiments. The new intervention will continue to be used, despite its "inferior" results to date, only if these results show that individuals to whom the new intervention will be administered can expect to benefit.

***Note also that the quality of life of the major early beneficiaries from the mammography-surgery treatment and their life expectancy would be lower than it was for the general population before this treatment was initiated. This suggests that naïve extrapolation of the benefits of the treatment assuming homogeneity among the surviving population would lead to an overestimate of the benefits. See Shepard and Zeckhauser (1975) for extensive discussion on this point.

need to engage in long-term follow-up studies and to search for possible surprising results will be particularly important. (See Cochran et al. (Chapter 11) and McPeek et al. (Chapter 10).)

The major implication for policy choice may unfortunately prove negative in many circumstances. Many surgical interventions, such as coronary artery bypass surgery, that provide gains in life quality or short-term reductions in mortality probably provide their major benefits to individuals who were initially at high risk relative to their age and sex cohorts. These individuals most likely remain at higher than average risk. Therefore, these interventions are accomplishing less than we might naïvely estimate from the improvements they generate in short-term indicators.

HETEROGENEITY AND POLICY CHOICE

This analysis has concentrated on the implications of heterogeneity in relation to decisions to promote the welfare of the individual patient. These are decisions that the physician faces every day. By contrast, the policymaker who allocates health resources, whether he be granting a certificate of need to construct a hospital, developing a state-sponsored program of malpractice insurance, or setting reimbursement rates for Medicaid, is simultaneously affecting the welfare of many individuals. We cannot conclude without mentioning briefly the way heterogeneity might enter his considerations—considerations which are necessarily directed to large groups of individuals or indeed to the population as a whole. The policymaker's decision to support one health-promoting program in preference to another that requires an equivalent outlay of resources should reflect society's valuations of the benefits that are produced, perhaps in a very indirect fashion, by the two programs. In assessing these valuations, explicit consideration of heterogeneity may provide useful information. It can help determine the expected benefits any particular patient will receive from an intervention. Moreover, if there is significant individual-to-individual variability in the likelihoods of requiring, seeking, and obtaining treatment, the heterogeneity concept can be employed, in analyses parallel to those considered here, to help predict those likelihoods. These different predictions can be merged to produce estimates of the distributions of benefits that alternative health-promoting programs will generate in the population.

Information on the distribution of benefits may facilitate decision-making. Society may possibly, and quite appropriately, wish to distinguish between an extra year of life for a 75-year-old as opposed to one for a person of 35. In comparing benefits for individuals of the same age, a year in intermittent pain for one person may be assigned a lower value than a year of full relief for another. (See Zeckhauser, 1975.)

On the other hand, this information may make some allocation decisions more sensitive politically. This is likely to occur when the information indicates that some programs are particularly helpful to certain ethnic, social, or economic groups, or to collections of individuals with particular diseases or symptoms. Sometimes society may feel more comfortable because certain issues involving fundamental values are not addressed explicitly when resource allocations are made. And indeed, if only an isolated, relatively small-scale decision is involved, society may benefit by blurring the trade-offs made between the benefits for different individuals or groups of individuals.

But there are countless major resource decisions affecting health that our society must make. If trade-off rates were permitted to vary significantly from decision to decision, gross inefficiencies would result. Moreover, if no grand tallies were kept, certain groups might end up grossly disadvantaged. We believe that for purposes of both equity and efficiency, policy choices should be grounded in the most accurate possible assessments of the distributions of benefits that the policies can be expected to produce. Attention to the heterogeneous nature of the potential patient population should assist in making these assessments.

Acknowledgments

We thank the editors of this volume, and Arthur Elstein, Howard Frazier, M.D., Duncan Neuhauser, William Stason, M.D. and Edith Stokey for helpful comments and suggestions.

References

Chiang CL: Introduction to Stochastic Processes in Biostatistics. New York, John Wiley and Sons, Inc., 1968

Cochran WG: The planning of observational studies of human populations. J Royal Stat Society, Ser A 128 (Part 2):234, 1965

de Dombal FT, Leaper DJ, Staniland JR, et al: Computer-aided diagnosis of acute abdominal pain. Br Med J 2:9, 1972

Mann NR, Schafer, RE, Singpurwalla ND: Methods for Statistical Analysis of Reliability and Life Data. New York, John Wiley and Sons, Inc., 1974

Moses LE: Comparison of crude and standardized anesthetic death rates. Chapter VI-2 in The National Halothane Study: Report of the Subcommittee of the National Halothane Study. Edited by JP Bunker, WH Forrest Jr, F. Mosteller, et al.Washington, DC, Government Printing Office, 1969

Shepard DS, Zeckhauser RJ: The Assessment of Programs to Prolong Life, Recognizing their Interaction with Risk Factors. Public Policy Program, Discussion Paper No. 32D Cambridge, Mass., Kennedy School of Government, Harvard University, 1975

Staniland JR, Ditchburn J, de Dombal FT: Clinical presentation of acute abdomen: study of 600 patients. Br Med J 3:393, 1972

Zeckhauser RJ: Procedures for valuing lives. Public Policy 23:419, 1975

5

Cost-benefit analysis of surgery: Some additional caveats and interpretations

Jerry R. Green

It must be a rare reader who has progressed this far in the book without questioning the application of cost-benefit analysis on a broad scale. This brief essay emphasizes some special issues relevant to medical decision-making and indicates how classical assumptions sometimes lead to nonoptimal behavior. Some of the problems have been discussed by Amy Taylor and Nava Pliskin in Chapter 1, the methodological prologue. The reduction to dollar figures of inherently nonquantifiable entities such as death, lost time from work or leisure, pain, and suffering forms the greatest barrier to the implementation of these methods. Clark Abt's Chapter 3 addresses such issues, as does Weinstein, Pliskin, and Stason's Chapter 21.

We will not dwell on them any further. Concentrating on the purely economic side, this chapter will explore the extent to which it is appropriate to use the prices actually paid for medical goods and services as measures of their true worth as inputs into the surgical process. A variety of conflicting forces may enter the picture. Some point to market prices undervaluing the true worth of medical inputs, while others are likely to lead to overvaluation.

It is best to start with a review of the reasoning which implies, in the context of ordinary resource allocation or economic planning, that such market prices are appropriate guides to policy. In this way, we will uncover some implicit assumptions that are subject to challenge in the present context.

At first blush, selling an input on a market where every potential buyer would pay the same price is surely the best way to allocate a fixed quantity of the resource. In this way we would ensure that it is received by those for whom it is most valuable. There are, however, two related questions to be settled before we can justifiably rely on the price mechanism alone to allocate resources efficiently. The first is that the value of the item for an individual might not correspond to its value for society as a whole. Inoculation against contagious disease is a prime example. Second, we cannot be sure that the total quantity to be distributed is itself "optimal." Perhaps there can be too many vitamins as well as too few. A more detailed analysis of the situation is therefore necessary.

Before proceeding to address these matters, it is necessary to say what "optimal" means. An optimum may be taken to represent a situation in which no individual can be better off without hurting at least one other person. At an optimal allocation of resources, some individuals may, nevertheless, be much wealthier than others. We will have little to say regarding the problem of income distribution and equity. Is it true that because someone is otherwise disadvantaged, he should be entitled to superior medical care, or priority in receiving service, as society's way of evening things out? Most people would agree that there are better, less chancy, ways of administering redistributive policies, and therefore would accept the distribution of wealth as given for the purpose of allocating medical resources.

Our concern will be the attainment of an optimum in the above sense with respect to the allocation of medical resources. Since the economist's traditional prescription is for laissez-faire, it is valid to ask why we should have cost-benefit analysis at all. The reason is that many of the assumptions underlying this presumption are invalid in the medical context. Stopping at this point is not enough. Whether evaluation takes place by the "invisible hand" of the marketplace or directly using cost-benefit analysis, sooner or later prices will be used to estimate costs. We want to know if these prices accurately reflect true social costs, and if not, what is the direction of bias. The answer typically depends upon which of the economist's assumptions is being violated, and why.

The following characterize the traditional conditions under which the "optimality" of an economic equilibrium can be proven.

1. The economic world is static and perfectly certain. All choices to buy or sell can be made now, and will be executed without default.

2. Each individual, and every firm, treat prices as given and do not try, or expect, to influence them by his market action.

3. All firms maximize their profits and redistribute them directly to individuals for their own discretionary use in expenditure.

4. Individuals choose rationally from among the alternative consumption plans available to them. That is, given two observations on the individual's chosen plans when he was faced with two different lists of prices, it will never be the case that his choice in the first instance would also have been affordable in the second and that the second would have been within his means in the first. The rationality of his choice in one circumstance or the other would have then been contradicted. Moreover, no one would ever waste any resource by consuming less of it than the amount he purchased.

Of course, no one pretends that these assumptions are actually satisfied all the time. People and firms make mistakes, foresight is imperfect at best, and, indeed, the complete list of potentially relevant prices is not really ever known. Nevertheless, markets perform tolerably well if the broader ideas behind these assumptions are generally operative. What we want to discuss is the set of circumstances peculiar to the allocation of surgical resources which causes these conditions to be systematically violated, and thereby produces prices in the market that are way out of line with the valuations we would like to use in our cost-benefit analyses.

We will proceed as follows: We reconsider each of the assumptions, show how it is likely to be violated in the medical context, and discuss the nature of the error that would be produced by a cost-benefit analysis that valued medical inputs at the actual prices being paid for them.

It will be easiest if we organize the discussion along the lines of the four assumptions of standard economic theory presented above.

STATIC ECONOMIC ENVIRONMENT

In the real world, all buying and selling is not executed at one primeval instant, before the rest of economic activity takes place. Potential investors or suppliers of new medical technology, for example, know the current prices for the goods and services they might plan to supply, but by the time their investments bear fruit, the conditions in the market could be very different. There is no room for this in the standard economic model sketched above. In that model, when an investment is made, the resulting revenues are known with certainty and the decisions can never be retrospectively incorrect.

Particularly in the medical context, imperfectly foreseen technical progress can cause serious misallocations of resources or misjudgments of potential cost and benefit if current prices were to be used. For example, if a sufficient supply of paramedical personnel were to be trained, the costs of postoperative care might be reduced substantially in many cases. But whether this will take place and how large the cost saving will be are unknowns.

In many elective surgical procedures, one of the costs to be considered if it is not undertaken is the potential that it may have to be done at a later date (see, for example, Neutra's paper on appendicitis, Chapter 18, and Neuhauser's on hernia, Chapter 14, in this volume). However, if cost-saving techniques may be introduced in the interim, the cost-benefit analysis based on current market prices will overestimate the relative value of performing the operation immediately. On the other hand, it is possible that medical progress will be made more rapidly in other surgical areas. This would tend to increase the value of hospital beds for uses other than the operation in question and would lead to an underestimate of the value of doing it immediately, before this unanticipated increase in the cost of hospital beds takes place.

PRICE-TAKING BEHAVIOR

Another source of inefficiency and error is the possibility that suppliers of medical resources recognize the dependence of prices upon the quantity that they sell. This is particularly acute when the item is protected by patent which prevents other suppliers from competing with the original inventor. Society is then faced with a genuinely insoluble problem. Without protection by patent, inventive activity would be stifled since the extra profits would quickly be eliminated by competition. But with patent protection, some degree of monopoly power is inevitable. This is a highly complex issue on both the economic and legal levels. We will merely indicate why monopoly power might result in misallocation.

Let us suppose that the manufacturer of some complex medical instrument, which is necessary in a particular operation, can sell 400 of them per year for $1,000 each or 450 of them for $800 each. Suppose further, having already discovered the necessary technology, the cost of manufacture is $500 per unit. Assume that hospitals can either equip their operating rooms for this operation or not. At a price of $1,000 it may be worthwhile only at larger metropolitan hospitals that are more likely to encounter such cases. There may be only 400 such hospitals, so that the situation in which 400 items are produced and sold is an economic equilibrium. It is better from the manufacturer's point of view than cutting the price to $800 and producing 450 of them, because that would give a total profit of $135,000 instead of the $200,000 that could be made by restricting supply.

However, from the social point of view, it would clearly be better to induce the extra supply. The cost of the last 50 units is only $500 each, while the benefits to the hospitals involved are all between $800 and $1,000. Therefore, although the cost-benefit analysis that would be performed by these 50 hospitals using the price of $1,000 would be correct in indicating that they should not purchase it separately, it would lead to an incorrect surgical policy in the health-care system as a whole. This is another example of how market prices can be misleading guides to social values.

PROFIT MAXIMIZATION

Perhaps even more serious than the two problems outlined above is the fact that many institutions in the medical sector have goals other than profit maximization in mind. It may seem paradoxical that more socially oriented objectives might lead to worse results than selfish profit maximization. Specifically, the prices that would emerge in a system with nonprofit maximizing behavior would no longer serve as correct guides in cost-benefit analysis. The following hypothetical example will serve to illustrate this point. Suppose that all hospitals increased the number of beds up to the point where profits were zero. That is, they go beyond the point of maximal profits to a larger scale of operations in the attempt to serve more patients. Even though each hospital takes the potential revenue from every extra bed as a constant (so that we avoid the problems mentioned above), the equilibrium price of each bed is lower than it would be if profit maximization were followed. This can be depicted as shown in Figure 5-1.

The upper diagram presents these calculations as they might be made by such a hospital. The downward slope of the curve labeled "price for bed depending on total available" is a result of the fact that progressively less urgent needs will be accommodated as the hospital expands. The curve for "cost of one more bed depending on the number available" depends upon factors such as crowding,

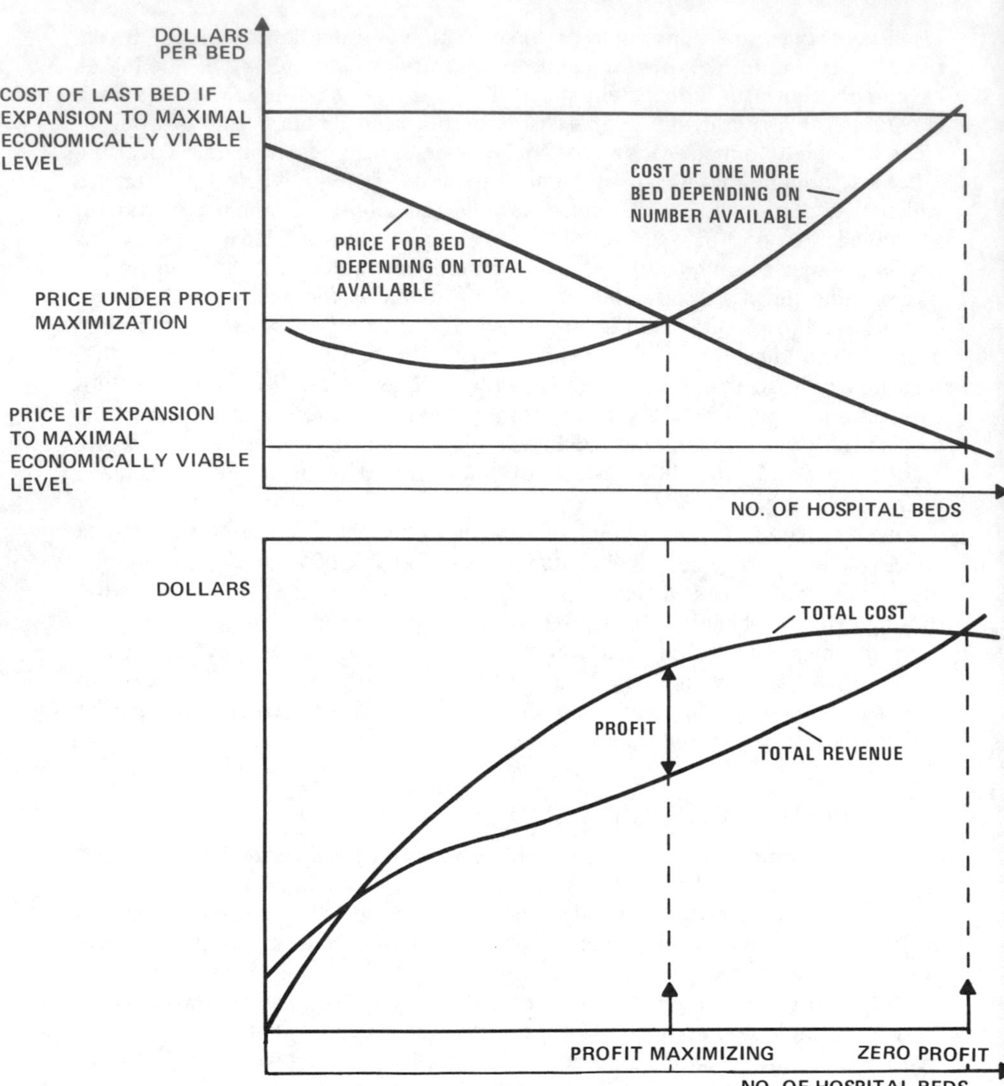

Figure 5-1. Determination of actual and profit-maximizing levels of hospital beds and related social cost calculations.

The upper figure plots the price and the social marginal cost per bed against the number of hospital beds. The curves cross at the number of beds maximizing profit.

The lower curves plot total cost against total revenue. The curves cross at the breakeven or zero profit point.

support services such as labs and outpatient clinics, etc. It will be decreasing when the hospital is smaller than its efficient scale, perhaps too small to justify having its own lab or specialized units of various types. The rising portion reflects crowding, increased administrative costs, and other costs which tend to increase more than proportionately with size.

In the lower graph the same data have been represented as the total cost and revenue corresponding to a given number of beds, rather than the cost and revenue of the last bed. The profit maximization point and size maximization point, subject to a no-losses constraint, are easily depicted.

Now consider in this milieu the problem of surgical versus medical treatment for some illness. The price of a hospital bed will be lower than its true social cost, and lower than it would be if hospitals were profit-maximizers. Therefore surgical treatment might be preferred on the basis of a cost-benefit analysis that used the equilibrium price of hospital beds as taken from market data, whereas a true social cost calculation would prefer the medical treatment.

RATIONALITY

Although it is hard to think of someone purposely acting against his own self-interest, this may arise in some completely unintentional ways because of the nature of medical decision-making and the bearing of the ensuing costs. I will restrict myself to two instances in which the formalization of rationality as non-contradictory behavior, which we have taken in assumption 4, can give rise to misleading and highly biased results.

The first is especially acute in situations of serious, relatively rare illnesses. It is sometimes referred to as the problem of the neglect of small probabilities. Typically, individuals will be quite inaccurate in their assessments of probabilities less than 1/50. When the incidence of a disease or other complication is orders of magnitude below this, they will tend either to neglect the possibility entirely or greatly overstate its frequency. Their demands generated by this, say for preventive medical services, will therefore accord with their prior beliefs but will be unrelated to the true social benefits to be derived. If a life-saving technique such as an intensive-care unit, would be economically viable only if used at a certain minimum intensity, personal expectations would be unreliable guides to the efficacy of acquiring it. Such information should be gathered directly, which is another point at which public policy guided by expert medical knowledge will outperform the market system.

Finally, we come to the issue of insurance. Medical insurance is so widespread, and problems related to it have been so well documented, that we need only make the briefest mention of it here.* Medical insurance is surely not "irrational." However, it does induce a violation of the rationality hypothesis at a later stage in the decision-making process. Notice that the hypothesis of rationality implicitly assumes that the individual is personally paying for any care he receives out of his own income. When economists speak of insurance, they

*The interested reader is referred to Arrow's "Uncertainty and the Welfare Economics of Medical Care," *American Economic Review*, 1963.

typically do not refer to the type of contract that reimburses the insured for his expenses. Rather, insurance in the standard economic model is a payment based on the medical condition alone, which can be allocated by the insured in any way he desires, independent of the medical costs he incurs. Insurance in the real world, however, has the feature that once the illness insured against is found present, the insurance company will cover medical costs (up to some maximum and perhaps with some deductibility provisions). This removes the incentive for the individual to act "rationally" with the insurance company's money. It also counteracts some of the incentive to take proper preventive care and to undergo screening procedures. These problems–known in the insurance literature as "moral hazards"–are not irrational in the ordinary sense, but they do violate the hypothesis of rationality as used in the proof of the optimality of market equilibrium. They create the potential for the individual to make apparently contradictory choices with the money he is to allocate among its alternative uses, the reason being that it is not *his* money and that the amount of it as his disposal depends on the choice he makes. In typical cases, once an individual knows that he is covered by insurance he does not economize on his medical costs. In this way the prices of some medical services are pushed up beyond their social value, since the only role left for prices is to allocate the existing supplies among the larger set of demanders. National Health Insurance Systems such as those in England or Canada must feel this phenomenon even more acutely. Cost-benefit analysis that uses such prices as estimates of social value of the procedures will err in this way.

SUMMARY

In this brief chapter I have tried to outline some of the reasons why one should be cautious in estimating values and costs of medical inputs by the prices at which transactions are made. Biases can be in either direction and there are few general principles to guide us. It is important, therefore, to ascertain in each case the structure of the markets for medical services relevant to the treatment of the particular condition under study. The studies that follow in this volume have tried to cope with these difficulties and have shown that cost-benefit analysis can be an effective aid, when carefully applied. But the problems are difficult and the reader is cautioned that the answers presented can depend critically, as we have shown, on the economic hypotheses employed because they form an integral part of the analysis.

Acknowledgment

I am grateful to the editors for their helpful comments on earlier drafts.

6

The value of diagnostic aids in patients with potential surgical problems

Barbara J. McNeil

How we measure the value of our diagnostic and therapeutic regimens in medical care is one of the central questions of contemporary medicine and surgery. The benefits of our efforts derive from the identification and effective treatment of patients with disease, while the associated costs are both life and financial–life costs relating to the hazards of diagnosis and therapy, and financial costs relating to the monies expended for these purposes. Comparison of benefits and costs for various diagnostic and therapeutic strategies depends strongly upon the disease in question, the complexity of diagnostic tests necessary for its identification, and the efficacy of various alternative treatment regimens.

In some clinical situations a single therapeutic regimen is considered superior to others and, in these cases, the benefits of diagnosis are directly related to the success of this therapy. Therefore, accurate identification and treatment of patients with disease and exclusion of those without disease are of paramount importance in affecting morbidity and mortality and in determining resulting financial expenditures. Other clinical situations may be more complex, however, because of the possibility of varying therapeutic alternatives with different financial costs and different requirements as to the specificity of information which must be known about the underlying pathological process. For example, one therapeutic regimen may be a symptomatic one not requiring such information, whereas another may be a specific one directed at and requiring knowledge of the etiology of the disease process itself. In these cases, therefore, diagnostic tests designed to elucidate the etiology of the disease process have an impact on health and financial costs and benefits only if large differences in outcome exist between the two therapeutic alternatives.

These two clinical situations are the broadest categories of interest in cost-effectiveness analyses of medicine and surgery. The diagnosis of pernicious anemia and its subsequent treatment with vitamin B_{12}, the diagnosis of pulmonary embolism and institution of anticoagulation, and the diagnosis of Stage I lung cancer followed by surgery illustrate the first situation. The identification of patients with either renovascular disease or coronary artery occlusive disease as appropriate candidates for subsequent reconstructive surgery rather than medical therapy exemplifies the second situation.

In this chapter we study one example from each category. The first example relates to patients suspected of having pulmonary embolism. Cost-effectiveness calculations for this type of disease process are limited primarily to determination of the cost of finding a patient with pulmonary embolism and to the cost of saving a life by medical intervention. The second example, the identification and treatment of hypertensive patients suspected of having renovascular disease, is much more complex. In this case, the calculations relate not only to the cost of identifying a patient with renovascular disease and to the cost of saving a life by surgical intervention but also to the evaluation of differences between empirical treatment (medicine) and disease-specific treatment (reconstruction of renal arteries). Comparison of the results of these two therapeutic strategies in terms of mortality, morbidity, and financial costs must be undertaken before the value of finding a patient with renovascular disease can be determined.

The general structure of these two discussions is: (1) an introduction and description of the data base used for the studies; (2) determination of the sensitivity* and specificity* of various diagnostic aids in the search for patients with disease; (3) the financial costs of case finding and life saving; and, in the case of the second example, (4) the value of determining the etiology of the disease in question and, therefore, of instituting specific rather than general therapy.

PULMONARY EMBOLISM

In order to study the contribution of various diagnostic aids to the detection of patients with pulmonary embolism, we used data collected over the past four years by the Department of Radiology at the Peter Bent Brigham Hospital (McNeil et al., 1974; McNeil et al., 1976; McNeil, 1976). We evaluated both nonspecific, inexpensive screening aids (i.e., the history, physical examination, laboratory tests, and noninvasive radiographic studies) as well as more specific and more expensive tests (i.e., pulmonary ventilation-perfusion scanning and pulmonary angiography).

The former modalities were evaluated in a young patient population suspected of pulmonary embolism, specifically patients under forty years of age presenting with pleuritic chest pain. These patients were studied on the assumption that they would not have a large percentage of abnormal findings deriving from long-standing chronic disease. The data derived from this analysis were expected to

*See Appendix for definitions.

indicate the maximum usefulness of individual findings in detecting patients with this disease. Because most institutions follow these inexpensive screening tests with perfusion and ventilation lung scanning, we then determined the accuracy of these examinations in identifying patients with pulmonary embolism (PE+) and in distinguishing them from patients without pulmonary embolism (PE–). These calculations led to criteria which allowed for the diagnosis of pulmonary embolism with varying degrees of certainty.

Calculations of the financial cost of case finding and life saving rested on several assumptions about therapy and its results: (1) Once the diagnosis of pulmonary embolism is made, anticoagulation is begun. Surgery is reserved for patients who either re-embolize on adequate anticoagulation or who have a medical contraindication to anticoagulation (Ebert, 1974). (2) Anticoagulation diminishes the risk of death in patients with pulmonary embolism from 25% to 8% (Dexter and Dalen, 1974; Thomas, 1973). (3) The risk of death from complications of anticoagulation with or without pulmonary embolism is .01% (Manchester, 1957; O'Sullivan, 1972; Barritt and Jordan, 1960).

These results of therapy dictated the assumptions underlying the diagnostic strategy: (1) Anticoagulation is begun without angiography if there is no medical contraindication and if the probability of pulmonary embolism on the basis of the lung scan is greater than 80%. This probability was chosen because it includes only a small percentage of patients without pulmonary embolism. (2) If the probability of disease on the basis of lung scan is less than 11%, no therapy is instituted and no further diagnostic tests are done unless additional symptoms develop. (3) If the probability of disease is between these extremes, pulmonary angiography is performed.

Accuracy of Diagnostic Tests in Patients Suspect for Pulmonary Embolism

In young patients several inexpensive diagnostic aids were extremely valuable in detecting pulmonary embolism (McNeil et al., 1976). When certain critical features were extracted from the history, physical examination, and chest radiograph on the basis of high likelihood ratios* and were plotted in the form of a receiver operating characteristic (ROC) curve (i.e., a plot of the true positive ratio versus the false positive ratio), there was a monotonic increase in the percentage of patients detected as the diagnostic evaluation proceeded in a logical manner (Fig. 6-1, triangles). For example, from history alone, 65% of patients with pulmonary embolism** were identified on the basis of previous venous disease (including pulmonary embolism) or recent surgery; at the same time, 16% of patients without pulmonary embolism were also included. When the results of a physical examination were introduced (i.e., new venous disease) along with these historical findings, and either a postoperative history or old or new venous

*See Appendix for definition.

**In this study the diagnosis of pulmonary embolism was confirmed by angiography in 70% of patients. In the remaining 30% the diagnosis was made by the patient's physician on the basis of other criteria. There were no differences in any of the historical, physical, laboratory, or radiographic findings in these two groups (McNeil et al., 1976).

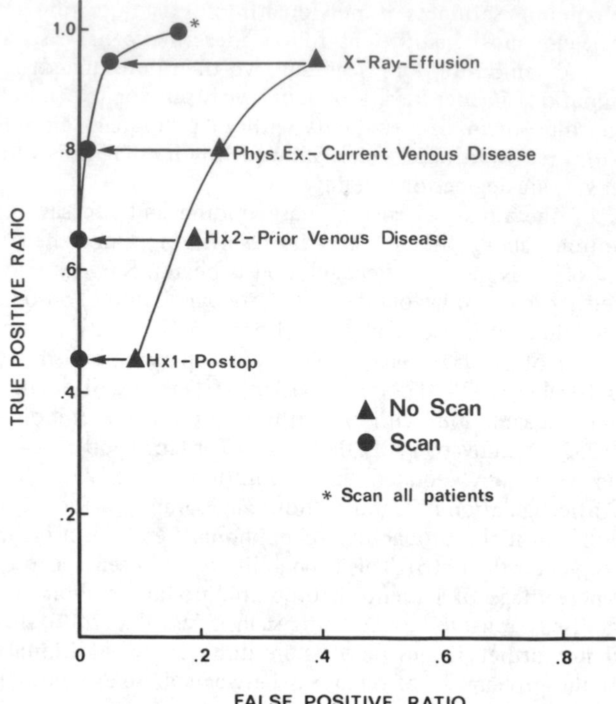

Figure 6-1. Receiver operating characteristic (ROC) curve.
On the vertical scale is the true positive ratio and on the horizontal scale, the false positive ratio. The triangles indicate, for successive stages of the diagnostic workup, the most discriminating variables useful in identifying patients with pulmonary embolism. The circles indicate the improved sensitivity when lung scans were performed only on patients having one or more of the indicated abnormal findings (see text). Reprinted by permission from the *Journal of Nuclear Medicine,* 17:163, 1976.

disease was present, 80% of patients with pulmonary embolism were detected. When the presence of unilateral or bilateral pleural effusions on chest radiograph was considered in addition to the above, the detection rate increased to 95%; at the same time, 40% of patients without pulmonary embolism were also included in the group having one or more of these above findings. Thus, on the basis of the history, physical examination, and chest radiograph a large percentage of patients with pulmonary embolism in a young age group was detected. None of the conventionally employed laboratory tests (e.g., arterial gases, serum enzymes) or the presence of associated cardiac abnormalities was useful in either identifying young patients with pulmonary embolism or in distinguishing these patients from those with other diseases.

Detection of all young patients with pulmonary embolism could not be achieved by any of the above inexpensive screening procedures, but all patients

Table 6–1. Percent of patients with and without pulmonary embolism having lung scans associated with varying probabilities of pulmonary embolism.

	% of Patients with	
Probability of PE+	*PE+*	*PE–*
0%*	0	25
1– 10%	0	42
11– 80%	21	29
81–100%	79	4
	100	100

*Normal lung scan

were identified when lung scans were performed in all patients suspect for this disease. When lung scans were performed on patients with abnormalities detected by the above inexpensive procedures, the same percentage of patients with pulmonary embolism was identified, but the number of false-positive diagnoses decreased (Fig. 6–1, circles).

The same information from the history, physical examination, and chest radiograph that was useful in detecting young patients with pulmonary embolism was not as discriminating in older patients, undoubtedly because of the high likelihood of these findings on the basis of nonembolic disease. Lung scanning was therefore the most productive screening examination in this group. In this context lung scanning means perfusion lung scanning in all patients, and ventilation studies in patients in whom the procedure can technically and beneficially be performed (about 50% of patients with abnormal perfusion studies). All patients with pulmonary embolism had abnormal lung scans, and the probability of disease varied with the perfusion and ventilation patterns observed (Table 6–1) (McNeil, 1976). Among patients with pulmonary embolism, 79% had examinations estimating the probability of disease at over 80%. Only 4% of patients without pulmonary embolism fell in this category. The proportion of patients with pulmonary embolism requiring pulmonary angiography was 21%; the proportion of patients without pulmonary embolism requiring angiography was 29%.

Cost of Case Finding in Pulmonary Embolism

The costs of case finding depended upon whether the patient population was young and presented with a single symptom (i.e., patients under forty years with pleuritic chest pain) or older and presented with a variety of complaints. In the former situation, the incidence of pulmonary embolism was 20% and in the latter, 10%. In both situations, costs were calculated assuming the following prices for radiographic procedures: chest radiograph, $25; perfusion lung scan, $125; ventilation study, $35; and pulmonary angiography, $300 (Interspecialty Committee, 1971). Costs for laboratory tests and physicians' services were not included.

Table 6–2. Cost of finding a young patient with pulmonary embolism using actual financial data obtained on 97 patients with pleuritic pain (20 with pulmonary embolism).

100% of patients with pulmonary embolism detected (20 of 20 patients)	
97 chest radiographs	$ 2,425
97 perfusion scans	12,125
22 ventilation studies	770
15 pulmonary angiograms	4,500
	$19,820 or $991 per patient found
95% of patients with pulmonary embolism detected (19 of 20 patients)	
97 chest radiographs	$ 2,425
50 perfusion scans	6,250
16 ventilation studies	560
7 pulmonary angiograms	2,100
	$11,335 or $596 per patient found

For young patients, the average costs of case finding varied with the percentage of patients found. Detection of all patients with pulmonary embolism required lung scans on all patients and resulted in a cost per patient found of nearly $1,000. When only a subgroup of the population had lung scans and, therefore, only 95% of patients with disease were detected, then the cost per patient found was 40% less–$600. Under these circumstances, the cost of finding the last patient with pulmonary embolism by these techniques was $8,500 (Table 6-2).

For an older, more heterogeneous patient population the cost of finding all patients with pulmonary embolism was over $2,000 per patient found. This increase resulted from the lower incidence of pulmonary embolism in an unselected heterogeneous population.

The financial cost of saving a life by identifying and treating a patient with pulmonary embolism was calculated for the *entire* patient population considering both the gain in lives by proper anticoagulation (true positive patients) and the loss in lives by unnecessary anticoagulation (false positive patients). It was approximately $11,300 per life saved.

RENOVASCULAR DISEASE

For evaluation of radiologic examinations in the search for patients with renovascular disease we analyzed data collected by the Cooperative Study of Renovascular Disease on over 1,000 hypertensive patients (McNeil et al., 1975; McNeil and Adelstein, 1975). These patients all had intravenous pyelography (IVP) and/or renography (RG) followed by renal arteriography. The results of arteriography distinguished those with renovascular disease (RVD+) from those without renovascular disease (RVD-) and therefore allowed determination of the sensitivity and specificity of the screening modalities. Calculation of financial costs for case finding and life saving rested on several assumptions: (1) The American hypertensive population numbers 23 million, 90% of whom have an unidentifiable cause of their hypertension ("essential") and 10% have an identifiable cause (Stokes et al., 1973). For this analysis we have assumed that all 10% have renovascular disease, although the actual prevalence may range from less than 1% to more than 10%. (2) All patients with an abnormal screening examination (IVP or renogram) have renal arteriography for further definition of their disease. (3) The mortality of angiography is 0.1%, the average surgical mortality rate is 7%, and average surgical cure rate is 50% (McAfee, 1971; Franklin et al., 1975; Foster et al., 1975).

Accuracy of the IVP and Renogram

Intravenous pyelograms were called abnormal when there were one or more abnormalities in the appearance time, calyceal concentration, or kidney length (Bookstein et al., 1972a; Bookstein et al., 1972b). By these criteria, 78.2% of patients with renovascular disease and 11.4% of patients without renovascular disease had abnormal studies. To put it another way, in a hypertensive population, 7.8 of 10 patients with renovascular disease were found by the IVP and 9.9 of 90 patients without disease were falsely included. Therefore renal angiography was needed by 17.7 of 100 patients for further definition of the disease process.

Iodohippuran renograms were analyzed according to the method of Burrows and Farmelant (McNeil et al., 1975; Farmelant et al., 1964; Farmelant et al., 1970). The degree of functional symmetry between the kidneys was graded from 0 to 1 with symmetrical function associated with a value near 1, and asymmetric function with varying grades less than 1. Most hypertensive patients without renovascular disease had symmetrical function (that is, values between 0.9 and 1.0) whereas patients with renovascular disease showed a much greater range of asymmetry in renal function.

The degree of asymmetry in renal function accepted as normal by this technique influenced markedly the sensitivity and specificity of the renogram. When mild asymmetry in renal function was called abnormal, most patients with renovascular disease were discovered, but a high percentage of patients without renovascular disease were also included. If a high degree of asymmetry in renal function was necessary before the examination was called abnormal, then a smaller percentage of patients with renovascular disease were discovered, but at the same time a smaller percentage of patients without renovascular disease were included.

For our calculations, we calculated the effects of considering two different degrees of functional asymmetry as normal. The first criterion, a sensitive one, called mild asymmetry in renal function abnormal and, as a result, 85% of patients with renovascular disease and 10% of patients without renovascular disease had abnormal renograms. The second, or specific criterion, said that only severe degrees of asymmetry were abnormal and resulted in detection of 62% of patients with renovascular disease and only 3% of patients without renovascular disease. Thus, in a hypertensive population, use of the former criterion resulted in the discovery of 8.5 of 10 patients with renovascular disease, and 9.0 of 90 without renovascular disease. With the latter criterion, the number of patients

Table 6-3. Cost considerations in the diagnosis and surgical therapy for patients with renovascular disease

Screening Modality	*% Pts With RVD+ Found*	*Cost Per Pt Found ($)*	*Total Cost for Detection and Surgery ($)*	*Cost Per Pt Cured Surgically ($)*
Intravenous Pyelogram				
TP ratio = 0.78	78%	1915	12.5×10^9	15,100
or				
Renogram				
TP ratio = 0.85	85%	1948	13.6×10^9	14,100
TP ratio = 0.62	62%	2151	10.2×10^9	15,700

found dropped to 6.2 of 10, but the number of patients falsely identified also dropped to 2.7 of 90. The number of patients requiring renal angiography with these two criteria were 17.5 and 8.9, respectively.

Cost of Case Finding in Renovascular Disease

The total and average costs of detection and surgical intervention in renovascular disease depended upon the costs of the screening examination (IVP and RG), renal arteriography, and surgery. The costs used in this study were derived from the Massachusetts Relative Value Scale and were $83 for the hypertensive IVP, $100 for renography, and $375 for renal arteriography (Interspecialty Committee, 1971; McNeil et al., 1975). The cost of surgery, derived from figures at the Peter Bent Brigham Hospital, was $5,000. The total cost of diagnosis (including the cost of the primary screening modality and subsequent arteriography) was equal to the number of patients screened times the cost of screening plus the number of patients undergoing arteriography times the cost of arteriography. The cost of identifying one patient with renovascular disease by these diagnostic modalities was this total cost of diagnosis divided by the number of patients with renovascular disease found by the diagnostic modality under consideration. The total cost for surgery also included the number of patients undergoing surgery times the cost of surgery.

Table 6-3 summarizes the financial costs relating to both detection and surgery (McNeil et al., 1975). Thus, the average cost for detecting a patient with renovascular disease was approximately $2,000, and the average cost for curing one was seven to eight times higher. The total costs for diagnostic evaluation of the entire American hypertensive population with surgery on appropriate candidates would be astronomical–billions of dollars.

The Value of Case Finding in Surgical Treatment

Determination of the value of finding patients with renovascular disease and of subsequent surgical intervention depends upon how well patients with reno-

STRATEGY 1

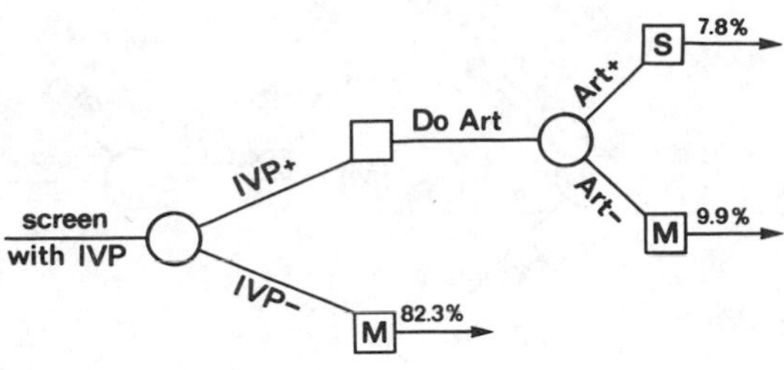

STRATEGY 2

do not
screen
M
100%

Figure 6-2. Decision flow diagrams for treatment of patients with hypertensive disease.

Strategy 1: Screening is performed on all patients with hypertension. If the intravenous pyelogram (IVP) is abnormal (IVP+), arteriography (Art) is always performed. When the IVP or arteriogram is negative, medical therapy (M) is followed. When the arteriogram is positive, surgical treatment is chosen (S). The outcomes of operation and medicine are shown in Figure 6-3. Strategy 2: No screening intravenous pyelography is done, and all patients are treated medically (M).

vascular disease would have done had their hypertension been treated medically instead of surgically. Surgical therapy requires extensive diagnostic screening to identify potential surgical candidates, whereas medical therapy does not.

These two strategies can be expressed explicitly in the form of decision flow diagrams (Figs. 6-2 and 6-3). For example, in the screening situation discussed above, all patients with an abnormal IVP undergo arteriography, and all patients with renovascular disease then found are treated surgically. All other patients are treated medically. Those patients treated surgically either live or die postoperatively, and those patients surviving the operation are either cured or not cured. Those not cured by surgery may be either improved or unchanged; in either case they receive medical therapy which results in medical cure, improvement, or failure (node C_1, Fig. 6-3). If the initial treatment is medical, either because screening was not performed (Strategy 2) or because the patients screened were not suitable surgical candidates, then the results are also cure, improvements, or failure (node C_2, Fig. 6-3). For both strategies, the chance node at the end of each branch of the decision diagram indicates the patient's state: he is well, he has suffered a nonfatal morbid event (complications of coronary heart disease or a cerebrovascular accident), or he is dead.

We compared the results of the two strategies by calculating the numbers of

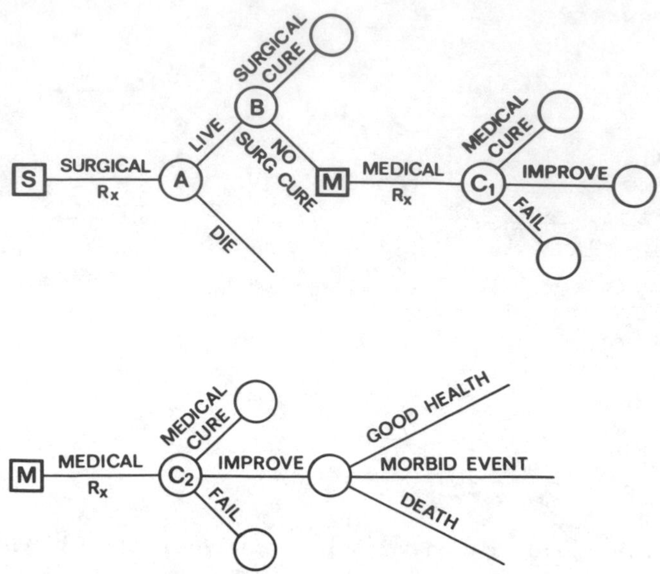

Figure 6–3. Outcomes associated with the surgical and medical regimens. The results of surgical management of patients with renovascular disease are detailed at chance nodes A and B. Results of primary or supplemental medical therapy are expressed at nodes C_1 and C_2. All the terminal chance nodes are associated with three possible outcomes: well, morbid event, or die.

well patients, patients having nonfatal morbid events, and patients dying from these events in these two groups for varying initial diastolic blood pressures (90 to 135 mm Hg) and for two rates of compliance with medical therapy, 50% and 84% (McNeil and Adelstein, 1975). The 50% compliance rate is probably the most common one in a typical American population and indicates that 50% of known hypertensive patients are lost to follow-up, 25% are cured (a drop in diastolic blood pressure to 90 mm Hg or less), and 25% are improved (a drop in diastolic blood pressure 10 to 15%) (Stokes et al., 1973; Borhani and Borkman, 1968; Schoenberger et al., 1972). The 84% compliance rate is an unusual one found only in specially designed hypertensive programs where 84% of the patients are cured and 16% are lost to follow-up (Finnerty et al., 1973; Charman, 1974). We used data collected by the Framingham Study on Cardiovascular Disease to estimate the probabilities of fatal and nonfatal morbid events and calculated these outcomes assuming a 16-year follow-up, the longest time period for which such data were available (Kannel and Gordon, 1970a; Kannel and Gordon, 1970b).

Figure 6–4 indicates the differences in outcome between the two strategies. When deaths were enumerated, medical therapy appeared better than surgical therapy in nearly all instances. However, extrapolation of original data revealed that at high diastolic blood pressures (> 135 mm Hg), surgical therapy resulted

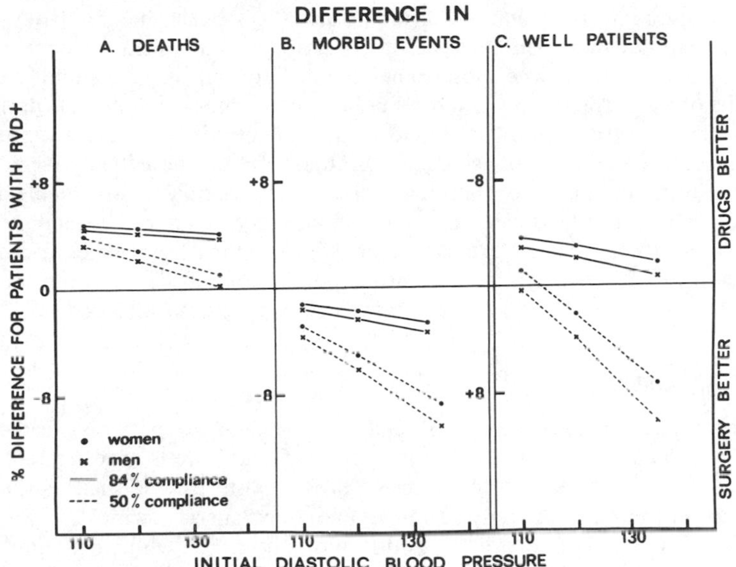

Figure 6-4. Difference in the number of deaths (panel A), nonfatal morbid events (panel B), and well patients (panel C) as a function of sex, compliance, and initial diastolic blood pressure.

The vertical scale represents the difference between the results of surgical and medical therapy in 100 patients with renovascular disease, either fibromuscular (FM) or atherosclerotic (AS). Negative differences in deaths or nonfatal morbid events favor surgical treatment, and negative differences in well patients favor medical therapy.

in fewer deaths. When nonfatal morbid events were enumerated, on the other hand, surgery was always better regardless of initial diastolic blood pressure or compliance (middle panel). When the number of well patients were considered, medical therapy was better at high compliance rates and surgical therapy at low compliance rates. In all cases, however, it is important to note that the maximum difference between the two strategies was about 10% for the patients with renovascular disease. This figure extrapolates, assuming an incidence of renovascular disease of 10%, to a difference in only 1% for the total hypertensive population.

These results demonstrate that there is some potential benefit to the identification and surgical treatment of patients with renovascular disease but that the mode of treatment contributes much less to ultimate prognosis than does initial diastolic blood pressure or compliance. The total financial costs for discovering the patients with renovascular disease in the American hypertensive population is of the order of billions of dollars, the average cost of finding a patient with renovascular disease is approximately $2,000 per patient found, and the cost of a surgical cure is $15,000. These costs result in changes of less than 1% in morbidity and mortality for our hypertensive population.

These analyses on the value of diagnostic aids (historical, physical, laboratory, and radiographic) in patients suspect for pulmonary embolism or renovascular hypertension emphasize the close dependency between diagnosis and therapy on results of cost-effectiveness analyses in both medicine and surgery. Determination of the value of therapy must either assume perfectly accurate diagnostic tests or must correct for inaccuracies in these tests. The effect of errors in individual tests within the overall diagnostic scheme is increased if the incidence of disease is low and thus can lead to an unnecessary number of secondary tests of higher specificity. These tests also usually have a higher associated morbidity and mortality. All of these factors must be considered in determining the cost and the effectiveness of various diagnostic and therapeutic strategies.

SUMMARY

The health and financial values of diagnostic testing in patients suspect for either pulmonary embolism or renovascular disease were investigated. The diagnosis of pulmonary embolism in young patients can be made with high sensitivity but poor specificity from several inexpensive diagnostic aids. The specificity is markedly improved by addition of a lung scan which concomitantly increases the cost of diagnosis by 40%. Because of the high mortality of untreated cases of pulmonary embolism, case finding in this disease is closely related to life saving. In diagnosing renovascular disease, relatively inexpensive screening tests can also be used to diagnose the disease with high sensitivity but relatively poor specificity. This specificity can be increased to 100% by a renal angiogram. Because of the marginal differences in life saving associated with diagnosing this disease and then treating it surgically instead of treating it empirically with medicine, this case finding is not closely associated with improved mortality figures.

APPENDIX

Diagnostic tests are characterized by four ratios. These ratios derive from the decision matrix which tabulates test outcomes (negative, positive) with the clinical or pathological outcomes (no disease, disease).

		Clinical State	
		Disease	*No Disease*
Test Result	Positive	a	c
	Negative	b	d
		$a + b$	$c + d$

In this notation the four test characteristics of interest are:

1. The true positive (TP) ratio or the proportion of positive tests in patients with disease, $a/(a + b)$. This is the *sensitivity* of the test.

2. The false positive (FP) ratio is the proportion of positive tests in patients without disease or $c/(c + d)$.

3. The true negative (TN) ratio is the proportion of negative tests in patients without disease, or $d/(c + d)$. This is the *specificity* of the test.

4. The false negative (FN) ratio is the proportion of negative tests in patients with disease, or $b/(a + b)$.

Another ratio of interest which can be derived from these is the *likelihood ratio*. This is the ratio of the true positive ratio to the false positive ratio, $a(c + d)/(a + b)c$. Tests with high likelihood ratios are better discriminators of disease than those with low likelihood ratios.

References

Barritt DW, Jordan SC: Anticoagulant drugs in the treatment of pulmonary embolism: a controlled trial. Lancet 1:1309, 1960

Bookstein JJ, Abrams HL, Buenger RE, et al: Radiologic aspects of renovascular hypertension. I. Aims and methods of the radiology study group. JAMA 220:1218, 1972a

Bookstein, JJ, Abrams HL, Buenger RE, et al: Radiologic aspects of renovascular disease. II. The role of urography in unilateral renovascular disease. JAMA 220:1225, 1972b

Borhani NO, Borkman TS: Alameda County Blood Pressure Study. Berkeley, California, Department of Public Health, 1968

Charman RC: Hypertension management program in an industrial community. JAMA 227:287, 1974

Dexter, L, Dalen JE: Pulmonary embolism and acute cor pulmonale, The Heart, Arteries and Veins. Third edition. Edited by JW Hurst, RB Logue, RC Schlant, et al, New York, McGraw-Hill Book Company, 1974, p 1264

Ebert PA: The role of surgery in the treatment of pulmonary thromboembolism. Surg Clin North Am 54:1107, 1974

Farmelant MH, Lipetz CA, Bikerman V, et al: Radioisotopic renal function studies and surgical findings in 102 hypertensive patients. Am J Surg 107: 50, 1964

Farmelant MH, Sachs C, Burrows BA: Prognostic value of radioisotopic renal function studies for selecting patients with renal arterial stenosis for surgery. J Nucl Med 11:743, 1970

Finnerty FA Jr, Shaw LW, Himmelsbach CK: Hypertension in the inner city. II. Detection and follow-up. Circulation 47:76, 1973

Foster JH, Maxwell MH, Franklin SS, et al: Renovascular occlusive disease: results of operative treatment. JAMA 231:1043, 1975

Franklin SS, Young JD Jr., Maxwell MH, et al: Operative morbidity and mortality in renovascular disease. JAMA 231:1148, 1975

Interspeciality Committee: Special service and billing procedures. Massachusetts Relative Value Study, 1971, Massachusetts Medical Society, Boston, Mass.

Kannel WB, Gordon T: The Framingham Study: an epidemiological investigation of cardiovascular disease. Section 26. Some characteristics related to the incidence of cardiovascular disease and death: Framingham Study, 16-year follow-up. Washington, DC, Government Printing Office, 1970a

Kannel WB, Gordon T: The Framingham Study: an epidemiological investigation of cardiological disease. Section 25. Survival following certain cardiovascular events. Washington, DC, Government Printing Office, 1970b

Manchester B: The value of continuous (1 to 10 years) long-term anticoagulant therapy. Ann Intern Med 47:1202, 1957

McAfee JG: Complications of abdominal aortography and arteriography. Angiography, Vol. 2. Edited by HL Abrams. Boston, Little, Brown and Company, 1971, p 717

McNeil BJ: A diagnostic strategy using ventilation-perfusion studies in patients suspect for pulmonary embolism. J Nucl Med, 17:13, 1976

McNeil BJ, Adelstein SJ: Measures of clinical efficacy. The value of case finding in hypertensive renovascular disease. New Engl J Med 293:221, 1975

McNeil BJ, Hessel SJ, Branch WT, Bjork L, et al: Measures of clinical efficacy. III. The value of the lung scan in the evaluation of young patients with pleuritic chest pain. J Nucl Med 17:163, 1976

McNeil BJ, Holman BL, Adelstein SJ: The scintigraphic definition of pulmonary embolism. JAMA 227:753, 1974

McNeil BJ, Varady PD, Burrows BA, et al: Measures of clinical efficacy. Cost-effectiveness calculations in the diagnosis and treatment of hypertensive renovascular disease. New Engl J Med 293:216, 1975

O'Sullivan EF: Duration of anticoagulant therapy in venous thrombo-embolism. Med J Aust 2:1104, 1972

Schoenberger JA, Stamler J, Shekelle RB, et al: Current status of hypertension control in an industrial population. JAMA 222:559, 1972

Stokes, JB III, Payne GH, Cooper T: Hypertension control—the challenge of patient education. New Engl J Med 289:1369, 1973

Thomas DP: The anticoagulant therapy of venous thromboembolism. Pulmonary Thromboembolism. Edited by KM Moser, M Stein. Chicago, Yearbook Medical Publishers, 1973, p 271

7

On the incidence of tonsillectomy and other common surgical procedures

Alan M. Gittelsohn
John E. Wennberg

The tonsils and adenoids have been subjected to a widespread, uncontrolled, therapeutic experiment over the past half-century. At times and in certain segments of the society, less than half the children have reached adulthood with the organs intact. While the operation was recorded in ancient history, its popularity is associated with the advent of modern surgery and anesthesia (Bakwin, 1958). Tonsillectomy began to increase in frequency early in the century with a precipitous rise following World War I. Procedure rates have continued at high levels since the 1930's and only in the past decade has there been evidence of a decline. During the early 1970's, over one million tonsillectomies were performed each year in the United States at a total cost estimated to exceed $250 million (National Center for Health Statistics, 1966). It continues to be the most common surgical procedure performed in the United States and Canada and is the main reason for the hospitalization of children.

Glover (1938) commented on the wide variation in the incidence of tonsillectomy in different geographic regions of England. Over a decade later the Registrar General of England and Wales recorded that a child in Rutlandshire was 19 times as likely to have a T&A as one in neighboring Cambridgeshire, and that the operative rate in Boxhill was 27 times greater than in Northern Birkenhead (Registrar General's Statistical Review, 1954). A similar situation pertains to the United States and Canada, where numerous reports have described large variations in tonsillectomy rates between different communities and between socioeconomic classes within the same community.

This chapter is partially supported by Public Health Service Grant PHS-RMO303.

An examination of case loads of short-term hospitals in New England, Liverpool, and Sweden revealed marked variations in the rates for common surgical procedures including appendectomy, cholecystectomy, hysterectomy, and prostatectomy (Pearson et al., 1968). A comparison between the United States with its predominant cost reimbursement financing and England under the National Health Service indicates that surgery rates of all types except appendectomy are twice as high in the former as in the latter (Bunker, 1970). Under the provincial health plans in Canada with universal coverage for all citizens, surgery rates involving removal of tonsils, gall bladders, appendices, prostates, and uteri are 50% to 150% higher than corresponding rates experienced in the United States. Among Federal employees the risk of female surgery and most other common surgical interventions is about double for subscribers of fee-for-service plans as for subscribers of salaried capitation plans (Perrot, 1971). Variations have also been documented among geographic subdivisions of states. For Blue Cross subscribers living in different sections of Kansas, Lewis (1969) found two- and threefold variations in rates of six common surgical procedures.

The present article is concerned with the variation in tonsillectomy rates between Vermont areas. Based on records of over 6,000 tonsillectomies, we compare practices between different communities, institutions, and individual physicians. The impact on resident populations is characterized in terms of varying expenditures and probabilities of receiving tonsillectomy.

Material and Methods

The data set on which the present report is based has been described in a prior publication (Wennberg and Gittelsohn, 1973). Patient discharge abstracts have been collected for all Vermont residents hospitalized in Vermont short-term facilities and in referral hospitals of the neighboring states of New York and New Hampshire. No attempt has been made to collect data in more distant institutions for reasons of feasibility. The estimated underreporting thereby resulting is under 5%.

Vermont is organized administratively into 251 towns averaging 37 square miles in area and ranging in population from 10 up to 35,000 persons. The hospital record is coded by town of patient residence. Each town has been classified as belonging to a hospital service area on the basis of the plurality of the hospitalizations of its residents. For towns containing the hospital or located nearby, the percent of use of the single facility is high in contrast to that for towns located between two hospitals where utilization tends to be divided. The service areas have been constructed to provide for geographic contiguity. The criterion for including a town in a hospital's catchment area is that at least 60% of its admissions be to that hospital. Towns dividing admissions between two or more facilities, and towns primarily feeding cases to out-of-state hospitals, have been excluded from the analysis. The resulting 13 hospital catchment areas include 175 towns and 88% of the total population of the state.

Eleven of the areas are served by a single community hospital. One area has two facilities in the same city, and a second area contains both a community and a 500-bed university hospital. Over 85% of all admissions of residents took place in the facility serving the catchment area. Maternities, general surgery, and most medical conditions comprising the majority of admissions tend to be highly localized. Thus, there is a close correspondence between the medical community of an area and the residents hospitalized from that area. For the common surgical procedures, about 90% were performed in the local hospital.

The 1970 Census populations for each town have been aggregated into hospital service area populations which serve as the basis for computing rates of surgical procedures. The numerators include all resident surgery cases no matter where the procedures were performed. Because the 1970 Census classified college students by locations of the institution regardless of permanent residence and because hospitals tend to use billable address for patient residence, the estimated number of nonresident students has been removed from the population. The adjustment is of importance in two of the catchment areas with Census age structures seriously distorted by the presence of colleges and universities. Without correction, the crude and age-adjusted surgery rates would be understatements because of inflated denominators.

The age-adjusted surgery rate has been utilized to permit direct comparison of populations with differing age structures. The age-adjusted rate is the weighted average of the age-specific rates where the weights are based on the proportions of persons in each age group for the total population of the 13 hospital catchment areas. For nonrepetitive surgery involving organ removal, the populations have been adjusted downward to account for prior surgery at all earlier ages. Such adjustment is an attempt to estimate the population at risk of surgery and is necessitated because the Census includes persons with organs removed prior to enumeration. The disparity between Census counts and persons at risk in a given population may be considerable. Fully half of the children resident in Area #7 are tonsillectomized by age 12 and thus should not be included in the denominator of the tonsillectomy rate after age 12.

A second type of measure used to describe the incidence of nonrepetitive surgery is the cumulative probability of organ survival to age x and its complement, the probability of organ loss by age x. These are conditional on survival of the individual to age x. Standard actuarial methods (Chiang, 1968) have been employed to convert the age-specific surgery rates to age-specific probabilities which have been combined to form cumulative probabilities of surgery from birth to age x. The proper interpretation of organ survival and loss probabilities requires the assumption of constancy through time of underlying surgery rates, i.e., if physicians and patients continue present behavior into the future, the proportion of persons attaining age x with the particular organ intact will be estimated by the cumulative probability of organ survival. In addition, it is necessary to assume that life expectation is not affected by the procedure. Letting r_x be the age-specific rate for a given operation between age x and $x + n$, the probability of organ removal by age $(x + n)$ given the organ is present at age x is estimated by:

$$q_x = \frac{nr_x}{1 + \frac{1}{2}nr_x}$$

with $p_x = 1 - q_x$, the age-specific organ survival probability; the cumulative survival probability from birth to age t is the product

$$P_{0t} = \prod_{x=0}^{t-1} p_x.$$

Few data are available for the study of long-term trends. For tonsillectomy, the popularity of the procedure appears to be declining. Perrot (1971) reports that tonsillectomy rates among dependents of Federal employees covered by Blue Cross/Blue Shield have fallen by 25% over the past decade. A similar reduction has been noted in Canada. Rates for other common procedures during the period have remained stable.

The Vermont data set consists of patient records obtained from 20 participating hospitals. Multiple procedures may be performed for a single admission and reporting practices vary between institutions. For example, in one hospital the operations are listed in chronological order on the face sheet of the medical record, and biopsies tend to precede definitive surgery. For records with more than one surgery code, the procedure with the highest California Relative Value Index value is selected as the major operation. When two procedures cannot be distinguished by their relative values, an anatomy rule is invoked whereby the procedure consistent with the major diagnosis is selected. Thus, a case with appendectomy and cholecystectomy and a diagnosis of cholelithiasis is assigned to the gall bladder removal because of consistency of the diagnosis with the latter procedure. All cases resulting in a nondecision are referred to the surgical consultant for review.

An indirect approach has been used to estimate dollar expenditures for T&A throughout the state because cost and charge data are not included in the hospital abstract record. Using Blue Cross/Blue Shield figures covering per-day domiciliary charges in a semiprivate room, the total domiciliary charge is given by hospital days times the day charge. Physician, operating room, and charges are based on the California Relative Value Index for the procedure times a factor of $35. The approach understates the total charges per case by not including ancillary services which, for uncomplicated T&A, would add less than 10% to the bill.

RESULTS

Adenotonsillectomy

The incidence of tonsillectomy and adenoidectomy by age and area of patient residence is shown in Table 7-1. For the 5,315 operations performed on persons under age 26, more than two-thirds of the patients were under age 10. Correcting for tonsil removals at earlier ages, the age-adjusted rates for the 13 areas range between 4 and 41 per 1,000 children per year. The highest rates were recorded in Area #7 where 446 tonsils or adenoids were removed from a population of 5,000 age 25 and under. Area #13 with a similar sized population

Table 7-1. Tonsillectomies and adenoidectomies per 1,000 children per year by age and area of residence, 13 hospital service areas, 1969-71.

Area	*Number of Cases*	*Cases per 1,000*[1]									
		All Ages[1]	*< 2*	*2-3*	*4-5*	*6-7*	*8-9*	*10-11*	*12-13*	*14-15*	*16-25*
Total	5,315	11	2	14	28	27	16	10	7	6	5
1	218	17	–	17	35	41	28	20	12	6	6
2	130	5	1	2	8	12	7	6	5	5	4
3	141	15	1	7	41	41	30	20	6	7	6
4	262	14	3	10	29	35	27	11	12	10	8
5	351	12	3	24	33	23	15	8	9	6	6
6	429	10	–	10	29	27	13	9	5	5	4
7	446	41	2	70	94	76	61	39	27	26	35
8	253	9	–	6	17	24	18	10	6	8	5
9	306	17	–	16	50	36	21	21	12	10	7
10	692	11	3	12	27	30	18	10	5	5	6
11	888	14	–	17	32	36	23	12	9	8	6
12	1,146	8	3	10	21	20	9	6	5	5	3
13	53	4	2	1	11	11	6	5	2	2	1

[1]For each area, the rate for "all ages" has been adjusted by age distribution of the total Populations corrected for estimated T&A's removed at earlier ages

recorded 53 T&A's. Annual rates for 4- and 5-year-olds range from below 1% in Area #2 to almost 10% in Area #7.

Probability of Organ Loss

The conversion of age-specific T&A rates to probabilities is illustrated in Table 7-2. Here the cumulative removal probabilities by specified ages are shown for the 13 hospital catchment areas. For the entire state, 1 in 5 (22%) will have a T&A by his or her twentieth birthday at current procedure rates. In essence, the statistic expresses the risk of T&A assuming the persistence of present physician and patient behavior. The risk varies widely over the state from a low of 9% in Area #13 to a high of 60% in Area #7. The latter corresponds to the experience in Canada and in other sections of the United States. The estimated probability of 60% for Area #7 is to be contrasted with values of 11%, 19%, 20%, and 27% in four directly adjacent communities, which, for the most part, are served by different groups of physicians operating in different hospitals. The 5 communities are similar in population density, topography, and per capita income; and it is unlikely that the differential tonsillectomy rates can be related to variations in the incidence of tonsillitis, recurrent sore throat, or otitis media. Rather, the major source of variation appears to be in differing attitudes by physicians as to indications for the procedure.

Age and Sex Differences

The age and sex incidence of tonsillectomy for the total of the 13 communities is displayed in Table 7-3. While the rates for males and females are the same over

Table 7–2. Proportion of children with tonsillectomy and adenoidectomy by area of residence and age, 13 hospital service areas, 1969–71.

Area	*Person-years (1000's)*	*Number of Cases*	*Probability of T&A Removal by Given Age*					
			4 yrs.	*8 yrs.*	*12 yrs.*	*16 yrs.*	*20 yrs.*	*24 yrs.*
Total	535	5,315	.03	.13	.18	.20	.22	.23
1	16	218	.03	.17	.25	.27	.31	.33
2	26	130	.01	.04	.07	.09	.11	.12
3	10	141	.02	.17	.24	.26	.29	.30
4	22	262	.03	.14	.20	.24	.28	.29
5	32	351	.05	.15	.19	.21	.24	.26
6	48	429	.02	.13	.16	.18	.20	.21
7	16	446	.13	.38	.50	.55	.60	.63
8	29	253	.01	.09	.14	.16	.19	.20
9	21	306	.03	.19	.25	.28	.32	.33
10	68	692	.03	.13	.18	.20	.22	.23
11	71	888	.03	.16	.21	.24	.27	.28
12	162	1,146	.03	.10	.13	.14	.16	.17
13	14	53	.01	.05	.07	.07	.09	.09

Table 7–3. Incidence of tonsillectomy and adenoidectomy by age and sex, 13 Vermont hospital service areas, 1969–71.

	Cases per 1,000 Children per Year[1]			*Number of Cases*			
	Both Sexes	*Male*	*Female*	*Both Sexes*	*Male*	*Female*	*Percent Male*
Total	11	11	11	5,315	2,648	2,667	50%
< 2	2	2	1	72	52	20	72
2– 3	14	16	11	548	327	221	60
4– 5	28	31	25	1,215	684	531	56
6– 7	27	29	25	1,200	655	545	55
8– 9	16	17	16	685	357	328	52
10–11	10	8	12	396	160	236	40
12–13	7	6	8	267	118	149	44
14–15	6	4	8	231	76	155	33
16–17	8	5	11	274	85	189	31
18–19	7	4	10	190	55	135	29
20–21	5	4	6	121	39	82	32
22–23	3	2	3	66	19	47	29
24–25	2	2	2	50	21	29	42

[1] Age-specific rates based on estimated populations at risk.

the entire 26-year age span, boys predominate at ages under 10 years, and girls predominate at all ages above 10 years. Girls comprise two-thirds of the T&A cases performed on teenagers and persons aged 20 through 25 years, while 60% of the preschool tonsillectomies are performed on boys. In terms of the mean age of T&A cases, boys average 8 years and girls nearly 10 years, a pattern which is consistent from area to area of the state. The 2-year delay in tonsillectomizing girls, compared with boys, may represent a sex difference in the occurrence of chronic sore throat, otitis media, or hypertrophied tonsils, which is reversed after age 10. Other possibilities might include parental tendencies to protect young girls. There are no additional items of data in the system capable of shedding light on the age-sex question.

The incidence of T&A by age is low in infants, rises rapidly to a peak at 5 or 6 years, and trails off gradually through the elementary and high school years. The pattern is consistent for communities with high and with low overall rates, the incidence curve being displaced upward or downward, but maintaining the same general form. Area #7, with the highest incidence in the state, reaches a peak at age 4, an age at which nearly 10% of the available children are tonsillectomized in a single year.

Type of Procedure

Of the 6,359 procedures carried out in persons 25 years and under in the 20 participating hospitals, 74% entailed removal of both adenoids and tonsils, 18% of tonsils alone, and 8% of adenoids alone with most of the latter operations performed in the two referral hospitals (Table 7-4).

The patient ages of the adenoid cases were similar in distribution to the T&A cases, both averaging about 7 years. By contrast, the tonsils-only cases had a mean age of 16 years. While tonsillectomy exhibited a general decline in the state as well as in other regions of the nation over the three years (Table 7-5), the isolated adenoidectomy appeared to be gaining in acceptance, the harbinger being its growing popularity in the university hospitals. In terms of the major diagnoses associated with the cases, 90% were ascribed to hypertrophied tonsils, 5% to chronic otitis media, and the remaining 5% to all other categories. Otitis media was reported as the major diagnosis in 16% of the referral hospital cases. A related phenomenon was the increased performance of myringotomy as a secondary procedure in the latter two facilities.

Expenditure Rates

Table 7-6 for T&A cases under age 26 exhibits estimated community expenditures for residents of the 13 hospital service areas during the 3-year period 1969 through 1971. The total dollars expended on the procedure was in excess of one million. The average charge per case ranged between $164 and $220,

Table 7-4. Number of T&A's performed on persons under 26 in 21 hospitals serving Vermont, 1969–71.

		Number of Cases		
	Total	*Teaching*	*Community*	*Mean Age at Surgery*
	6359	1854	4505	8.91
Tonsils	1168	225	943	16.12
Adenoids	482	388	94	7.22
T&A	4709	1241	3468	7.30

Table 7-5. Number of T&A's by hospital and year, Vermont, 1969–71 (under 26 years of age).

Hospital	*Number of Cases* 1969	1970	1971	*Percent Change ('69–'70 vs. '71)*
Total	2162	2250	1947	-12%
1	616	581	431	-28
2	7	20	62	+359
3	69	75	86	+19
4	47	40	47	+8
5	81	85	57	-31
6	25	18	17	-21
7	10	8	4	-56
8	204	179	159	-17
9	269	301	322	+13
10	97	57	48	-38
11	4	5	1	-78
12	83	127	132	+26
13	69	78	60	-18
14	114	126	104	-13
15	144	193	128	-24
16	224	234	185	-19
17	35	44	21	-47
18	64	79	83	+16
19	0	0	0	–
20	0	0	0	–
21	0	0	0	–

around the state average of $195, the major source of variation being associated with differing average lengths of hospital stay, which varied between 1.2 and 2.4 days. The annual T&A dollars per capita represents an estimate of community expenditures for the procedure among persons 25 years and under. The estimate ranges from 63¢ in area #13 to $5.69 in the highest T&A area #7.

Physician Case Loads

A total of 92 physicians performed one or more of the 6,356 T&A procedures in persons age 25 and under during the 3-year period (Table 7-7). Thirty-six physicians did 10 or less, accounting in the aggregate for only 90 of the cases. More than 80% of the procedures were carried out by two dozen practitioners and more than half of all cases were accounted for by 10 physicians. The highest numbers of T&A operations recorded per physician were 373, 389, 395, 429, and 462, the efforts of these 5 individuals representing over one-quarter of the total case load. For the most part, T&A's are not referred, with nearly 90% of the cases performed by local physicians in the hospital serving the residence community. The tonsillectomy rates in the smaller communities of the state thus primarily reflect the decision processes and efforts of a small number of physicians practicing in the local hospital. Such localization is the key to understanding the wide variance in tonsillectomy rates in the 13 hospital service

Table 7-6. Estimated dollars expended on T&A's for persons under 26 years of age, 13 hospital service areas, 1969–71.

Area	*Number of Persons under 26 (1,000's)*	*Number of T&A's*	*Total Dollars Expended (× 1,000)*	*Mean Cost per Case*	*Dollars per Capita*
Total	535	5,315	$1,038	$195	$1.94
1	16	218	46	212	2.92
2	26	130	26	198	.98
3	10	141	31	220	3.02
4	22	262	55	210	2.51
5	32	351	73	205	2.28
6	48	429	78	183	1.65
7	16	446	90	203	5.69
8	29	253	49	195	1.72
9	21	306	67	219	3.14
10	68	692	144	208	2.11
11	71	888	181	204	2.55
12	162	1,146	189	164	1.16
13	14	53	9	167	.63

Table 7-7. Tonsillectomy and adenoidectomy cases in persons under age 26 by number of procedures per physician, Vermont hospitals, 1969–71.

Number of T&A's per Physician	*Number of Physicians*[1]	*Number of T&A's*	*Percent of Cases*	*Cumulative Percent*
Total	92	6356	100	–
< 10	36	90	1	1
10–	16	329	5	7
30–	9	360	6	12
60–	7	539	9	21
90–	8	862	13	34
120–	6	934	15	49
180–	3	595	9	58
240–	1	240	4	62
300–	1	359	6	68
360–	3	1157	18	86
420+	2	891	14	100

[1]Three cases excluded because of unknown M.D.

areas. The rate of 409 tonsillectomies per 10,000 children per year recorded in Area #7 is nearly four times greater than the state rate of 111 and more than ten times greater than the rate observed in Area #13.

There are major differences in procedure rates, types of procedures performed, and diagnostic labeling between areas served by teaching and community hospitals. Towns, primarily feeding patients into teaching hospitals, experience low overall rates, while there is a wide variance in rates between the community hospital areas. The teaching hospital case loads are characterized by increased use of adenoidectomy without tonsillectomy, of myringotomy performed in conjunction with T&A, and of chronic otitis media as the major reason for surgery. By contrast, the community hospital case loads are predominantly tonsillectomy with and without adenoidectomy performed because of hypertrophied tonsils on children nearly one year older than those in the teaching facilities. The latter effect is associated with increased use of tonsillectomy without adenoidectomy in older teenagers which, in several of the community hospitals, comprises more than one-third of the T&A cases.

Incidence of Common Surgical Procedures

The occurrence rates for several common surgical procedures are exhibited in Table 7-8 which includes comparable data for Saskatchewan (Saskatchewan Hospital Services Plan, 1970), the United States, England and Wales, and Federal employees covered by group plans and Blue Cross/Blue Shield.

The rates are expressed as cases per 10,000 population adjusted to the age distribution of Vermont to account for differing age structures. For the non-repetitive procedures involving organ removal, the rates are understatements as the populations include individuals with prior surgery and not at risk. The extent of the understatement is small except for tonsillectomy and other procedures performed at rates exceeding 5 per 1,000 per year.

Table 7-8. Surgical procedure rates per 10,000 population, 13 Vermont hospital service areas, 1969–71, selected populations (all ages).

Area	*T&A*	*Appendectomy*	*Prostatectomy (males)*	*Inguinal Hernia (males)*	*Mastectomy (females)*	*Hysterectomy (females)*	*Cholecystectomy (females)*
1	66	15	32	50	29	39	27
2	23	15	15	38	16	30	19
3	63	20	29	38	22	30	29
4	54	14	25	38	20	33	30
5	54	25	23	52	24	32	30
6	41	21	21	45	35	48	38
7	135	30	27	54	22	41	53
8	41	31	22	45	27	51	25
9	69	18	28	47	24	60	29
10	46	18	23	47	22	41	32
11	60	25	24	49	22	40	24
12	31	14	32	41	18	43	28
13	16	23	20	51	20	30	18
Vermont	46	19	25	45	22	41	29
Saskatchewan	87	32	27	34	21	63	56
U.S.A.	63	20	20	51	26	52	na
England & Wales	32	22	9	29	15	21	na
U.S. Employees							
BC/BS	75	22	23	48	28	49	na
Group	20	10	11	30	19	24	na

Age-adjusted rates computed without decrementing population for prior removals.

For most of the procedures the Vermont rates tend to approximate or to be slightly lower than United States rates. With the exceptions of repair of inguinal hernia and mastectomy, Saskatchewan rates tend to exceed all but the extreme rates recorded in any Vermont hospital service area. A more direct comparison without geographic confounding is recorded in the experience of Federal employees covered by capitation and fee-for-service plans (Perrot, 1971). For each procedure listed, the Blue Cross/Blue Shield rate is about double that for group-plan members.

In Vermont, hysterectomy ranges between 30 and 60 cases per 10,000 women per year. The highest Vermont area approximates the Saskatchewan experience, and the lowest area approximates the hysterectomy experience of prepaid group-plan members. A similar circumstance pertains to cholecystectomy, where the Vermont rates range between 19 and 53 cases per 10,000 women. For both of the latter procedures, the highest Vermont area is approximated by Saskatchewan and the lowest Vermont area by England and by United States members of group health plans.

Vermont appendectomy rates vary over the 13 hospital service areas from 14 to 31 cases per 10,000 per year and are bracketed at the low end by United States employees with group health insurance and at the high end by Saskatchewan. In Hannover of the Federal Republic of Germany, the incidence of appendectomy is 60 per 10,000, more than double the highest rates recorded in most other countries (Lichtner and Pflanz, 1971). Within Hannover, the rate for white collar workers is 95 as contrasted with a rate of 30 for blue collar workers. No data are presented which suggest that these variations are related to differential disease incidence. Rather, three out of four cases are ascribed to recurrent scarred appendicitis, neurogenic appendicitis, and chronic appendicitis, terms which the authors state "practically represent normal status."

Hospital patient day rates, reflecting the multiplicative effects of admission rate and medical decisions concerning length of hospital stay, vary by as much as an order of magnitude over the 13 Vermont service areas (Table 7-9). Tonsillectomy days per 10,000, adjusted for age, range between 19 and 289. Appendectomy days vary between 74 and 188, prostatectomy between 232 and 569, hysterectomy from 295 to 670, and mastectomy from 87 to 209. Cholecystectomy days vary by more than threefold between areas. For each procedure except mastectomy, the Saskatchewan day rate, resulting from high admission rates and long hospital holding times, exceeds all but the highest Vermont areas and is about double the state average.

DISCUSSION

The rates at which particular types of medical interventions occur in different communities depend on a complex series of transactions between patient and physician, the nature of the population being served, and characteristics of the predominant medical organization. One might envision a simple model where the process is initiated by an individual seeking a physician's consultation as a result of a perceived change in health status, perhaps involving discomfiture, pain, or other types of distress. Because of large individual variation in pain

Table 7-9. Patient days of hospitalization per 10,000 population, 13 Vermont hospital service areas, 1969–71 (all ages).

	Days per 10,000 per Year						
Area	*T&A*	*Appendectomy*	*Prostatectomy (males)*	*Inguinal Hernia (males)*	*Mastectomy (females)*	*Hysterectomy (females)*	*Cholecystectomy (females)*
Vermont	91	123	405	273	146	439	372
1	151	110	569	326	188	447	309
2	50	115	270	221	119	384	216
3	145	145	497	287	182	284	478
4	117	98	379	230	151	356	438
5	95	135	345	349	207	327	433
6	84	142	364	329	209	544	535
7	289	187	477	325	133	421	651
8	88	188	429	259	109	516	279
9	160	128	374	361	173	670	386
10	92	122	528	344	158	496	436
11	124	171	356	262	131	396	270
12	49	74	410	190	112	421	352
13	19	144	232	261	87	295	208

thresholds and in beliefs concerning efficacy, the decision to seek care ranges widely among persons confronted with a particular condition. Given that a positive decision has been made, access to treatment is importantly conditioned by the availability of physicians and health facilities as well as by financial means. Given that care has been sought and an appointment obtained, the probability that a particular diagnostic label is assigned to the patient and a particular modality of care recommended depends on the individual practitioner, his diagnostic acumen, his medical specialty, and his belief in the appropriateness of the approach. The various transition probabilities involved in the steps leading to the observable event of surgery are rarely the object of investigation. The relation between disease incidence and the initiation of specific therapy is obscured by the intermediate transitions.

Suppose that the following denote the conditional probabilities of interest:

S_k	Probability of intervention type k
P_{hi}	Probability of disease h in individual i
q_{ij}	Probability individual i seeks care from physician j
$r_{jk(h)}$	Probability physician j recommends therapy k for the condition h.

The probability S_k for a particular procedure k may then be represented as the sum over all disease states h, physicians j, and individuals i,

$$S_k = \Sigma_h \Sigma_i \Sigma_j P_{hi} q_{ij} r_{jk(h)}.$$

The data based on hospital surgery do not permit direct measurement of the transition probabilities which govern the process. The relationship between the surgery rates S_k and the disease incidence probability P_h is difficult to investigate, requiring fine structure observations well beyond the scope of currently existing data systems. Generally, even the S_k are not available for population groups, the exception being enrolled members of certain health insurance plans. Except for a small number of intensively studied conditions, there are at best gross estimates of the P_{hi} such as the incidence of gall bladder disease which might lead to cholecystectomy, of uterine fibroids which might result in hysterectomy, and of appendicitis which might lead to appendectomy.

We have little knowledge of the access probabilities q_{ij}. Few systematic attempts have been made to study the differences in the $r_{jk(h)}$ which appear to be related to the physician's training and the particular discipline under which he practices. For the disease h = thyrotoxicosis during the 1950's, when at least two modes of therapy were prevalent, the conditional probability of thyroidectomy was largely dependent on whether the physician (j) was a surgeon or an internist who was more likely to recommend treatment with radio-iodine. An element of randomness in physician behavior regarding recommendations for tonsillectomy is illustrated by the so-called Glover phenomena (Glover, 1938). A group of children were independently assessed by N different physicians in terms of the desirability of removing their tonsils. The number of positive recommendations per child ranged randomly between none and N.

The suggestion that organization of practice plays an important role in determining the $r_{jk(h)}$ is contained in the experience of Federal employees and their dependents subscribing to salaried capitation plans such as Kaiser Permanente and to fee-for-service plans such as Blue Cross/Blue Shield. The S_k for the common procedures shown in Table 7-8 are about double for the latter as for the members of group plans. It is unlikely that the average underlying incidence probabilities P_h vary twofold between two groups of persons, both working for the Federal establishment in similar occupational circumstances, in the same geographic locations and differing ostensibly only in the decision to opt for one type of medical insurance or the other. Since no data have been collected on health status and outcomes under the two plans, it remains unclear whether either or both systems lead to overutilization or to underutilization.

An additional factor of possible importance in determining the intervention probabilities $r_{jk(h)}$ is the composition of the medical manpower supply itself. In England and Wales, with about half the number of surgeons per capita as in the United States, Bunker (1970) reports that about half as much surgery is performed. A similar circumstance pertains to the number of surgeons per capita among Kaiser Permanente subscribers as contrasted with populations in the same areas covered by reimbursement-type medical insurance. Irrespective of economic motivations, the type of training and specialization may condition significantly the form of therapy selected, since alternate modes are admissable in a wide variety of presenting circumstances. The additional effect of group practice organization with peer review and reduction in financial barriers to consultation may also be of importance in altering the $r_{jk(h)}$.

Within Vermont, the predominant financial base of medical practice is fee-for-service. As such, variations in the tonsillectomy rate S_k between medical communities of the state must be related to differences in incidence, access, and manpower. The most common indication for tonsillectomy is stated to be a hypertrophied organ (Bolande, 1969). Over 90% of Vermont cases had a final diagnosis explaining admission of hypertrophied tonsils. Since tonsil size is gauged in relation to pharyngeal size, and relative tonsil size is reported to be at a maximum between 4 and 6 years of age, the judgment of hypertrophy appears to be most likely for children in that age group, where procedure rates are at a maximum. Harper suggests that 4-year-olds with larger tonsils become 7-year-olds with ordinary tonsils because of the relatively more rapid pharyngeal growth (Harper, 1962). A possible example of this phenomenon is the observation by Dods (1952) of 681 children for whom tonsillectomy was postponed because of a poliomyelitis outbreak. Over one-third were judged not to require the operation when re-examined 18 months later. In a sample of 1,000 New York school children 11 years of age, 60% had already been tonsillectomized. The remaining 40% were re-examined by school physicians who selected 45% for T&A. The children without T&A recommendation were re-examined by a second group of physicians, who recommended that 46% undergo the procedure. The third re-examination of the twice-rejected children led to tonsillectomy recommendations in 44%. After three successive evaluations, a total of 65 children were never recommended for tonsillectomy. The authors concluded that the process of recommendation depended principally on the physician rather than on the child's health status (American Child Health Association, 1934).

Access to physicians of children with conditions that lead to tonsillectomy cannot be directly appraised. But there is evidence that the annual contact rate of patients with physicians and the insurance and income status of residents living in different Vermont medical communities are similar and unrelated to variations in use of procedures. There is also evidence of variability in physician decision-making in recommending tonsillectomies (unpublished report on Vermont Health Utilization Survey, 1973). The principle of economy would suggest as a null hypothesis that the major element in the variability in occurrence of tonsillectomy between Vermont communities is the physician factor.

The situation for appendectomy and other common procedures is more obscure. For each surgical procedure except herniorrhaphy, the rates exhibit a significant threefold variation between communities of the state and tend to be bracketed on the low end of the scale by group practice and on the high end by Saskatchewan. The relation between the S_k over the 13 Vermont communities is not clear-cut, so that the total surgical load varies by between 49 and 69 cases per 1,000 per year. An area with a high level of female surgery may be low for other procedures. The high tonsillectomy and cholecystectomy area has low rates for hysterectomy and mastectomy.

Under the circumstance, there is no objective measurement of health needs in terms of the prevalence and incidence of the generic conditions associated with surgical intervention of the types under discussion. Demand, as measured by utilization, is defined and conditioned by supply. Above certain minimal levels, variations in utilization may be associated with either unmet health requirements or with characteristics of the providers. The data are consistent with both hypotheses.

SUMMARY

1. The rate at which adenotonsillectomy is performed in different Vermont communities varies between 4 and 41 cases per 1,000 children per year. The risk of T&A by age 20 varies between 9 and 60%.

2. Although rates for males and females are similar over the first 25 years of life, males have higher rates under age 10 and females after age 10. The peak incidence occurs between 5 and 6 years for both sexes.

3. Three-fourths of the cases involved removal of both tonsils and adenoids. The isolated adenoidectomy, representing 8% of the cases, appears to be gaining in acceptance, particularly in the university hospitals. On an overall basis, T&A incidence declined by 10% annually over the study period. The major diagnosis reported was hypertrophied tonsils in 90% of the cases.

4. The estimated annual expenditures per capita for T&A varies between 63¢ in the lowest incidence community to $5.69 in the highest incidence community.

5. T&A case loads for individual physicians ranged between 1 and 462 over the three-year period. Ten physicians performed one-half of the 6,356 procedures in the series.

6. The variation of T&A rates between Vermont communities is discussed in terms of differential incidence, access to medical care, and physician viewpoints as to indications for the procedure. The similarity of these communities in terms of demographic characteristics, medical insurance coverage, and physician visit rates suggests that the variation in physician attitudes is the major factor in producing population based T&A rates which range between 4 and 41 cases per 1,000 children each year.

Acknowledgment

The assistance of J. Senning and P. Hickcox in preparing the data for this report is gratefully acknowledged.

References

American Child Health Association: The Pathway to Correction in Physical Defects. New York, 1934, p 80

Bakwin H: The tonsil-adenoidectomy enigma. J Pediatrics 52:339, 1958

Bolande RP: Ritualistic surgery—circumcision and tonsillectomy. N Engl J Med 280:591, 1969

Bunker JP: Surgical manpower. A comparison of operations and surgeons in the United States and in England and Wales. N Engl J Med 282:135, 1970

Chiang CL: Introduction to Stochastic Processes in Biostatistics. New York, John Wiley & Sons, Inc., 1968

Dods L: Some aspects of Australian pediatrics. Pediatrics 10:364, 1952

Glover JA: The incidence of tonsillectomy in school children. Proc R Soc Med 31:1219, 1938

Harper P: Preventive Pediatrics. New York, Appleton-Century-Crofts, 1962

Lewis CE: Variations in the incidence of surgery. N Engl J Med 281:880, 1969

Lichtner S, Pflanz M: Appendectomy in the Federal Republic of Germany. Med Care 9:311, 1971

National Center for Health Statistics (HEW, unpublished material). 1966

Pearson RJC, Smedby B, Berfenstam R, et al: Hospital caseloads in Liverpool, New England, and Uppsala: An international comparison. Lancet 2:559, 1968

Perrot G: The Federal Employees Health Benefit Program (Community Health Services, HEW). 1971

Registrar General's Statistical Review of England and Wales, Part I, 1954

Saskatchewan Hospital Services Plan. Annual Report, 1970

Unpublished report on Vermont Health Utilization Survey, 1973 Survey Research Program, University of Massachusetts and Joint Center for Urban Studies, Massachusetts Institute of Technology and Harvard University, 1973

Wennberg J, Gittelsohn A: Small area variations in health care delivery. Science 182:1102, 1973

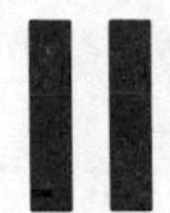

SURGICAL INNOVATION AND ITS EVALUATION

Surgical innovation may result from the insights and judgments of gifted and experienced individual surgeons or it may be the end product of complex, costly, and time-consuming laboratory and clinical investigations that synthesize past experience and the results of controlled clinical trials.

Before the advent of anesthesia and aseptic techniques, in themselves remarkable innovations by surgeons, surgery was a rough and ready art in which experience and anatomic knowledge were the surgeon's only guides. Pain during an operation and septic complications afterwards confined the surgeon to rapid and limited procedures, except when major interventions were a grim alternative to virtually certain death. Surgical knowledge, apart from anatomy, was as primitive as the medical sciences of those times. From these circumstances arose a tradition (which permeates surgery even today) that places a premium on effective, simple measures, directly tested by the surgeon's immediate observations. In current parlance, surgery is an "invasive" technique, and until the end of the nineteenth century such invasions had to be justified by both simple execution and simple logic.

Toward the end of the nineteenth century innovations became more far-reaching as the scope of surgery rapidly expanded in the wake of the new anesthetic and aseptic techniques. In Chapter 8 Barnes reviews some of the less fortunate innovations in American surgery between 1880 and 1942 to gain insight into their origin and how they were evaluated. In this period, the earliest innovations were largely recorded in statements by individual surgeons, without reference to the work of their colleagues. Citations of other papers were rare or absent, and therefore innovations had to have an intrinsic appeal. During the 60 years following 1880, the recording of innovations changed radically as the necessity for relating them to previous laboratory experiments and clinical work became apparent. The accelerated growth of medical science and of medical publications made this improvement inevitable. Yet the need to evaluate innovations was commonly unappreciated.

Today it is expected that new therapies will be validated by controlled clinical trials. Gilbert, McPeek, and Mosteller examine, in Chapters 9 and 10, surgical innovation between the years 1964 and 1972, as reflected in published reports. They focus attention on the general process of assessment of new surgical procedures and clearly demonstrate the importance of rigorous experimental design. The authors provide, in addition, documentation of current progress in surgery and anesthesia, including innovations that offer important gains for patient care; and, in Chapter 10, they review the need for long-term studies of the effects of surgery on the quality of life, including subjective as well as objective measures of outcome.

The practical demands of randomized trials in the field and the precautions required for their successful execution are illustrated by three examples presented in Chapters 11, 12, and 13. Chapter 11 by Cochran and his coauthors examines the comparative evidence on the treatment of duodenal ulcer by two slightly different operations, vagotomy with pyloroplasty on the one hand, and vagotomy with antrectomy on the other. The purpose in choosing this particular problem for analysis is to consider in detail the requirements for an experimental design where the expected differences are small, where the operation is important, and where past studies have sometimes omitted important steps required for a convincing experimental design. Chapters 12 by Miao and 13 by Barsamian describe the successful performance of randomized clinical trials to assess the efficiency of gastric freezing as a treatment for duodenal ulcer and of internal mammary artery ligation to relieve angina pectoris. Each treatment had been introduced with enthusiasm and each had been widely acclaimed on the basis of uncontrolled trials. Controlled clinical trials showed that the true effect of both procedures was a negative one.

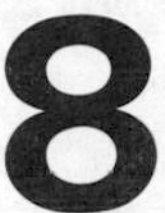

Discarded operations: surgical innovation by trial and error

Benjamin A. Barnes

In his presidential address to the American Surgical Association in 1889, the distinguished Boston surgeon Dr. D.W. Cheever stated, "I believe that we are warranted in saying that the future of surgery is without limit." After reviewing the accomplishments of surgery, he ended by quoting Sir Francis Bacon: "Lean not on authority; the test of truth is time" (Cheever, 1889). In this chapter we consider past efforts to evaluate innovations in surgical therapy and examine certain truths that emerged with time. We present evidence pertaining to the need for prompt and careful evaluation of surgical procedures. Our selection of nonbeneficial operations is drawn largely from the first part of the twentieth century. It is our hope that by knowing something of their origins, acceptance, and final discard we may learn lessons of value for the future evaluation of surgical innovations.

In considering innovations in American surgery, one naturally turns to the *Transactions* of the American Surgical Association, which have recorded yearly since 1880 the deliberations of the most prestigious and notable gathering of American surgeons. The *Transactions* represent a saga of American surgery as set forth by its academic leaders and its distinguished practitioners in papers carefully prepared and selected for the annual meeting (Sparkman, 1974). For the present purpose, the *Transactions* were reviewed from 1880 through 1942 to obtain examples of surgical innovations and therapies which were subsequently judged to be worthless. The review was not carried beyond 1942 because it seemed likely that some procedures considered since that time have yet to receive definitive evaluation, whereas procedures performed in the more remote past may be considered more dispassionately for the purposes of this chapter.

Articles advocating new or improved methods of therapy were reviewed in detail; from these, reports were selected which in general contained a series of cases given a specific treatment for a specific diagnosis. Single case reports were usually not selected because of their more limited implications. Diagnoses and operations were drawn from general surgery, including vascular and peripheral nerve surgery. Contributions on surgical techniques were not considered.

The process of selection was designed to provide papers concerning surgical therapies subsequently proved to be without benefit. These papers represent less than 5% of the *Transactions,* which during the same period also contained many outstanding and significant advances in surgery. We cite, for example, the early anatomic studies by Warren (1885 and 1887) on the healing of ligated arteries or anastomosed bowel; the explicit and enduring account by Richardson (1894) of the management of extra-uterine pregnancy and pelvic hemmorhage; the imaginative and fundamental exposition by Matas (1901) on artificial respiration by direct intralaryngeal intubation; the symposium on diseases of the stomach and duodenum presented by Moynihan, Mayo, Deaver, and others in 1908; and, at the end of our period of interest, the widely acclaimed first report of the surgical management of the patent ductus arteriosus by Gross (1939). While these are examples of the achievements of surgery, we deliberately focus our attention on discarded procedures because of our interest in the process of evaluation leading to rejection. A useful complementary study would be one to analyze the process of evaluation leading to the acceptance of enduring concepts and procedures.

No adverse criticism of the authors is intended or implied. Surgeons caring for patients ninety years ago exercised their skills in a different environment. Understanding of disease, diagnostic measures, and anesthesia were rudimentary, and appreciation of experimental design was primitive or nonexistent. For example, x-ray diagnosis was unavailable in 1889, and patients were operated upon for relief of typical renal colic on the presumption that they had a urinary tract stone. When a stone could not be found at operation, the surgeon not unreasonably wished to carry out some procedure which might be helpful to the patient already subjected to the risks of anesthesia and surgical exploration. Such appears to be the genesis of a report of 21 cases suggesting that the capsule of the kidney be divided for relief of "nephralgia" (Tiffany, 1889).

At a time when modern principles of biology had not been established, it is not surprising that surgeons might attempt an operation that would be considered inappropriate today. Often the incentive for innovation was an effort to improve an otherwise desperate situation, and a report on the transplantation of pedicle skin flaps from one individual to another (Finney, 1909) is an example of what today we call "parabiosis." This attempt to heal a chronic ulcer by transfer of tissue from one individual to another followed within only a few years the basic discovery by Karl Landsteiner in 1901 and Jan Janský in 1907 of the major blood groups. The system they characterized is simple compared to the system of histocompatibility antigens and antibodies that we confront in tissue transplants from one individual to another. It is not with such self-limited innovations, innocent as they may seem from our present vantage point, that we are concerned here. Rather, we consider examples from the past of the persistent and uncritical application of a surgical procedure over many years by different surgeons before the rationale for it is discredited and the procedure judged to be without merit. If such examples occurred in the past, perhaps we have a problem in the evaluation of surgical innovations today. We must at least consider the possibility that our knowledge, compared with that which our surgical heirs will have, is as incomplete and as short of the ultimate truth as the knowledge of earlier surgeons in relation to our present understanding.

Although record systems were primitive and follow-ups incomplete by modern standards, the *Transactions* of the American Surgical Association provide ample evidence of the concern and interest of the membership in end results. For a noteworthy example, a study over sixty years ago examined psychological sequelae of major surgery (Mumford and Hartwell, 1908) and included a 10-item questionnaire to investigate the quality of postoperative life. The remainder of this chapter will be devoted in the main to follow-up studies in four areas of surgical activity as recorded in the *Transactions:* (1) surgery for ptosis which was practiced between 1890 and 1928 with a peak of interest around 1910; (2) surgery for constipation which was practiced between 1909 and 1933 with a peak of interest around 1920; (3) surgery of endocrine glands starting in 1895 and continuing after 1942 with special interest in the 1930's; (4) surgery of peripheral and autonomic nerves for nontraumatic disease which was initiated in 1888 and continued after 1942 with special interest around 1930.

Surgery for ptosis

Between 1890 and 1928 there were 11 major papers on this topic. By the definition of the period, ptosis was a condition characterized by an abnormal, dependent position of internal organs, particularly the viscera of the abdominal cavity. Ptosis and its relation to the condition of neurasthenia were given the most extensive theoretical treatment by Reynolds (1910), lacking, however, any convincing experimental details. His theory attempted a unified, anatomic approach to the interpretation and interrelation of such diverse matters as posture, position of internal organs, neuroses, menopausal symptoms, low back pain, and so forth. At the start of the century the diagnosis of neurasthenia embraced a large spectrum of neuropsychiatric disorders that were probably the counterpart of those that demoralized individuals experience today and attempt to relieve through psychiatry. In 1910 it fell to the surgeon and general practitioner to care for such conditions. Discrete well-documented abnormalities of body composition or anatomy were inconsistent or absent. The diagnosis of surgically treatable ptosis was made in women five to seven times as often as in men (Keen, 1890; Harris, 1901). When the kidney was alleged to be in too low a position, this explained why patients were neurotic, had dragging back pain, constipation, fetid breath, occasional attacks of vomiting, cardiac symptoms, disturbances of the reproductive organs in the female, and exacerbation of the symptoms at the time of menses. It was stated that the elevation of the kidney to the proper position often required removal of the 11th and 12th ribs followed by four weeks of bed rest to allow adhesions to develop.

Operations for ptosis were repeated two or three times if necessary, and approximately half the patients were thought to be cured (Keen, 1890). For a condition of "simple dilatation of the stomach and of gastroptosis," the stomach was sutured to the upper abdominal wall, and the author concluded that operations on the stomach alone would probably "not be sufficient, but should be assisted by right nephrorrhaphy, hepatorrhaphy, . . .[and in] . . . women similar supporting operations will be necessary upon the genital organs as well. . ." (Curtis, 1900).

The concept of ptosis evidently gave surgeons a general license to stitch abdominal organs into improved positions. These positions were in accord with the surgeon's understanding of conventional anatomy learned at the dissecting table or on the anesthetized supine patient, where the normal effects of gravity on organs could not be appreciated. In 1910 several papers favorably evaluate operations for the relief of neurasthenia and associated visceral ptosis (Blake, 1910; Smith, 1910; Polk, 1910; Kelly, 1910). A review of 51 female patients noted that 29% were completely relieved of their neurasthenia following pelvic surgery, and the remainder were equally divided between those improved and those remaining unchanged. At the height of interest in surgical relief of neurasthenia, the Boston surgeon Dr. M.H. Richardson stated "that neurasthenic symptoms reappeared just the same [after several operations], as soon as the glamour of the operation was lost and the patient had returned to the humdrum of home from the professional atmosphere of the operating-room and clinic, in which great interest was shown in her case and in which she herself felt a stimulated interest" (Richardson, 1910). Here are the words of an experienced surgeon expressing implicitly the limitations of surgery in the treatment of the so-called neurasthenic, young female at the start of the century.

Other less perceptive criticism of treating neurasthenia by correction of visceral ptoses also appeared. Gastrointestinal symptoms were allegedly caused by "putrefaction" and "auto-intoxication" secondary to an abnormal length of large bowel. In selected cases of neurasthenia surgeons performed the Lane operation, in which the ileum was transplanted into the left colon with excision of the right and transverse colon (Blake, 1910). Ultimately it was pointed out that many patients were not improved by these operations and that the symptoms returned with discouraging frequency (MacLaren and Daugherty, 1911; MacLaren, 1916). MacLaren's second report probably had considerable effect in discouraging such operations.

As a last note in this account of visceral ptosis and its surgical correction, one report advanced an elaborate theory asserting that chronic appendicitis is due to an interference with cecal peristalsis (Smith, 1928). In a series of 571 cases with the diagnosis of acute or chronic appendicitis, 151 patients were found to have acute or subacute appendicitis, an incidence of 25% of all patients explored for presumed diseases of the appendix. In the 420 patients with the diagnosis of chronic appendicitis, 202 underwent appendectomy, and in the remaining 218 a procedure was performed to free up the cecum and to sever adhesions and bands that had allegedly prevented normal cecal peristalsis. Thus, as far as the cecum was concerned, reasoning had adopted a diametrically opposite position—from regarding its abnormal mobility as a cause of disease to regarding its abnormal fixation as a cause of disease as well. For the nonsurgical reader it should be noted that today operations for neurasthenia have disappeared and that the diagnoses of visceroptosis or chronic appendicitis are very rarely considered.

Surgery for Constipation

Between 1909 and 1933 there were eight major papers on this topic. The general style for these surgical interventions to correct "chronic intestinal stasis" was rather imaginatively established by Mr. Arbuthnot Lane, a visiting surgeon from England who participated in the annual meeting of the American Surgical Association in 1909. He presented his vision of an elaborate pathology of abdominal bands and adhesions running between the abdominal viscera and causing sharp angulations leading to intestinal stasis. He did not consider associated pathological findings limited to the abdominal cavity, and he claimed the breasts commonly had cystic degeneration leading to carcinoma, kidneys were mobile, patients had small amounts of subcutaneous fat, skin was frequently stained, respiration was chiefly diaphragmatic, cold extremities were consistent with poor circulation, and muscles were small. Lane presented further observations on cystic degeneration in the breasts stating that this degeneration was not usually seen in women having regular intercourse and that more frequent cystic changes were noted in the left breast as a consequence of secondary damage to the left (*sic*) ovary and of ovarian cystic changes caused by bands to the sigmoid colon. Patients' symptoms included headache, lassitude, inability to perform ordinary duties, mental distress, migraine headaches, laziness, and poor temper control. Various abdominal pains with a diminution in libido were thought to be a consequence of "auto-intoxication" (Lane, 1909). He recommended the operation, bearing his name, of lysis of all adhesions and of ileosigmoidostomy with resection of all the colon proximal to the anastomosis.

Following Lane's precedent and the authority imparted by his standing in British circles of surgery, a series of papers appeared. Some advocated a large incision so that the surgeon could identify fibrous bands, adhesions, ptotic viscera, "Lane's kink" in the terminal ileum, "Jackson's membrane" being a fold of peritoneum holding the right colon in what is today regarded as a normal retroperitoneal position, and so forth. Excision of a redundant sigmoid colon was recommended to relieve chronic constipation caused by angulation of the sigmoid, an entity distinct from volvulus of the sigmoid colon (Delatour, 1913).

Another approach to intestinal stasis was based on the assumption that the ileocecal valve was in spasm causing stasis of the small bowel contents, cecal stagnation, dilatation, and sagging. This was thought to require a plastic procedure to eliminate the culpable valve (Martin, 1914). A modification of the Lane operation proposed by Ochsner (1917) recommended that, in addition to an ileosigmoidostomy, the terminal ileum just proximal to the cecum be brought out as an end ileostomy and that the sigmoid just above the ileosigmoidostomy be transected with the proximal end brought out as an end colostomy. This permitted flushing of the intervening cecum, ascending, transverse, and descending colon to eliminate auto-intoxication and intestinal toxemic symptoms. In one series of 36 cases to relieve "intestinal torpor" and "coprostasis" a number of procedures were performed including severing peritoneal adhesions, appendectomy, and various bowel resections. There were two deaths (Ross, 1921).

Other surgeons were concerned with cecal atony, mobile cecum causing tension on the superior mesenteric vessels and duodenal obstruction, and ileocecal obstruction associated with appendicitis. These presumed abnormalities were held accountable for constipation, toxic symptoms of headaches, chronic invalidism, and an unbalanced nervous system. Appendectomy, plastic operations on the wall of the cecum, and resection of the cecum and terminal ileum were advocated (Starr and Graham, 1922; Speese and Bothe, 1930).

Finally, in 1933 concerns about duodenal stasis and obstruction emerged again with a new term for a class of patients requiring duodenojejunostomy. They were thought to suffer from the "habitus enteropticus." The authors (Pool et al., 1933) state that "since the diagnosis of duodenal stasis is made upon the symptoms and signs of abnormal physiology without directly demonstrating an organic lesion, it requires the most careful coordination of findings by the internist, roentgenologist, and surgeon." This admission of the absence of objective signs and the subsequent statement by the authors that "the findings at operation are often not conclusive, as duodenum may be collapsed at the time" indicate the subjective aspects involved in making the diagnosis. However, 17 patients were given the benefit of a duodenojejunostomy to short-circuit the obstruction. For the nonsurgical reader it should be noted that today operations for chronic constipation (in sharp contrast to operations for intestinal obstruction), for auto-intoxication or Lane's kink or Jackson's membrane, have disappeared together with Lane's pathological explanations and diagnostic entity of chronic intestinal stasis.

Surgery of Endocrine Glands

Between 1895 and 1934 there were eight major papers on this topic. As the physiology of the endocrine glands became known, it was to be expected that disorders attributed to hyperfunction would be considered amenable to extirpative surgery. Operations for partial or complete removal of endocrine glands were proposed and became safer procedures when replacement hormone therapy was developed and could support those patients who had morbid hypofunctional states postoperatively. Such replacement therapy was a late development and prior to its availability surgeons were intrigued with the possibility of transplanting endocrine glands to make up for hormonal deficiencies. Some provocative innovations are considered in this section.

A report of 111 patients with benign prostatic hypertrophy recommended double castration to diminish the size of the prostate gland and to eliminate obstruction of the bladder outflow (White, 1895). In the following year a careful comparison of castration and prostatectomy for this condition was presented with the conclusion that mortality was greater following castration because it did not immediately provide free urinary tract drainage and because of postoperative depression (Cabot, 1896). The comment on depression of the nervous system unquestionably was prompted by the well-known demoralization and loss of manhood that males may sense following removal of the testes. These two papers are evidence of an early interest in extirpative endocrine gland surgery and offer a rare example of the presentation and conclusive rejection of a surgical procedure in two successive years. Contemporaneous with this interest was the publication in 1895 of a Swiss series of 1,000 patients undergoing thyroidectomy by Theodor Kocher, one of the earliest contributors to endocrine surgery.

The thymus gland was thought to be the cause of respiratory tract obstruction, frequently in infants with enlargement followed by stridor and dyspnea. This condition was known as "status thymolymphaticus." Excision of the gland was recommended with the citation of previous experience where 42 thymectomies for respiratory tract obstruction resulted in 54% cures, 36% deaths, and 10% not relieved (Mayo, 1912). Status thymolymphaticus was mysterious inasmuch as it was claimed that the enlargement of the thymus gland causing death by suffocation could subside and disappear completely by the time an autopsy was carried out. In the days before chest x-rays and before sophisticated understanding of respiratory physiology such absurdities were accepted. The thymus gland, relatively larger in infants than in adults, had at that time no recognized function, and it was singled out as the scapegoat for obstructive respiratory disorders. In retrospect we note at earlier autopsies the thymus in patients dying after prolonged illness was incorrectly interpreted as a gland of normal size (in fact, shrunken by chronic depletion of lymphocytes), and by comparison, the finding of a "large" thymus in patients dying abruptly was incorrectly interpreted to be acute enlargement of the gland (in fact, normal in size).

Thyroid surgery was advised for the treatment of dementia precox, and one report presented four cases where this condition was associated with only minor changes in the size and form of the thyroid gland and with no evidence of thyrotoxicosis (Eastman, 1922). Each had a hemithyroidectomy, and all were improved according to the surgeon. The mounting interest in endocrine gland surgery made the year 1928 a propitious one for a statement in this field comparable to the paper by Leriche (*vide infra*) given at the same meeting on surgery of the autonomic nerves. The concept was advanced that there existed a force known as the "kinetic drive" seen in certain diseases such as epilepsy, neurasthenia, hypertension, endarteritis obliterans, hyperthyroidism with hypertension, etc. To control this drive giving rise to abnormal function and pathological states, operations were designed to accomplish "dekineticization." Opinion suggested that adrenalectomy, sympathectomy, and thyroidectomy were needed to achieve dekineticization, and twenty-nine such operations were performed. (Crile, 1928). The author recommended unilateral adrenalectomy for hypertension and thyrotoxicosis.

These theories and operations consistent with them remained viable for seven years, and in 1934 a second paper presented results of dekineticization in 326 patients (Crile, 1934). It was restated that diseases with excessive activity of the brain-thyroid-adrenal-sympathetic system would benefit. Such disorders as neurocirculatory asthenia, hyperthyroidism, peptic ulcer, and possibly diabetes were thought to benefit from this therapeutic intervention. Specific indications were listed for bilateral adrenal gland denervation including neurocirculatory asthenia, hyperthyroidism associated with neurocirculatory asthenia, or for hyperthyroidism if the patient were a singer or a preacher where damage to a recurrent laryngeal nerve could cause a serious handicap in speaking. Furthermore, it was noted that peptic ulcer occasionally responded to unilateral adrenal gland denervation and that bilateral adrenal gland denervation would decrease the severity of epileptic attacks because the "rhythmic hyperactivity of the entire energy system, muscular system and glandular system" would be modified. Finally, polyglandular disease, succinctly described as the presence of hirsutism and obesity, would likewise benefit from this operation.

In 1934 two papers presented patients treated with transplants of thyroid, parathyroid, and adrenal cortical tissue (Stone et al., 1934; Beer and Oppenheimer, 1934). These abortive attempts at transplantation were performed prior to any understanding of the allograft reaction and the role played by histocompatibility antigens. The results were inconclusive concerning growth of endocrine grafts, and the surgeons were unaware of the complex situation with which they were tinkering. For the nonsurgical reader it should be noted that today the thymus gland is known to be an essential organ in the maturation of the normal immunological apparatus and is accountable only under the most unusual circumstances for respiratory tract obstruction. Endocrine surgery for dementia precox, epilepsy, and the concept of "dekineticization" were never justified by any conclusive data, and on the basis of what we now know, the early transplants of endocrine glands could not have succeeded.

Surgery of peripheral and autonomic nerves for nontraumatic disease

Between 1888 and 1932 there were eleven major papers on this topic. Once the anatomy and physiology of the peripheral nervous system that coordinates involuntary activity was established, inevitably certain disorders thought to be caused by hyperactivity of these nerves, or by an imbalance between normally functioning nerves and hypoactive nerves, were treated by simple surgical section. Involuntary activity such as the control of blood vessel diameter, blood pressure, heart rate, gastric secretion, intestinal peristalsis, uterine contractions, and secretory functions of the adrenal medulla, to mention a few, are modulated by these autonomic nerves, also called sympathetic nerves. Early efforts to use surgical interruption of these nerves in the therapy of a wide variety of conditions are considered in this section.

Nerve stretching was practiced following a report in 1872 of this procedure by an otherwise unidentified physician named Nussbaum. With citation of this solitary precedent a paper by Dandridge (1888) presented results of nerve stretchings and concluded that in central nervous system disease, paralysis, and tetanus it was of no value although it appeared to be useful in persistent neuralgia and in restoration of sensation to the extremities. Nutrition of the limbs improved following nerve stretching with the disappearance of ulcers and tubercles, and because of this alleged phenomenon the paper has been included with others concerned with the autonomic nervous system since it is conceivable that the stretching of a peripheral nerve at times may have resulted in a peripheral sympathectomy with consequent vasodilatation. Benefits of stretching the sciatic nerve were alleged to extend to the opposite leg, and the author used the procedure in epilepsy where one may identify the peripheral nerve that supplies a region localized by the aura of an epileptic attack.

Ambitious applications of surgery of the automatic nerves followed as their physiology became more widely understood through the works of Otto Loewi, Walter B. Cannon, and other physiologists after 1920. Based on Sir Thomas Clifford Allbutt's theory that angina pectoris was secondary to spasm of the first portion of the aorta and associated with aortitis, it was suggested that section of the nerves going to the wall of the aorta might relieve the painful spasm permanently and beneficially since nitrate salts provided only temporary relief. The original suggestion made by J.B. Herrick in 1912, which we now know to be correct, that angina pectoris is a symptom of ischemic heart disease secondary to occlusive lesions in the coronary arteries was not generally appreciated even ten years later. The reflex arc to the aorta was interrupted by dividing all sympathetic nerves going to the heart on the left side, by division of the depressor nerve from the vagus nerve, and by division of the left superior cervical ganglion or left superior cardiac nerve (Kerr, 1925). Two of eight patients had bilateral operations. Two-thirds of patients received complete or partial relief, but there was a reported mortality of 17%.

Two years later a paper cited 10 examples from the surgical literature of bilateral recurrent nerve palsy following operations to remove the superior cervical sympathetic ganglion for control of angina pectoris. With this complication the distressing symptoms of angina pectoris were replaced or accompanied by dyspnea—equally distressing due to the obstruction to ventilation occasioned by the paralysis of the vocal cords (Seelig, 1927). Seelig made the disturbing comment that "many patients with angina pectoris not subjected to operation experience spontaneous and lasting freedom from pain. . . ." The disquieting doubts about the logic and evaluation of the operation introduced by this disclosure of the natural history of the disease were apparent, and a healthy discussion followed. In it the results of sympathetic ganglionectomies for the treatment of insane epileptics were reported as never curing a case (Mayo, 1927). The rationale of this procedure was not given but it may well have been erroneously assumed that epilepsy is caused by local vascular spasm in the cerebral circulation and that this spasm could be prevented by a local sympathectomy.

In 1928 the distinguished French surgeon Professor René Leriche, attended the annual meeting of the American Surgical Association and did for surgery of autonomic nerves the same service as Lane did for surgery for constipation at the 1909 meeting and as Crile did for surgery of endocrine glands at the 1928 meeting (*vide supra*). Each of these master surgeons provided an unchallenged entitlement for other surgeons to copy their example and to be clear of doubt and criticism from less prestigious sources. Leriche presented a paper that set forth the most inclusive justifications for operations on the sympathetic nervous system with the authority granted visiting European surgeons of the highest rank. Although he stated "we do not know the exact significance of the branches we cut . . .[and] we are ignorant, as a rule, of the cause and the exact mechanism of the diseases which we wish to cure. . ." nevertheless the following conditions were stated as being benefited by autonomic nerve section: angina pectoris, asthma, hyperthyroidism, dysmenorrhea, sclerocystic ovaries, vulvar kraurosis, pelvic cancer with pain, painful extremity syndromes, scleroderma, traumatic arterial lesions, beginning ischemic gangrene, phlebitic ulcers, varicose eczema, pain and cramps of old phlebitis, chronic ulcers secondary to varicose veins, to third degree burns, to fractures of superficial bones, to amputation stumps, etc., Volkmann's contracture, nonunion of fractures, and osteoporosis secondary to trauma.

Illustrative of the logical difficulties that arise for Leriche in evaluating the results of an operation for a particular disease is the statement that "in true Raynaud's disease, simple periarterial sympathectomy done on both sides produces a permanent cure" (Leriche, 1928). The implication of this statement in practice is that if the operation is not successful, the fault is with the diagnosis. The possibility that the operation may not be effective in all patients with this disorder (as we now know to be the fact) is excluded by a definition of a disease based in part on the successful response to a particular operation. With Leriche's ingenious example it is not surprising that other operations were improvised—such as division (*sic*) of the vagus nerve for the treatment of pylorospasm (Mayo, 1928). This condition was thought probably to precede the development of a peptic ulcer; and since we now know that the vagus nerve relaxes the pylorus, it is unfortunate this surgeon's experience was not more extensively presented.

Lumbar sympathetic ganglionectomy and ramisectomy were recommended for congenital ideopathic dilatation of the colon (Judd and Adson, 1928). The rationale, incorrect according to curent knowledge, for the operation stated that the dilatation of the colon was secondary to spasm of the distal colon caused by excessive sympathetic nerve activity. Commenting on the end results of periarterial sympathectomy for many of the conditions that Leriche had identified, one surgeon concluded after a review of the clinical results in 72 patients on whom 90 operations were performed to interrupt their sympathetic nerves that 35% of the patients had a successful result (Müller, 1928). He adds perceptively that "the reports in literature vary from the recording of utter failure to miraculous cure and apparently something in the individual case determines the result, something which we are unable to foresee or predict." This surgeon undoubtedly would have been delighted to learn about chi square statistics! Another surgeon also recommended section of the sympathetic nerves for the treatment of Hirschsprung's disease and for certain types of constipation (Rankin and Learmonth, 1930; Robertson, 1931).

Finally, in 1932 a report was made of removing cervical sympathetic ganglia for the treatment of epilepsy on the basis that such nerve excisions were likely to increase the blood flow to the brain (Mayo, 1932). This is five years after the report mentioned above citing the indifferent results following this operation. For the nonsurgical reader it should be noted that autonomic nerve surgery, unlike surgery for ptosis and constipation, has an established place in current surgical practice. It is largely restricted today to lumbar and cervical sympathectomies to achieve vasodilatation in vascular disorders where there is little or no organic obstruction, such as caused by an atheromatous, calcified, arterial wall plaque. The number of lumbar sympathectomies to improve circulation to the lower extremities sharply decreased following the early brilliant successes of reconstructive arterial surgery. Vagus nerve section is also well established in the treatment of peptic ulcer disease. Most of the indications claimed by Leriche were never proved to be of value.

DISCUSSION

As noted above many of the concepts justifying operations were subsequently proved incorrect, but the purpose of this chapter is not to emphasize surgical errors as these are inevitable when energetic and ambitious minds attempt to treat poorly understood disease. However, an important point is the duration of acceptance of the faulty concepts before final discard. For ptosis the quoted papers extending over a 38-year period suggested a peak interest in this condition around 1910, and the surgical maneuvers required to correct the presumed faulty position of organs in the abdominal cavity were of minimal technical complexity and could be completed by surgeons in that period with low morbidity and mortality. For constipation, papers extending over a 25-year period suggested a peak interest at about 1920, and the operations recommended were more complex than those for ptosis since they often demanded resections of the bowel and gastrointestinal anastomoses. Improvements in surgical technique and anesthesia were responsible for a low morbidity and mortality. Surgery for control of endocrine function appeared earlier than that concerned with the autonomic nervous system presumably because understanding of endocrine function and its clinical implications occurred decades earlier than the advances in neurophysiology that contributed to the identification of autonomic nerves to be removed or sectioned to correct diseased states. The abandonment of the futile operations on endocrine glands was less swift than the abandonment of the futile operations on the autonomic nerves, and we would like to think, but cannot prove, that the more rapid discard of these later operations is a consequence of the emergence of a healthy skepticism in sophisticated surgical circles concerning the evaluation of end results. For example, some of the surgery recommended on the autonomic nerves appeared and disappeared within a few years around 1930.

Possibly the most critical and central defect in these cited studies of innovative surgical therapy is the lack of control experience. The concept of controls appeared to be totally unknown to the surgeons of this period, although the references cited indicate they were puzzled by spontaneous cure rates and by the glaring inconsistencies in results following some operations receiving the *imprimatur* of experienced colleagues. Additional examples of unusual surgical innovations in specific diseases needing controls for prompt evaluation and subsequent acceptance or discard are numerous. Tuberculous peritonitis was treated by exploratory laparotomy and removal of ascitic fluid, and furthermore, irrigations with normal salt solution were advised on the basis of the experience of the noted English surgeon, Spencer Wells, and of Franz Koenig in Germany (Abbe, 1896; Ochsner, 1902). Ochsner reported 32 cases treated surgically where the advanced state of tuberculous peritonitis after failure of medical treatment was the indication for exploration of the peritoneal cavity, removal of ascitic fluid, and "admitting air to the peritoneal cavity." After this therapeutic ventilation the peritoneal cavity was closed, and, significantly, the patient was placed on medical therapy for an indefinitely long period (Ochsner, 1902).

Another example is the Talma operation for cirrhosis of the liver (Vander Veer, 1912). This operation was carried out for the relief of ascites, a complication seen in patients suffering with cirrhosis of the liver. A portion of the omentum was removed on a vascular pedicle from the abdominal cavity through a short incision and placed in the subcutaneous tissues of the abdominal wall to facilitate, by mechanisms undefined, the resorption of ascitic fluid. The procedure was endorsed "despite the fact that it does not seem quite rational in theory" (Vander Veer, 1912). This simple and technically trivial operation was carried out for many years before it was dropped from clinical practice.

Also in need of control experience was the therapeutic ligation of accompanying veins in the treatment of ischemic conditions of the lower extremity or elsewhere secondary to traumatic interruption of the arteries or to arteriosclerotic occlusion (Pemberton and McCaughan, 1932; Brooks, 1934). Treatment of patients with arterial insufficiency is complex with many confounding variables in the disease process, in the extent of the collateral circulation, in the status of the coagulation mechanism, and in the presence of associated disease such as diabetes, hypertensive cardiovascular disease, and so forth. The therapeutic ligation of a major vein, when the arterial supply had been impaired by chronic disease or acute trauma, was recommended for a few years before complete abandonment. This apparently was the consequence of common sense and of gross evaluation of clinical results rather than of any controlled experiment.

A final example of the need for control experience is the attempt to prevent peritoneal adhesions by papain described in a paper citing an experience of 231 cases given papain intraperitoneally following operations (Ochsner and Storck, 1936). As with patients suffering from ischemic lesions of extremities, the group of patients developing peritoneal adhesions and secondary complications is a heterogeneous one. It is well known that peritoneal adhesions are extremely common and rarely cause any symptoms whatsoever. Furthermore, the prospects of the surgeon for identifying adhesions putatively causing symptoms are diminished by the fact that frequently adhesions must be cut in order for the surgeon to obtain a proper exposure of other adhesions perhaps causing some complication such as partial small bowel obstruction. There are numerous reports where adhesions are severed by a surgeon with complete and permanent cure of symptoms, on the one hand; and, on the other, with equally distressing symptoms returning shortly after the operation. This appears to be a situation impossible to sort out lacking appropriate controls.

In addition to the absence of proper experimental design as judged by the standards of 1977, with appropriate controls in the evaluation of a new procedure, five major grounds for the prolonged acceptance of some ineffectual operations in the past were identified: (1) uncritical acceptance of established dogma or conventional wisdom in surgery as dictated by established leaders in the field; (2) primitive comprehension of the standards for adequate follow-up including such details as sample bias, duration of follow-up, and objectivity of observations; (3) casual acceptance by the surgeon that a discrete disease requiring treatment was present when, in fact, there was none, e.g. ptosis; (4) unjustified confidence of some influential surgeons in their understanding of human pathology, (5) virtual absence of ethical constraints demanding the greatest economy in human morbidity and mortality in the development and application of new treatments, e.g., operations on patients with epilepsy and dementia precox. Unstated, but pervasive, ingredients that influenced these five considerations must have been the strong, emotional orientation and fervent, personal involvement with which many surgeons of the past approached their challenging tasks. This may have been the consequence of their more solitary position in meeting major responsibilities, of past operations being an act of faith in the absence of scientific validation in many instances, and of the negligible medical support of patients by anesthetists and internists thirty or more years ago. In contrast, the superb and remarkably productive collaboration practiced today between surgeon, anesthetist, and internist has broadened the base for professional judgments and responsibilities and has reduced to a significant degree the individualistic and singlehanded characteristics of surgical performances in earlier times. In recent years substantial advances have taken place in the experimental design of clinical investigations, and the ethics of these investigations are today a matter of general concern. These welcome developments are noted in many other chapters, and although the process of review of surgical innovation is not perfect, it is vastly improved and will continue to improve in the future.

SUMMARY

A review of the *Transactions* of the American Surgical Association between 1880 and 1942 discloses operations that were accepted and later discarded. The acceptance and rejection of these procedures are reviewed to gain information about the process of evaluation of surgical innovations in the past. Examples of operations to treat ptosis, constipation, endocrine abnormalities, and autonomic nerve dysfunction provide instructive lessons for the future.

References

(TASA = *Transactions* of the American Surgical Association)

Abbe R: Tubercular peritonitis. TASA 14:117, 1896

Beer E, Oppenheimer BS: Transplantation of the adrenal cortex for Addison's disease. TASA 52:278, 1934

Blake JA: What are the end results of surgery or surgical operations for the relief of neurasthenic conditions associated with various visceral ptoses? To what extent do they improve the neurasthenic state itself? TASA 28:494, 1910

Brooks B, Johnson GS: Simultaneous vein ligation. TASA 52:57, 1934

Cabot AT: The question of castration for enlarged prostate. TASA 14:189, 1896

Cheever DW: The future of surgery without limit. TASA 7:1, 1889

Crile GW: Clinical studies of adrenalectomy and sympathectomy. TASA 46:150, 1928
Crile GW: Indications and contra-indications for denervation of the adrenal glands. TASA 52:312, 1934
Curtis BF: The surgical treatment of simple dilatation of the stomach and gastroptosis. TASA 18:124, 1900
Dandridge NP: Nerve-stretching. TASA 6:491, 1888
Delatour HB: Angulation at the sigmoid–a cause of intestinal stasis. TASA 31:598, 1913
Eastman JR: Thyroid surgery and the dementia precox syndrome. TASA 40:430, 1922
Finney JMT: The transplantation of skin flaps from one part of the body to another and from one individual to another. TASA 27:298, 1909
Gross RE: Surgical management of the patent ductus arteriosus: with summary of four surgically treated cases. TASA 57:8, 1939
Harris ML: Movable kidney: its cause and treatment. TASA 19:457, 1901
Judd ES, Adson AW: Lumbar sympathetic ganglionectomy and ramisectomy for congenital idiopathic dilatation of the colon. TASA 46:159, 1928
Keen WW: Nephrorrhaphy. TASA 8:181, 1890
Kelly HA: Movable kidney and neurasthenia. TASA 28:513, 1910
Kerr HH: Operative treatment of angina pectoris. TASA 43:485, 1925
Lane WA: Chronic intestinal stasis. TASA 27:23, 1909
Leriche R: Surgery of the sympathetic system. Indications and results. TASA 46:129, 1928
MacLaren A, Daugherty LE: A study of pyloroptosis; gastric atony as the original cause of neurasthenia, and its cure. TASA 29:316, 1911
MacLaren A: Chronic appendicitis and its relation to visceroptosis. TASA 34:478, 1916
Martin E: The ileocolic valve as a factor in chronic intestinal stasis; operative treatment. TASA 32:175, 1914
Matas R: Artificial respiration by direct intralaryngeal intubation with a modified O'Dwyer tube and a new graduate air-pump in its applications to medical and surgical practice. TASA 19:392, 1901
Mayo CH: Division of the vagi for pylorospasm. TASA 46:359, 1928
Mayo CH: Surgery of the sympathetic nervous system. TASA 50:1, 1932
Mayo CH: Surgery of the thymus gland. TASA 30:528, 1912
Mayo CH: In discussion of "A critique of the operative therapy of angina pectoris based on a case of vocal-cord paralysis following sympathectomy" by MG Seelig. TASA 45:159, 1927
Moynihan BGA, Mayo WJ, Deaver JB, et al: Symposium on diseases of the stomach and duodenum. TASA 26:129, 1908
Müller GP: End results of periarterial sympathectomy. TASA 46:154, 1928
Mumford JG, Hartwell JB: Psychical end-results following major surgical operations. TASA 26:628, 1908
Ochsner A, Storck A: The prevention of peritoneal adhesions by papain. TASA 54:263, 1936
Ochsner AJ: The safe elimination of the colon for the relief of uncontrollable intestinal stasis. TASA 35:172, 1917
Ochsner AJ: The surgical treatment of tuberculous peritonitis. TASA 20:191, 1902
Pemberton J deJ, McCaughan JM: Traumatic lesions of arteries: indications for therapeutic ligation of veins. TASA 50:521, 1932

Polk WM: The end results of surgical operations for the relief of neurasthenia associated with the various visceral ptoses. TASA 28:507, 1910

Pool EH, Niles WL, Martin KA: Duodenal stasis:duodeno-jejunostomy. TASA 51:107, 1933

Rankin FW, Learmonth JR: Section of the sympathetic nerves of the distal part of the colon and the rectum in the treatment of Hirschsprung's disease and certain types of constipation. TASA 48:279, 1930

Reynolds E: The etiology of the ptoses and their relation to neurasthenia. TASA 28:473, 1910

Richardson MH: Extra-uterine pregnancy and pelvic hemorrhage: cases and remarks. TASA 12:299, 1894

Richardson MH: In discussion of "Movable kidney and neurasthenia" by HA Kelly. TASA 28:513, 1910

Robertson DE: Treatment of megalocolon by sympathectomy. TASA 49:256, 1931

Ross GG: The altered anatomy and physiology of the cecum and ascending colon, the result of adhesions. TASA 39:39, 1921

Seelig MG: A critique of the operative therapy of angina pectoris based on a case of vocal cord paralysis following sympathectomy. TASA 45:159, 1927

Smith R: Chronic appendicitis. TASA 46:368, 1928

Smith R: What are the end results of surgery or surgical operations for the relief of neurasthenic conditions, associated with various visceral ptoses? To what extent do they improve the neurasthenic state itself? A consideration of the various factors involved and an opinion as to what we may and should expect. The end results after two years in fifty-one cases. TASA 28:502, 1910

Sparkman RS: A saga of American surgery: the Transactions of the American Surgical Association. Ann Surg 180:705, 1974

Speese J, Bothe FA: Ileocaecal obstruction associated with appendicitis. TASA 48:290, 1930

Starr FNG, Graham RR: Cecal atony and mobile cecum. TASA 40:260, 1922

Stone HB, Owings JC, Gey GO: Transplantation of living grafts of thyroid and parathyroid glands. TASA 52:262, 1934

Tiffany LM: Free division of the capsule of the kidney for the relief of nephralgia. TASA 7:167, 1889

Warren JC: The healing of arteries after ligature. TASA 3:141, 1885

Warren JC: The process of repair after resection of the intestine and intestinal suture. TASA 5:141, 1887

White JW: The results of double castration in hypertrophy of the prostate. TASA 13:103, 1895

Vander Veer EA: Talma operation for cirrhosis of the liver, with report of cases. TASA 30:136, 1912

9

Progress in surgery and anesthesia: benefits and risks of innovative therapy

John P. Gilbert
Bucknam McPeek
Frederick Mosteller

I. INTRODUCTION

For the last three decades the public has shown strong interest in medical research and given it considerable support. Although part of this effort has been directed at theoretical problems, most of it looks toward better therapies and cures for specific diseases. When these attempts have been successful, as in the Salk vaccine or the development of successful organ transplantation, the outcome is one of our society's major victories. An important fraction of the gross national product, 0.2% (Walsh, 1972), goes into this effort to improve health care in the nation, and a special bureaucratic structure directs and stimulates this research.

This study is concerned with the effectiveness of new therapies in their clinical setting. In our review we strive for insights about the general process rather than the specific therapies in our sample. Thus, we come to a knowledge of the forest by looking at the properties of a selection of trees, and the reader should be constantly on guard against distraction by the specifics of individual items in

This chapter was facilitated by Grant GM-15904 from the National Institute of General Medical Sciences to Harvard University, by National Science Foundation Grant GS-32327X1 to Harvard University, and by the Miller Institute for Basic Research in Science, University of California-Berkeley.

the selection. Most of us are not accustomed to this general outlook on methodology, and so the viewpoint may be difficult to maintain.

To study the recent process of producing more effective therapies, we have reviewed a sample of 107 published papers concerned with appraising surgical and anesthetic treatments as used on human subjects. We ask of these therapies that are sufficiently promising to be tested in patients what proportion has proved to be substantial improvements over the existing ones, what proportion has been moderately successful, and what proportion has been found to be less effective than existing alternatives.

Using these papers, we estimate the probability distribution of the percentage improvement an innovation is apt to make, as well as the chance that it will turn out to have been an improvement at all. Thus, our aim is to describe the effectiveness of the crop of new proposed therapies in comparison with the effectiveness of the treatments they are designed to replace. By doing this, we hope to clarify the role of clinical trials in the process of identifying and documenting successful innovations as well as their role in protecting society from innovations that are not as effective in practice as the therapies we have in hand. Existing therapies have been tested over time and are still in use because they have been judged to be better than existing alternatives. Thus, we do not expect every new therapeutic idea to pay off.

Except for some major breakthrough comparable to the introduction of antibiotics, we have little reason to suppose that the general course of development of new therapeutic ideas will change drastically. Consequently, one may assume that the distribution of successes and of failures in the near future will not change very much. The results presented here should give realistic expectations, at least for the short term.

The plan of this chapter is first to describe how we chose the papers and to give some limitations of the sample. Section III presents three ways of looking at the performance of innovations: one qualitative and two quantitative ways based on new statistical methods. The methods of Section III may be useful in other circumstances as well.

In Section IV we mention incidental findings about methods of randomization and reporting on ethical issues. The general conclusions and discussions are given in Section V. Brief summaries of the individual papers and the more technical statistical matters are given in the appendices. In Chapter 10 we discuss issues of quality of life and long-term follow-up in light of the papers in this sample.

II. METHODS

IIA. Materials

We have drawn a sample of 107 papers from the medical literature in surgery and anesthesia. We wanted an objective sample of papers evaluating different treatments actually given to patients. To get such a sample, we turned to the National Library of Medicine's MEDical Literature Analysis and Retrieval System (MEDLARS) (Cummings, 1975; Day, 1974). Computer-produced bibliographies can be retrieved from this data base which, since January 1964, has provided an exhaustive coverage of the world's medical literature.

Almost all MEDLARS users want to study a particular biomedical subject. This system is designed to help readers locate papers on specific topics and diseases and is not oriented to retrieve articles on the basis of the *design* of the study reported in the papers, such as "a series" or "a randomized clinical trial." By searching the system for "prospective studies" of specified surgical operations or anesthetic drugs, we gathered papers whose authors used patients to evaluate surgical and anesthetic treatments. The papers appeared between 1964 and 1972.

We discarded papers in languages other than English because of our own language disabilities, and papers describing trials or series with fewer than 10 patients in a group because we wanted to study large investigations rather than case studies. The bias and sample selections, then, result from peculiarities of the MEDLARS indexing system and contents at the time of the search rather than from our prejudices.

We call these papers collected from the MEDLARS system **the sampled papers**, and their titles appear together in the bibliography, separate from the papers we otherwise refer to in the course of this discussion. We refer to the sampled papers by a number, and to the others by author and date.

Our sampled papers reported on three basic types of studies: **randomized controlled trials**, **nonrandomized controlled trials**, and **series**. We use the term "randomized controlled trials" when the investigator compared two or more treatment groups and patients were assigned to the groups by a formal randomization process. The nonrandomized controlled trials did not have such a formal randomization process and varied from comparing groups treated concurrently in the same institution to comparing patients treated previously by one method with patients treated currently with another. The papers reporting on series described a set of patients treated in some specified manner but with no specific referent for comparison except possibly other reports in the literature dealing with similar patients. We do not discuss series further, except in Section IV and in Chapter 10.

All areas of surgery* were not given a chance to be sampled, though the more popular areas were. Further, a search may not uncover all papers of a given type. Consequently, we cannot use these data to investigate rigorously questions about the comparative amounts of human research or clinical trials being done in the different fields, though we do get strong hints about the considerable popularity of certain kinds of investigations during this period. For example, when we find 16 cancer, 11 ulcer, 12 orthopedic, and 7 portacaval shunt studies out of 107, and no studies of craniotomies or of tonsillectomy and adenoidectomy, even though these topics were included in the search, we get a strong impression that during this period the first four types of studies are more common than the latter ones. (From another source, Sarah Brown,

*From now on we shall use the generic terms *surgical* and *surgery* to include both surgery and anesthesia.

(personal communication), we know of at least one controlled study (Mawson, 1967) of tonsillectomy and adenoidectomy during the period, but our MEDLARS search did not find it.)

One might suppose that if our MEDLARS approach were perfect and produced all the papers we would have a census rather than a sample of the papers. To adopt this model would be to misunderstand our purpose. We think of a process producing these research studies through time, and we think of our sample—even if it were a census—as a sample in time from the process. Thus, our inference would still be to the general process, even if we did have all appropriate papers from a time period.

IIB. Distribution and Degree of Success among Innovations

When surgical therapies are compared for effectiveness, what happens? How often does an innovation appear to be superior to its competitors? In appraising the results of comparative investigations, we take several simplifying actions.

First, for our conclusion we lean hard on the summary of the investigator.

Second, we classify each therapy as either an **innovation** or as a **standard**. Some diseases have a widely recognized standard therapy against which all other treatments are measured. A good example of this has been (the standard) radical mastectomy for cancer of the breast. In such fields the standard is easy to recognize; all others can be considered as competing innovations regardless of the time of their introduction.

In other instances, this distinction between standard and innovation is not so easy to make. When a well-known remedy is to be tested in a slightly different milieu, is it to be called a new remedy? We do so. We have used the letter I to denote the treatment we regarded as an innovation and the letter S for the standard. In (39) and (8) we use P for a placebo.

Third, we speak of a pair of competitive therapies as having three possible relations: about equal ($S = I$), the first preferred to the second ($S > I$ or $I > S$); and the first *highly* preferred to the second ($S >> I$ or $I >> S$). We tried to report on this scale what we think the original investigators would have reported. Usually their words make this clear, and a quotation from their article (Appendix 9-I) commonly indicates direction and degree of preference. Naturally others may have somewhat different views from those we give.

Fourth, we have divided studies of therapies into two classes: (i) **primary**, those therapies intended to cure or ameliorate the patient's primary disease, and (ii) **secondary**, those therapies dealing with improvements intended to prevent or treat such complications as infection or thrombo-embolic disease, or improvements in anesthesia or postoperative care. Again we found the distinction to be informative, although not always easy to make. The basic 107 studies included 36 randomized clinical trials, of which 21 deal with primary therapies and 15 deal with secondary therapies. Thus, in our sample the randomized trials split roughly equally between the two kinds. Not all studies could be used in the more quantitative analysis because some did not fit these patterns.

Fifth, for each study we provide in Appendix 9-I a brief summary statement of the findings restricted to the comparison of performance of therapies.

One randomized trial (31) of a primary therapy was set aside because, as carried out, the number of cases was too small for its complicated design to lead to conclusions. A second (35) was set aside for reasons indicated in the summary, leaving us 34 papers. One paper (8), a large study of cancer of the prostate, described *two* studies, each involving results for more than one stage of the disease: the first study compared four different surgical treatments, and the second compared four dosage levels of estrogen. Thus, the number of pairs of treatments available for comparison in this paper dealing with a set of primary therapies could have swamped the counts from the other studies. We treat this study separately in Subsection IIIB-4 and in the Brief Summary of (8) in Appendix 9-I and in Appendix 9-IV, part 2, and we included one comparison from the second study in Table 9-1.

Qualifications and Discussion. As an alternative methodology, each paper might have been evaluated by experts to find out whether they thought the paper strong enough to support its conclusions, as was done by Cochran et al. in Chapter 11, but in the present study we stop with the original investigators' views.

Table 9-1. Summary for innovations in randomized clinical trials.

		Primary	*Secondary*	*Total*
$I >> S$:	Innovation highly preferred	1	4[a]	5
$I > S$:	Innovation preferred	5	2	7
$I = S$:	About equal, innovation a success (see Section IIIA-1)	2	2	4
$I = S$:	About equal, innovation a disappointment (see Section IIIA-1)	7[a]	3	10
$S > I$:	Standard preferred	3	3	6
$S >> I$:	Standard highly preferred	1	3	4
	SUBTOTALS: Comparison	19	17	36
	Papers	18[e]	14[b]	32
$I_1 >> I_2$		2[a]	2	4
$I_1 = I_2$		2	1	3
$S_1 >> S_2$		–	1	1
	TOTALS: Comparison	23	21	44
	Papers	19[f]	15[g]	34

[a]One paper provided 2 such comparisons.
[b]Three papers provided 2 comparisons.
[e]One paper provided 2 comparisons.
[f]Two papers provided 3 comparisons.
[g]Three papers provided 2 comparisons, and one paper provided 3 comparisons.

Although this section concentrates on the findings in the comparisons of therapies, much additional valuable information is present in every study, such as advice about the execution of the therapy, what population the paper deals with, findings on the course of the disease, and special advice about management and treatment, in addition to literature reviews and scientific findings.

III. RESULTS

IIIA. Qualitative Analysis

We base the analyses given in this section on the randomized clinical trials and on the controlled trials in our sample of papers. We give a review of the qualitative findings in the next two subsections and give more quantitative analyses in Sections IIIB and IIIC. The studies are further subdivided into those that deal with primary therapies and those that deal with secondary therapies within each of the above-mentioned types of trials.

IIIA-1. Randomized Controlled Trials

In most studies at least one innovative (*I*) therapy is compared with one standard (*S*) therapy; and in a few studies where two innovations are evaluated, innovations can be compared as well. Similarly, a paper that compares an innovation with two standard therapies provides a basis of comparison between the two standard treatments.

Innovations compared with standards. Referring to Table 9-1, we see that 34 papers reported on randomized trials and that 32 papers provided 36 comparisons between an innovation and a standard. In 5 of these, or about 14%, an innovation was highly preferred to a standard. In 16 comparisons, including the previous 5, about 44%, the new therapy was regarded as successful, sometimes because it was no worse than a standard and thus became available as an alternative.

In 10, or 28%, the equality of an innovation with a standard could be regarded as a disappointment because, although more trouble or more costly or more risky, it did not perform better. In 20 comparisons, about 56%, a standard was preferred (counting innovative disappointments) to an innovation.

Innovation versus innovation. In 3 comparisons, one innovation turned out to be about as successful as another innovation. In 4 comparisons, one innovation was highly preferred to another. Thus, occasionally, competing innovations differ markedly in their performance.

Standard versus standard. One paper provided a comparison of two standards. One of the standards was highly preferred to the other. (Surprisingly, "no treatment," an innovation, was highly preferred to both standards.)

Discussion. Overall, Table 9-1 shows that innovations highly preferred to standard treatments are difficult but not impossible to find, and that almost half of the innovations provided some positive gain. It is worth reflecting on what our attitude might be toward extreme findings in either direction. Suppose nearly all studies, or even the lion's share, found the innovation to be highly preferred; one would have to conclude that standard therapies were fairly easy to improve on and indeed that the kind of medicine being appraised was in its infancy—or else that a sudden breakthrough had been made on all fronts, unlikely with so many different diseases and therapies as discussed here. At another extreme, if no substantial gains occurred, the suggestion is that the field has topped out, at least during the period of the study, and is awaiting some new insights.

IIIA-2. Nonrandomized Controlled Trials

In addition to the randomized clinical trials, 11 less well-controlled trials seemed appropriate for reporting. Results are shown in Table 9-2 in a manner similar to that used for the randomized trials. These split into 3 primary and 8 secondary studies.

Innovation versus standard. All 3 primary studies found innovations preferred or highly preferred, a rather more optimistic report than the randomized trials gave. The studies of secondary treatments had relatively fewer "equalities" (occasions when I=S) than the randomized studies, and the distribution leans by and large more favorably toward innovations. The pooled primary and secondary totals give about 58% of innovations preferred compared with about 44% for the randomized trials. For highly preferred innovations, the difference is even more striking: 42% for the nonrandomized trials against 14% for the randomized trials.

Discussion. This difference between randomized and nonrandomized trials is similar to that found in other reports (Chalmers, 1972; Grace, 1966; Miao, Chapter 12 in this book), where less well-controlled studies tend to give innovations a higher rate of success than do well-controlled studies. Whether this is

Table 9-2. Summary table for controlled but nonrandomized trials.

	Primary	*Secondary*	*Total*
$I >> S$	2	3	5
$I > S$	1	1	2
$I = S$		3[d]	3
$S > I$		1	1
$S >> I$		1	1
TOTALS: Comparisons	3	9	12
Papers	3	8	11

[d]In one study the innovation was a disappointment; in another, two innovations were disappointments. In addition to these, one comparison of two innovations found them about equal.

due to the lack of control or because the comparisons involved lead to large differences and thus lend themselves well to investigations with weaker control or for other reasons, such as sampling variation, is an open question.

IIB. Quantitative Comparisons

The comparisons of innovations with standards given in Tables 9-1 and 9-2 are more qualitative than quantitative. To get a more quantitative measure of the comparisons, we have taken the subset of 11 papers on primary therapies where survival seemed an appropriate measure of performance. Using these papers, we reviewed the distribution of differences in survival when innovation and standard are compared. These differences are presented in Section IIIB-1. In Section IIIB-2, a statistical calculation provides an estimate of the mean and variance of the underlying distribution, and in Section IIIB-3 a more sophisticated analysis provides a direct estimate of the cumulative distribution itself.

Parallel to this sequence of analyses, we analyze that subset of 11 papers on secondary therapies where freedom from a complication offers a measure of effectiveness. We have used the difference in the percentages of patients free of the complication as a measure of the gain for the innovation over the standard. (We have not analyzed the papers based on nonrandomized trials given in Table 9-2 because too few papers were available for this type of analysis.)

IIIB-1. Comparisons of Performance

Figure 9-1 plots the percentage of survivors for the standard therapy against that for the innovation. It summarizes 11 primary studies, 2 of which had 2 comparisons of a standard against an innovation, making 13 comparisons in all. The 7 points below the 45° diagonal line show the innovation performing better, the 6 points above show the standard performing better. The greatest observed gain shown by the point farthest below the line (coordinates 74%, 49%) comes from a study of therapeutic portacaval shunt (68). Curiously, the point farthest above the line (32%, 50%) corresponds to a study of prophylactic portacaval shunt (17), and its innovation was associated with the greatest apparent loss. The overall impression given by the figure is one of points hugging the diagonal line rather closely. The degree of scatter from the line depends in part upon the size of samples (number of patients used in the studies), and we explore this idea later.

Figure 9-2 shows 24 comparisons based on eleven secondary studies (five had 1 comparison, four had 2, one had 3, one had 8 [two sets of 4, one dealing with drainage, the other antibiotics]). The 15 points below the line indicate the innovation as an improvement over the standard treatment; the 8 above indicate the reverse; and the 1 on the line gives a tie. The greatest apparent gain observed for an innovation compared with a standard is from ampicillin to prevent wound infection (73). The greatest apparent loss shown by an innovation compared with a standard was wound breakdown following drainage used to prevent septic complication after appendectomy for a gangrenous appendix (58). The sample size for that study is rather small and so the observed difference may exaggerate (or underestimate) the true effect.

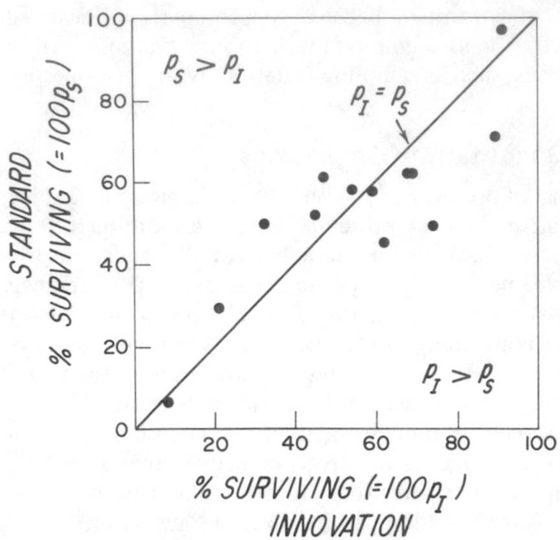

Figure 9-1. Comparison of performance of innovative therapies with standards for primary therapies.

Primary therapies—survival percentages. Points falling below the 45° line indicate higher survival rates for the innovation than for the standard. Primary therapies are intended to cure the patient's disease.

The overall scatter about the 45° line in Figure 9-2 is large, encouraging us to believe that larger percentage differences have been found here than in the studies of Figure 9-1. By and large, the changes in rate of complications are larger than the changes in survival rate. We make this more quantitative below.

Qualifications and Discussion

Primary Therapies: In considering primary therapies, when several survival periods were available (6 months, 1 year, 3 years, and so on), we chose a period for which the survival was near 50%.

Sometimes the data are not given by fixed length of follow-up, but rather on total survivors among all treated so far, and therefore length of observation varies among surviving patients. Then we computed the proportion surviving, even though the comparison is not as sharp, as if all patients had been followed for a fixed time period. If the treatments are randomly assigned, independently of time, to an incoming stream of patients, then this comparison of survival percentages does offer an index of the comparative strength of the therapies. The index could be misleading if the early survival rate were higher for one therapy and the later survival rate lower for the same therapy. The comparison is an average over the period reported, and we would rather use total survival to date than drop the study from the analysis.

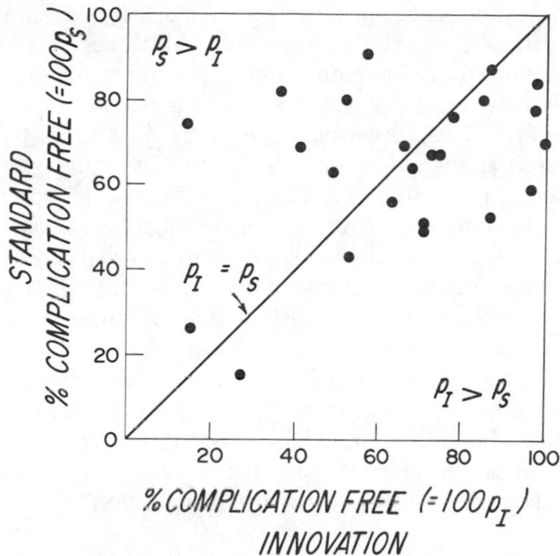

Figure 9-2. Comparison of performance of innovative therapies with standards for secondary therapies.

Percentages avoiding specific postoperative complications. Secondary therapies are intended to reduce the frequency of postoperative complications. Points below the 45° line indicate fewer complications of a specific sort accompanying the innovation than the standard. The innovations have 15 points below, 8 above, and 1 on the line.

Secondary Therapies: For most studies, one complication was regarded as especially important, and the percentage of patients not developing that particular complication is computed for both the standard and the innovation. In one study, we averaged results for 12 complications (3). In another, the results were estimated from graphs. Included here is the colon surgery dealing with everting vs. inverting in suturing (38) though its survival rates were included under primary therapies, because it seemed reasonable also to review its complications quantitatively.

In the graphical presentation given in Figures 9-1 and 9-2, we did not directly consider the effect of sample sizes on the uncertainty of the differences. The following two presentations take account of the effect of sample sizes and give estimates of the distribution of differences that would be obtained if many experiments of unlimited sample sizes could be performed. It frequently happens in statistical arguments, as here, that although we cannot know the truth for each investigation separately, we can estimate properties of the collection of investigations.

IIIB-2. Correcting for Sample Size

In the work reported so far, some innovations performed better than a standard, others worse. We next regard these outcomes as a sample from the population of all those innovations developed by our medical system and tested by randomized clinical trials. Every study has its uncertainties associated with sampling variability and other sources of unreliability. We allow for sampling variability in our description of the gains and losses. The general idea is that if we focus on a particular sort of performance, we may be able to gather strength from several studies even though they may deal with disparate operations. For example, among the primary studies we focus on those where the main hope from the operation is the extension of life. Then we might ask about the distribution (variety) of improvements actually achieved by this type of innovation.

If every study were based on an enormous sample of patients, reports of gains and losses alone would give us the distribution of differences in true performance in our sample of papers. In turn, that sample distribution would estimate the distribution of gains in the population—the overall process generating these studies and comparisons. But studies are of necessity limited in size, and in reports of small studies, differences vary more due to sampling error than in reports of large ones. We need to pool the results of such studies, large and small, in a way that will give an idea of the distribution of *true* gains and losses in the trials.

One such method is given in Appendix 9-II. The scheme is to allow for the sampling variability associated with specific trials and come up with a pooled figure. The observed difference may be thought of as having two additive components—the true difference plus the sampling deviation. Analysis of variance methods produce estimates of the mean and variance of the sample of true differences. Then, assuming that true differences are approximately normally distributed, we can estimate the frequencies of different gains.

It is important to understand that this method develops summary statistics for *true* gains and losses *across* studies. The statistics reported are: (a) the estimated average true gain, averaged across comparisons equally weighted; and (b) the estimated standard deviation of the true gain, averaged across comparisons equally weighted. If, for example, the average gain were 0% and the standard deviation of the gain 6%, gains of 10% or more could occur in about one-twentieth of the opportunities. It would still be true that the increment would be positive for about half the innovations and negative in half, in agreement with Table 9-1. It then becomes the goal of clinical research to identify the favorable and unfavorable innovations so that we may use the former with confidence and avoid the latter.

The following statistics summarize the results (for details see Appendix 9-II, Table 9-App. II-1):

	Estimated Mean Gain	*Estimated Standard Deviation of Gains*
Primary Therapies	1.3%	7.7%
Secondary Therapies	0.4%	20.6%

The mean for the primary therapies is not far from zero, a result that agrees with our more qualitative analysis of Table 9-1. A zero mean is consistent with some innovations having substantial improvements balanced by others having substantial losses. A large standard deviation of effects of innovations would support this interpretation, and indeed the standard deviations of true gains seem substantially different from zero. (A zero standard deviation would imply that all innovations give essentially the same amount of improvement.) And so, some innovations do produce substantial improvements.

These figures also yield a rough guess about the proportion of comparisons having true differences favoring the innovation as great as, say, 10%. For the primary therapies, the probability that a new therapy has a positive gain of at least 10%, if the sample represents the future well, is about 0.13.

Turning to the secondary therapies, a gain of at least 10% (a 10% reduction in a specific complication) has a probability of 0.32 for innovations tested by randomized clinical trials.

Occurring versus detecting. A caution is in order about a somewhat subtle point. Although we use the data here to estimate the proportion of studies or comparisons that offer gains of at least a given size, the possibility remains that in an actual experiment such gains may not be correctly recognized. This may happen because sample sizes must be limited and so sampling error is inevitable. This variation could be reduced, when practical, by using larger samples. Sampling error can go in either direction. Nevertheless, when we write of a 10% gain in this part of our discussion, we mean the gain that would be found if an unlimited sample were taken in each study.

Weights. In the current discussion, *comparisons* of paired therapies have equal weight. Other weights are possible and, for some purposes, preferable. For example, one could consider weights determined by the frequency of the disease or complication being studied; or perhaps frequency could be further weighted by importance or severity of the disease or complication. The data given in Appendix 9-IV make the option of using such weights available to the reader.

IIIB-3. Empirical Cumulative Distribution of True Gains

The procedure just used is rough and ready and leans hard upon the normal distribution in its calculation. An approach called "empirical Bayes" or "Bayesian" (Efron and Morris 1974; 1973a; 1973b) offers an alternative means of estimating the cumulative distribution (Appendix 9-III).

Empirical cumulative distributions of the true population of gains based on the methods of Appendix 9-III for the primary therapies (part 1 of Appendix 9-IV) and the secondary therapies (part 3 of Appendix 9-IV) are displayed in Figures 9-3 and 9-4.

Figure 9-3 shows the estimated cumulative distributions of the true gains in percentages for the primary and for the secondary therapies. Figure 9-4 shows the *same* information plotted on normal probability paper (Dixon and Massey, 1951). The vertical scale has been transformed. If the estimated cumulative

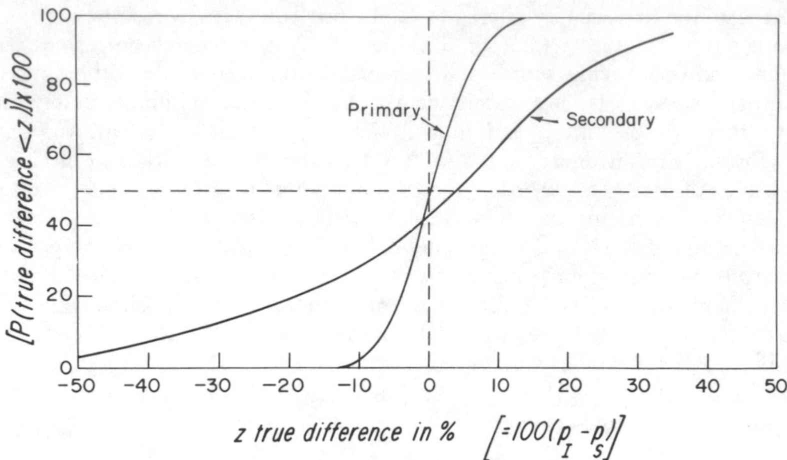

Figure 9–3. Cumulative distributions of improvements.

Empirically estimated cumulative distribution of improvements (innovation minus standard) as a difference in percentages. To find the probability of a difference in percentages less than a given number z, say $z = 10\%$, erect a perpendicular from 10% on the horizontal axis to the appropriate curve, and read its ordinate off the vertical axis, about 0.95 for the primary and about 0.6 for the secondary.

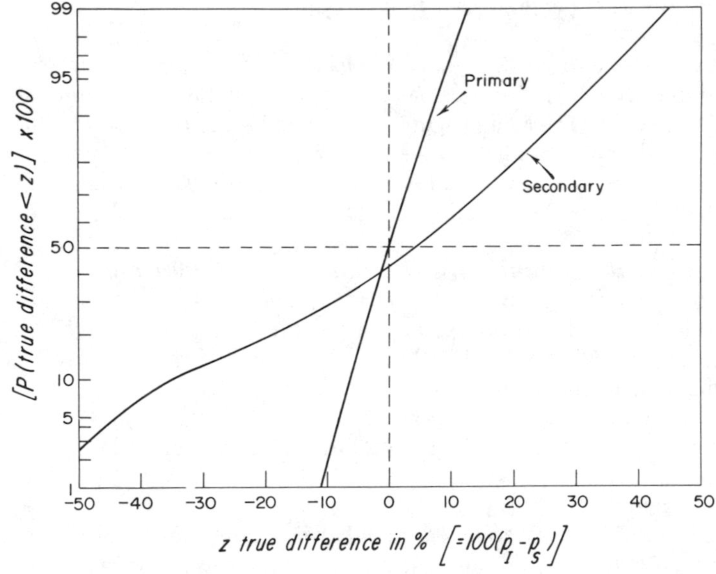

Figure 9–4. Empirically estimated cumulative distribution of improvements (innovation minus standard) as a difference in proportions. Normal Probability Paper.

distributions were exactly normal, the curves would appear as straight lines in Figure 9-4.

By plotting the curves on normal probability paper as shown in Figure 9-4, we find the straight line of the primary therapies meaning that their distribution of true differences is estimated to be approximately normal. But for the secondary therapies, the estimated distribution departs from normality.

By picking a gain in percentage, z, and reading an ordinate on the appropriate curve, one can estimate the probability of a new therapy producing a gain as small as or smaller than the chosen value.

For examples we have:

a. For primary therapies the probability (i) of a loss of 10% or more in survival is about 0.02; (ii) of a 0% loss or more is about 0.48; (iii) of a 10% gain or less is about 0.96—which means that the probability of a 10% gain or more is about 0.04. We regard this as a better estimate than that given in Section IIIB-2 (.13), because we prefer the method rather than because we prefer the answer.
b. For secondary therapies, the probability (i) of a loss of 10% or more in a specially chosen complication is estimated as 0.28; (ii) of a 0% loss or worse, 0.43; (iii) of a 10% gain or less, 0.62—implying that a 10% gain or more has an estimated probability of 0.38, which compares with 0.32 obtained in Section IIIB-2.

Table 9-3 gives details on both sets of estimates as, of course, do Figures 9-3 and 9-4. And so other estimates can be obtained from the table and these figures.

Discussion. This technique leans on Bayesian ideas, which require us to know the true distribution of the data given the true difference. Here the normal is a good approximation, provided the groups being compared are not too small.

Table 9-3. Estimated probability of the true difference in percentage, Z, being less than a given value, z, for comparisons of primary and of secondary therapies.

Primary		*Secondary*			
z	$P(Z < z)$	z	$P(Z < z)$	z	$P(Z < z)$
-15	0.001	-50	0.025	5	0.526
-12.5	0.004	-45	0.045	10	0.622
-10	0.018	-40	0.072	15	0.724
-7.5	0.060	-35	0.099	20	0.812
-5	0.154	-30	0.127	25	0.874
-2.5	0.302	-25	0.158	30	0.920
0	0.482	-20	0.193	35	0.953
2.5	0.664	-15	0.232	40	0.976
5	0.812	-10	0.279	45	0.990
7.5	0.909	-5	0.340	50	0.996
10	0.963	0	0.427		
12.5	0.987				
15	0.997				

This size assumption is satisfied because of the requirement of at least 10 patients before selecting a paper as part of our sample. In addition, for a Bayesian approach, one needs an assumption about the shape of the true distribution of true differences. Again, we take that as normal and carry out further calculations obeying this assumption. However, we regard this assumption as a sort of "smoothing device." Other shapes could be used. Lastly, we let the data decide on the form of the final estimate of the distribution of true differences, only somewhat constrained by the assumptions of normality in the two previous steps.

It would require a substantial study to decide whether the simple approach (Appendix 9-II) used earlier with a firmly assumed normal approximation applied at the end, or this approach (Appendix 9-III) with a release from the normal at the end, is more likely to be closer to the truth. We suppose, until such a study is done, that the approach presented in Appendix 9-III is the better. The reader should understand that we are using new statistical theory and that the methods presented merit further study.

IIIB-4. Possible Biases

Although we do not have a probability sample of the published papers, the sample is objectively chosen, and a rather good one for reflecting the sorts of differences analyzed here. What is less clear is how good a sample it is of therapeutic surgical research on patients generally during this period. First it is likely, and those we have talked with agree, that published papers are reports on better work on the average than that in unpublished research. Second, research that turns out well, our discussants agree, is more likely to be published. This reasoning suggests that the mass of unpublished research, insofar as it might produce measures comparable to those described in this paper, would have a lower average performance for innovations compared with standards than those in our sample. We suppose, then, that the innovations assessed by randomized clinical trials and reported in the surgical literature, and here, are biased upwards—that is, they present a more promising picture for innovation than if all innovations were subjected to randomized clinical trials. No doubt some innovations are so unsatisfactory that they are abandoned, along with whatever trials were initiated on them (47). These conjectures suggest that if one were to consider adjusting the distributions reported just above to report on all surgical innovations versus standards the mean of the distribution would be lower and the standard deviation would probably be larger to allow for more frequent large negative differences. We have no grounds other than speculation for the amount of such changes.

Prostate Study

As already mentioned in Section IIIA-1, we did not include the results of one paper in the preceding analysis. This paper (8) reported on two large studies of cancer of the prostate (described in the Brief Summary of Paper #8).

In the first study separate experiments were undertaken on patients with each of four stages of cancer of the prostate. Two therapies were compared in the Stage I and II patients, while four were compared in the two more advanced stages. This gave 14 comparisons between various pairs of 6 different treatments. In one group one treatment was much preferred to the other, while in another group of patients another therapy was less well liked than the other three tested in that group. All other comparisons were essentially equal.

In the second study three doses of estrogen and a placebo were tried in patients in Stages III and IV. The middle dose was preferred, but the main conclusion of the authors was that "treatment may be withheld until it is required for relief of symptoms or because of progression of the disease."

To summarize these prostatic cancer findings in the context of our findings for the other studies: fewer comparisons showed a preference for one therapy over another than we found in Section IIIA-1. It is not clear how to assign these treatments to *I* and *S*, but in any way that this might be done a plot of the results comparable to Figure 9-1 would show most of the points to be very close to the diagonal line.

If the cancer of the prostate study could have been analyzed using the methods of Sections IIIB-2 and IIIB-3, the results might have suggested that the data were consistent with a zero mean and a zero standard deviation. That is, we might not be able to reject the hypothesis of no differential benefit for any of the treatments in this study. Our caution in saying this derives again from the issue of orienting the *I* vs *S* differences and, since in this instance this is not clear, it is hard to tell what is appropriate. All told, the estimated distribution for primary studies would have a mean near zero and a smaller standard deviation if these studies were included.

IIIC. Perspectives on Gains from Innovations

In a recent review of randomized trials used in evaluating social programs (Gilbert, Light, and Mosteller, 1975), the authors concluded that many new programs do not work and the effects of those that do are usually small. In contrast to these findings in the area of social innovations, this review of innovations in surgery and anesthesia provides evidence for a more optimistic view of their rate of progress. Almost half of the innovations reported in this series of controlled trials were of at least some benefit, and a fair number of these show substantial effects. Thus, the analyses suggest that 4 out of 10 innovations in secondary therapy produce a reduction in complication rates of 10% or more, while 2 or 3 out of 10 innovations in primary therapy produce a 5% or greater increase in survival. These estimates are for the distribution of the underlying true effects of the innovations. In a sense these results describe the clinical judgment that chooses those innovations as promising enough to test. If innovations were successful in a high proportion of trials, it would suggest that new therapies were being delayed until we were absolutely sure of their success, while if almost none were it would suggest a scarcity of new ideas in the field. Thus, these distributions also describe research productivity and its effects on the development of better clinical care.

Another view is that this research process tries to reject all the innovations that produce losses and to keep the ones with gains. If this were done, then the median gain retained for the primary therapies would be about 4%, and that for the secondary therapies would be about 15%. Of course, this would be an idealized state, for we cannot hope to weed out *all* the losses and detect *all* the gains. But it gives an estimated upper limit to what could be accomplished.

This discussion applies only to those innovations in care that are evaluated by using the kinds of trial that we have examined in our sample. Thus, we are not in a position to discuss the distribution of the changes in therapy that are instituted without controlled trials. We are also not in a position to appreciate the role that laboratory and other basic research have played in the development of the kinds of new therapies that are evaluated through controlled clinical trials.

We emphasize further that to say that a proportion of new innovations is of substantial benefit does not serve to identify which they are. Reducing a death rate from 35% to 25% is an important improvement in patient care, but this does not mean that it will be easily identified in the everyday setting of clinical practice. Indeed, statistical theory shows that a well-run randomized controlled trial would need 223 patients in each group to be 75% confident of detecting such a difference at the one-sided 5% level of significance. Without a large formal trial, the uncontrolled effects of patient selection, of adjuvant therapies, and of other factors make the detection of such differences even more difficult.

IV. INCIDENTAL FINDINGS: REPORTING ON RANDOMIZATION AND INFORMED CONSENT

In reviewing the 36 randomized trials, we observed some problems both in the execution and reporting of the randomization which we discuss in Section IVA. Problems of ethics and informed consent loom large in clinical trials, and we describe in Section IVB the reports we found in the 107 studies.

IVA. Randomization and Its Reporting

In the bibliographic work, we have observed a substantial and potentially troublesome range both in methods of randomizing treatments in clinical trials and in care in reporting these methods. Although randomization has several purposes, protecting the investigation from unintended selectivity, that is, bias, stands at the top of the list. Often investigators so briefly report how they randomized that the reader cannot tell what they did.

Other investigators use methods that can readily lead to biases. When someone associated with the trial can personally choose who gets what treatment, he or she may do so, and thereby wreck the protection provided by randomization (for a classical example see Student, 1931). Knowing what treatment the next patient will get may influence the decision about eligibility and thus create bias. All schemes designed to balance cases partake of this weakness. (Eligibility should be decided separately from and prior to the randomization to treatment.) Further, when investigators use the method of alternate cases to assign patients to either of two treatments, they risk the possibility that two or more candidates appear essentially simultaneously and that some preferences or choices of the person assigning the treatment will affect the trial. If that person prefers, for example, women or young people for treatment A, more of them will get it. Sometimes we can readily believe that patients present themselves in a nearly random order and, were there no picking and choosing, the idea of using this method to assign treatments could work. But bunching will likely arise, and someone will likely influence the assignments, however unwittingly.

For example, one research study, not among the sampled papers, using "alternate assignments" wound up with about 150 in one group and 250 in the other, instead of numbers at most one apart. When a discussant of that paper complained of this, the investigator explained that it was a busy clinic and that mistakes were bound to be made, but that the woman who made the assignments knew nothing of medicine and, by implication, could not have biased the trial. Maybe not. But now each reader must weigh this aspect of the clinical trial instead of concentrating on the medical problems of the study.

Another way to randomize that lets the calendar introduce possible biases uses birth dates, say odd and even, to assign treatments. Someone knowing the birth date and the associated treatment can decide that the person is not eligible for the study and thus introduce a selection effect. The same objection applies to patients' file numbers in prospective studies (though not in retrospective studies). Let us note that the objection here is not to rules that disallow entrance into the study. Exclusion rules are often essential, but these rules should be insulated from the choice of treatment once one has established the patient's eligibility, though, of course, suitable safeguards must be used.

Although informal methods of randomization can be used effectively they are subject to abuse, such as "Let's flip again since we have already had four heads in a row." Informal methods such as coin-tossing are usually difficult to document so that they can be checked if questions arise later—as they do with astonishing regularity. The use of a published table of random digits makes it easy to keep a written record of which numbers were chosen and how the numbers were used to make the assignments.

As randomizing devices, marked slips of paper in envelopes sound good. But sometimes the envelopes are not opaque, especially when held against a bright light as they often are, and the assigner can shuffle envelopes, knowing the properties of the participant and the possible treatments.

By 1976 tables of random numbers were widely available and inexpensive to use (Fisher and Yates, 1963; Rand Corp, 1955). Even tables of random orders (random permutations) are fairly widely available (Moses and Oakford, 1963; Fisher and Yates, 1963; Cochran and Cox, 1968). No difficulty should arise, then, in finding excellent random numbers.

Although such damage to randomization may seem far-fetched, many find it wise to assume that things that can go wrong in an investigation are likely to. When the randomizing mechanism leaks, the trial's *guarantee* of lack of bias runs down the drain. And then what could have been firm becomes an added uncertainty for our conclusions. Of course, randomization alone cannot guarantee that we have done a proper experiment or will get correct answers or inferences, but it can help.

These remarks suggest that when expensive and delicate studies such as randomized clinical trials are carried out, the nuts and bolts, like the steps of randomization and the degree of blindness, need tightening and inspection, and that when the investigator carries out such quality control measures, they deserve careful reporting in much more than a phrase. Care here offers one indicator of the quality of the investigation. When such care has not been reported, some readers may uncharitably assume that it has not been taken.

IVB. References to Ethical Issues

Based upon the 107 sampled papers, we note that during the period 1964–72 discussions of ethics and informed consent were not common in research articles. The low frequency need not indicate that consent was not obtained or that ethics were not carefully considered in these investigations. It does mean that during this period investigators did not routinely take these matters up in the text of a research paper. We find ethics or informed consent mentioned in 13 papers. (See Appendix 9-VI.)

Most discussions of ethics or informed consent were associated with randomized trials which included about one-third of the studies. In reading through the papers, we occasionally noted what seemed to be a need for investigators of series to report on ethical problems such as when the patient may undergo additional tests beyond those required for the therapy. Perhaps their authors have obtained consent and reported less often.

Most references to ethics or informed consent are very short, often merely allusions or a word or two in a sentence or even an inference to be drawn from what was said. We may have missed a remark or two of this kind, although the papers were given a special reading with exactly this question in mind.

V. SUMMARY OF FINDINGS

In our selection of 107 research papers in surgery that involved patients, 36, about one-third, were based at least in part on randomized trials (with at least 10 patients in each of at least two treatment groups) while an additional 15 papers, about one-seventh, primarily reported less well-controlled trials (11 of these could be used in our comparative work of Table 9-2). The remaining 56 papers reported findings that depended upon a series of patients without any well-defined comparison group as part of the same study.

In reviewing those papers where a randomized trial compared an innovative therapy to a standard, the new treatment was found to be preferable by the authors of the original investigation, as we interpret their words and tables, in almost half of the papers. In a few cases the standard was "no treatment." (See Appendix 9-I.)

Quantitatively, when tested by randomized clinical trials, about 14% of innovations worked much better than the standard, and in about 30% more the innovation was regarded as successful. In about 44% of the comparisons the standard was somewhat preferred, and highly preferred in an additional 11%. Innovations among primary therapies (those intended to cure the patient's disease) were less often highly preferred than innovations in secondary therapies (those intended to reduce complications and speed recovery).

Figures 9-3 and 9-4 show the estimated distribution of gains obtained when consideration is given to the sample sizes of the individual studies. In this analysis primary therapies were assessed for percentage improvement in survival, secondary therapies for percentage of patients free of specific complications.

Continuing with Figure 9-4, innovative primary therapies showed gains of 0% or more in survival in about half the comparisons, and of 10% or more in about one-tenth of the comparisons. The innovative secondary comparisons got estimated gains of as much as 5% in reduction of complications about half the time, of as much as 20% about one-fifth of the time, and gains of as much as 30% for one-twentieth of the comparisons.

These findings give us an idea of the sorts of gains that can be made from selecting the better of pairs of therapies that are carefully tested. The left sides of the curves warn us also that innovations may lose rather than gain, and so evaluation is needed. For example, losses of as much as 20% in secondary therapies could occur about one-fifth of the time. These curves emphasize the size and frequency of the losses as well as the gains. Thus, as physicians well know, one cannot assume in advance that a new treatment is an improvement over an old one, even when it looks promising enough to warrant a clinical trial.

These distributions show that some innovations provide important gains for the clinical care of patients. In order to capitalize reliably on these better therapies, they must of course, be correctly identified through clinical trials. In the design of such trials, one must appreciate that what may constitute an important gain in clinical practice, such as reducing a death rate by 5%, is not a large effect from the numerical viewpoint and may not be large enough to be easily identified. Indeed, the distributions we have derived indicate that important yet hard-to-detect differences occur for most of the innovations in our sampled population.

Since relatively small, though important, numerical gains or losses are to be expected from most innovations, clinical trials must regularly be designed to detect these differences accurately and reliably. When a systematic trial of a new therapy is being considered initially, it is frequently subject to great optimism. The advocate for a new therapy may believe, for a number of specific reasons, that it will prove to be greatly superior to the standard and, indeed, preliminary informal experience may seem to provide good evidence for this. As our data show, this initial optimism though frequently warranted is often not justified.

More care in actual randomization of patients to treatments is required because looseness here sacrifices the protection the method gives. Further, more care in describing the randomization methods is required to assure readers that effective procedures have been used.

Discussions of the ethical issues surrounding the trials reported in these papers were infrequent and brief. This does not necessarily reflect either a lack of propriety or a lack of concern for these issues, but rather the custom in publications during the reporting period.

These papers taken as a group provide an optimistic picture of progress in surgery and anesthesia. This progress depends on a judicious combination of continued development of new therapeutic ideas and their evaluation by good-sized, unbiased clinical trials.

Acknowledgments

Several individuals and organizations have helped us complete this paper. We have had advice and helpful suggestions from many scholars, among them Benjamin A. Barnes, M.D., John P. Bunker, M.D., Garry Fitzpatrick, M.D., Rebecca Gilbert, Nan Laird, Walter S. Kerr, M.D., John Lamberti, M.D., Erich L. Lehmann, Lillian Miao, Eldred D. Mundth, M.D., Juliet P. Shaffer, George Prout, M.D., John Raker, M.D., Grant V. Rodkey, M.D., C.A. Wang, M.D.–all of whom have clarified and lengthened the paper considerably.

In getting and organizing the sample of MEDLARS papers, we have had the advice and support of Katherine Binderup at the Francis A. Countway Library of Medicine, Charlotte Kenton of the National Library of Medicine, and Mary B. Ettling.

In developing the statistical material, checking the work, and doing the computing, we have had help from Anne Bigelow, Gale Mosteller, Julie Norton, Lester Pennelly, and Keith Soper.

The manuscript has been prepared by Teresa Cunningham, Holly Grano, Marjorie Olson, and Karin Young.

Bradley Efron and Carl Morris have generously advised us on the analysis in Section IIIC and Appendix 9-III.

Our thanks are particularly owing to the authors of the original research papers and their editors. Without their contributions this study would not have been possible.

We have further benefited from participation in the Harvard University Faculty Seminar in Health and Medical Practices, 1973-75, facilitated by the Edna McConnell Clark Foundation. We have had helpful discussions with seminars in Statistics and Public Policy at the University of California at Berkeley and in Statistics at California State University at Hayward. Frederick Mosteller held a Miller Research Professorship at the University of California at Berkeley during much of the preparation of the manuscript.

References

Chalmers TC, Block JB, Lee S: Controlled studies in clinical cancer research. N Engl J Med 287:75, 1972

Cochran WG, Cox GM: Experimental Designs. Second edition. New York, John Wiley and Sons, Inc., 1968

Cummings MM: Your National Library of Medicine. JAMA 223:1359, 1975

Day M: Computer-based retrieval services of the National Library of Medicine. Fed Proc 33:1717, 1974

Dixon WJ, Massey FJ, Jr: Introduction to Statistical Analysis. New York, McGraw-Hill Book Company, Inc., 1951, p. 55

Efron B, Morris C: Data analysis using Stein's estimator and its generalizations. Santa Monica, California, Rand Corporation R-1394-OED, March 1974

Efron B, Morris C: Stein's estimation rule and its competitors: an empirical Bayes approach. J Am Stat Assoc 68:117, 1973a
Efron B, Morris C: Combining possibly related estimation problems. J R Stat Soc B 35:379, 1973b (with discussion pp 403ff)
Fisher RA, Yates F: Statistical Tables for Biological, Agricultural and Medical Research. Sixth edition. New York, Hafner Publishing Co., Inc., 1963
Gilbert JP, Light RJ, Mosteller F: Assessing social innovations: an empirical base for policy. Evaluation and Experiment: Some Critical Issues in Assessing Social Programs. Edited by CA Bennett and AA Lumsdaine. New York, Academic Press, 1975
Grace ND, Muench H, Chalmers TC: The present status of shunts for portal hypertension in cirrhosis. Gastroenterology 50:684, 1966
Mawson SR, Adlington P, Evans M: A controlled study evaluation of adeno-tonsillectomy in children. J Laryngology 81:777, 1967
Moses LE, Oakford RV: Tables of Random Permutations. California, Stanford University Press, 1963
Rand Corporation: A Million Random Digits with 100,000 Normal Deviates. New York, The Free Press, 1955
Student: The Lanarkshire milk experiment. Biometrika 23:398, 1931
Walsh RJ (ed): Socioeconomic issues of health. Am Med Assoc, Center for Health Services Research and Development, 1972

APPENDIX 9-I. BRIEF SUMMARIES

(The numbers and abbreviations at the close of the descriptions given in this Appendix refer again to the innovative and standard comparison.)

$I >> S$ Innovation highly preferred to standard
$I > S$ Innovation preferred to standard
$S > I$ Standard preferred to innovation
$S >> I$ Standard highly preferred to innovation
$I = S$ Standard and innovation perform about equally well

When more than one standard or innovation is compared, we use subscripts, S_1, S_2, I_1, I_2.

Primary Therapies (Randomized Clinical Trials)

Cancer of the lung (69/II-510)*
Innovation: radiotherapy in addition to surgery
Standard: surgery
Outcome: In treating cancer of the bronchus, radiotherapy "(*I*) gave . . . in terms of survival, a somewhat better result than surgery (*S*) . . . [among patients] judged to be operable."
Gain: 199 to 284 days of survival
R: $I > S$

*Reference numbers are given two ways: first to the reference number as used in the list in Appendix 9-V, then by the code number used for the paper during the work.

Cancer of the lung (23/XI–505)
Innovation: irradiation and chemotherapy with vinblastine
Standard: irradiation alone
Outcome: In lung cancer when irradiation and vinblastine chemotherapy (I) were compared with irradiation alone (S) "Survival up to 2 years gave no evidence of an improvement [owing to the dual treatment] and neither did measurement of such factors as tumor size and symptoms."
Gain: 1.4% in survival
R: $I = S$ (a loss for innovation)

Kidney transplantation (99/VIII–1101)
Innovation: treatment of kidney recipients with antithymocyte globulin (HATG)
Standard: no treatment with antithymocyte globulin
Outcome: In renal transplant recipients antithymocyte globulin (I) [HATG] "survival despite incompatibility is an exception to the general experience and is approximately 15% to 25% higher than with incompatible intrafamilial transplants. . . . There was no difference in transplant survival of cadaveric grafts whether or not HATG was administered." But HATG-treated cadaveric grafts produced fewer rejection and other episodes.
Gain: 15% to 25% fewer kidney transplant failures
R: $I > S$

Cancer of the prostate (8/I–6)

Study 1
Standard 1: estrogen therapy (5 mgm diethylstilbesterol)
Standard 2: surgery (radical prostatectomy)
Standard 3: surgery in addition to estrogen therapy
Standard 4: castration (orchiectomy)
Standard 5: castration in addition to estrogen therapy
Placebo: (P)
Outcome: This study included comparisons of treatments in each of four stages of the disease. The treatments were placebo (P), estrogen (S_1), radical prostectomy (S_2), radical prostectomy and estrogen (S_3), orchiectomy (S_4), and orchiectomy plus estrogen (S_5).
In Stage I: $S_2 >> S_3$
In Stage II: $S_2 = S_3$
In Stage III: $P = S_1 = S_4 > S_5$ (possibly $>$ is $>>$)
In Stage IV: $P = S_1 = S_4 = S_5$
The 5 DES estrogen (S_1) "revealed an unsuspected toxicity" and so a dosage study, Study 2, was undertaken.

Study 2
Innovation: estrogen therapy 1 mgm diethylstilbesterol
Standard: estrogen therapy, 5 mgm diethylstilbesterol
Outcome: A dose level of 1 mgm diethylstilbesterol (I) is believed as effective as 5 mgm diethylstilbesterol (S_1), and the authors recommend that it be delayed until patient's symptoms require relief.
Gain: (See Table 2, Appendix 9–IV)
R: $I > S$
(Part of Study 2 is included in Table 9–1; Study 1 is not.)

Cirrhosis of the liver (19/I–317)
Innovation: prednisone treatment
Standard: no treatment with prednisone
Outcome: In cirrhosis patients treated with (*I*) or without (*S*) prednisone "the death rates were the same in both groups, but when female patients without ascites were considered alone, the death rate of prednisone-treated patients was significantly decreased. By contrast in patients with ascites prednisone seemed to increase the death rate." (Today prednisone is ordinarily used to improve quality of life rather than survival.)
Gain: 0% in survival
R: $I = S$ (a success for *I*, since prednisone may be used without adverse affects on survival) (This paper presents some difficulties in classification because not only does it seem to lie on the borderline between surgery and medicine, but also on the borderline between primary and secondary therapies.)

Advanced cirrhosis of the liver with esophageal varices (9/II–511)
Innovation: surgery: prophylactic portacaval shunt
Standard: medical treatment, without surgery
Outcome: "In this type of patient from the lower socioeconomic group with poor nutritional habits, prophylactic portacaval shunt (*I*) does not exert a beneficial effect upon survival."
Gain: –4% in survival (not statistically significant)
R: $I = S$ (a loss for innovation)

Advanced cirrhosis of the liver with esophageal varices (17/XI–2007)
Innovation: surgery: prophylactic shunt
Standard: medical treatment
Outcome: The medical control group (*S*), had a better survival rate and fewer days in hospital than the prophylactic portacaval shunt group (*I*), even though the operative mortality was low.
Gain: Surgery group had 68% mortality vs 50% for medical treatment.
R: $S > I$

Advanced cirrhosis of the liver with esophageal varices (68/XI–1910)
Innovation: surgery: therapeutic portacaval shunt
Standard: medical treatment, without surgery
Outcome: ". . . preliminary data suggest the superiority of surgical [therapeutic portacaval shunt (*I*)] over medical treatment (*S*)." Test for acute hyaline necrosis is also proposed as a basis for excluding patients with unfavorable operative prognosis.
Gains: The estimated 3-year survivals are 70% (*I*) vs 35% (*S*).
R: $I \gg S$

Duodenal ulcer (51/II–509)
Innovation: selective vagotomy (at surgery cutting only those fibers of the vagus nerves supplying the distal stomach)
Standard: truncal vagotomy (cutting the vagus nerves as they enter the abdomen)

Outcome: "The main reason for adopting selective vagotomy has been the hope that diarrhea . . . would be eliminated. . . . There was no significant difference in the incidence of diarrhea one year after operation."
Gain: There were 6% fewer cases of severe diarrhea after the innovative operation, selective vagotomy (not statistically significant).
R: $I = S$ (a loss for I, as selective vagotomy is a longer, technically more difficult operation)

Duodenal ulcer (47/IV–708)
Innovation 1: surgery: vagotomy with pyloroplasty
Innovation 2: surgery: vagotomy with hemigastrectomy
Innovation 3: surgery: segmental gastric resection
Outcome: In a 3- to 6-year follow-up of three types of ulcer surgery, segmental gastric resection (I_3) gave such poor results—47% unsatisfactory on Visick grading—that it was abandoned. Vagotomy with pyloroplasty (I_1) is regarded as a safe operation, though vagotomy with hemigastrectomy (I_2) had better performance in survivors, no unsatisfactory Visicks compared with 9% in vagotomy with pyloroplasty.
Gain: I_1: 9% unsatisfactory Visick score
I_2: 0% unsatisfactory Visick score
I_3: 47% unsatisfactory Visick score
R: $I_1 = I_2 >> I_3$

Chronic duodenal ulcer (22/II–506)
Innovation: surgery: vagotomy with gastrojejunostomy
Standard: surgery: partial gastrectomy
Outcome: In an 8-year follow-up comparing "vagotomy with gastrojejunostomy (I) and partial gastrectomy (S) for chronic duodenal ulcer . . . the differences are small but favor vagotomy."
Gain: symptomatic score less by 24% for (I)
R: $I > S$

Duodenal ulcer (45/VI–1814)
Innovation: surgery: vagotomy with hemigastrectomy
Standard: surgery: vagotomy with pyloroplasty
Outcome: In a 2- to 10-year follow-up study, the overall results for vagotomy and pyloroplasty (S) vs vagotomy and hemigastrectomy (I) are said not to be very great.
Gain: the average number of unfavorable symptoms for (S) is 0.78 and that for (I) 1.34, but suggestively larger recurrence for (S).
R: $I = S$ (a success for I since in occasional cases one operation may be technically easier than the other)

Cancer of the head and neck (55/VII–1904)
Innovation: X-ray therapy followed by surgery
Standard: surgery alone
Outcome: Comparing preoperative irradiation (I) with surgery alone (S) for head and neck cancer, "no benefit . . . can be demonstrated in the irradiated group." Survival curves are similar, but if forced to choose, the irradiated group looks the least bit better and they have a slightly lower local recurrence rate.

Gain: no gain
R: $I = S$ (a loss for I)

Advanced cirrhosis of the liver without esophageal varices (82/V–1705)
Innovation: surgery: prophylactic portacaval shunt
Standard: medical treatment, without surgery
Outcome: "In the management of cirrhosis of the alcoholic in lower socioeconomic groups the prophylactic portacaval shunt should be abandoned."
Gain: The survival curve is slightly lower for surgery (I) than medical treatment (S), but they are very close.
R: $I = S$ (a loss for innovation)

Cancer of the breast (107/VIII–721)
Innovation 1: radical mastectomy with internal mammary lymph node dissection
Innovation 2: radical mastectomy with intra-arterial chemotherapy
Standard: radical mastectomy
Outcome: Five-year survival rates from three breast cancer operations, radical mastectomy (S), radical mastectomy with internal mammary node dissection (I_1), and radical mastectomy with intra-arterial chemotherapy (I_2) are all comparable (especially after adjusting for mix of positive and negative nodes).
Gain: 7%, 6% in survival (not statistically significant)
R: $S = I_1 = I_2$ (favorable to standard radical mastectomy since it is simpler)

Advanced cancer of breast (93/II–502)
Innovation: destruction of pituitary by implantation of radioactive yttrium-90 early in course of disease
Standard: standard palliation measures, not involving early pituitary suppression
Outcome: Early pituitary implantation of yttrium-90 (I) for control of advanced breast cancer turned out not to be beneficial and may be harmful, especially in cases with only local recurrence where 2-year survival went down from 50% to 20%.
Gain: 2-year survival 20% (I) vs 50% (S) in cases with only local recurrence
R: $S > I$

Cancer of the colon and rectum (29/II–607)
Innovation: chemotherapy with triethylenethiophosphoramide in addition to standard surgery
Standard: surgery without chemotherapy
Outcome: In a 5-year follow-up of surgery (S) for cancer of the colon and rectum, triethylenethiophosphoramide (I) did not improve and possibly reduced survival.
Gain: Innovation *reduced* survival 5% or 6%.
R: $S > I$

Large bowel surgery (38/II–507)
Innovation: everting suture technique for colon anastomoses
Standard: inverting suture technique for colon anastomoses
Outcome: "These experiences . . . provide a clear condemnation of the use of an everting technique of suture in the large intestine in clinical practice."

Gain: (*I*) produced 16% more wound infections and 34% more fecal fistulation.
R: $S >> I$

More Complicated Findings

Duodenal ulcer (49/II–508)
Innovation: surgery: vagotomy and antrectomy
Standard: surgery: vagotomy and drainage
Outcome: ". . . antrectomy (*I*) is superior to vagotomy and drainage (*S*) . . . for elective treatment for duodenal ulcer in the majority of patients because of its lower recurrence rate without . . . increased morbidity or mortality." If the risk with antrectomy seemed high, then the higher recurrence rate of vagotomy and drainage was regarded as acceptable, in fact 10 patients randomized to antrectomy were moved to the other operation.
Gains: recurrence rate 8% (*I*) vs 0% for (*S*)
R: $I > S$ (but . . .) (included in Table 9–1)

Finding Does Not Fit the Pattern Above

Aorto-iliac arteriosclerosis (35/VI–1815)
Standard 1: surgery: aortoileofemoral thromboendarterectomy
Standard 2: surgery: aortofemoral bypass graft
Outcome: Both aortoileofemoral thromboendarterectomy (TEA) (S_1) and bypass graft (BPG) (S_2) were operations used for aortoiliac arteriosclerosis. Too early to tell which operation works better, but TEA is harder to do and probably not wise to use in a teaching situation, the authors say.
R: S_1 ? S_2 (? means relationship unclear)

Secondary Therapies (Randomized Clinical Trials)

Postoperative venous thrombosis (34/X–1302)
Innovation: heparin treatment
Standard: no heparin treatment
Outcome: "The results of this study confirm that small doses of heparin (*I*) given before and after elective surgery significantly reduce the postoperative frequency of venous thrombosis." It also appeared effective for emergency operations and for high-risk medical patients.
Gain: thrombosis 2% (*I*) vs 16% (*S*)
R: $I >> S$

Large bowel surgery (73/II–606)
Innovation: treating the abdominal wound with topical ampicillin at surgery
Standard: no topical ampicillin treatment
Outcome: ". . . topical powdered ampicillin (*I*) in the main abdominal wound was associated with a significant reduction in wound sepsis. No side effects were noted."
Gain: wound sepsis reduced about 38%
R: $I >> S$

Large bowel surgery (74/I–1)
Innovation: treatment with neomycin and erythromycin
Standard: no neomycin-erythromycin treatment
Outcome: After using neomycin-erythromycin (N-E) (I) in colon surgery in addition to an oral antibiotic, the authors recommend adequate preoperative mechanical preparation and conclude (presumably from the literature) that the addition of routine systemic antibiotics appears to be an unwarranted and unrewarding measure. In the experiment, ". . . three of ten who received the mechanical preparation alone developed wound sepsis. . . There were no wound complications in the patients who received the combination of neomycin-erythromycin base." Although the study is small, adding N-E appropriately looks helpful.
Gain: (S) associated with 30% wound infection rate
R: $I > S$

Infection after radical surgery for ulcerative colitis and Crohn's Disease of the large bowel (3/I–407)
Innovation: prophylactic colomycin in addition to standard preoperative treatment
Standard: usual regimen of mechanical preparation of bowel and oral sulfonamides without colomycin
Outcome: In bowel preparation, "The addition of colomycin (I) to the standard regime (S) of mechanical preparation and sulphonamides conferred no benefit. . . ."
Gain: local complications reduced about 20%; general complications up about 9%
R: $I = S$ (a disappointment for I)

Gastric decompression after vagotomy for ulcer (70/XI–2002)
Innovation: no tube placed in stomach for decompression
Standard 1: gastrostomy tube decompression
Standard 2: nasogastric tube decompression
Outcome: "Significantly fewer patients with no decompression developed respiratory infections postoperatively." The nasogastric tube was more often reported as "distressing" (70%) than the gastrostomy tube (18%), but no corresponding discomfort report is available for patients with no tube (perhaps it is hard to ask the questions).
Gain: innovation associated with about 50% fewer chest infections.
R: $I >> S_1 >> S_2$

Traumatic liver injuries (57/III–704)
Innovation 1: cholecystostomy plus standard drainage
Innovation 2: choledochostomy plus standard drainage
Standard: standard surgical drainage of injured area
Outcome: Results for biliary drainage in hepatic trauma suggest that standard drainage only (S) is both simpler and at least as good as standard drainage plus cholecystostomy (I_1), and apparently better than standard drainage plus choledochostomy (I_2) at least for small wounds–(study for large wounds still under way).
Gain: choledochostomy (I_2) associated with about 50% more complications
R: $S > I_1 >> I_2$

Infection after cardiovascular surgery (39/I–301)
Innovation 1: prophylactic penicillin and streptomycin
Innovation 2: prophylactic oxacillin
Standard: placebo, no prophylactic antibiotic
Outcome: In a study of prophylactic antibiotics and heart surgery, placebo (P), penicillin-streptomycin (I_1), or oxacillin (I_2) was administered. The antibiotics had about equal percentages of wound infections. (The placebo was terminated halfway through.)
Gain: I_1 vs P, 6% reduction; I_2 vs P, 7% reduction
R: $I_1 = I_2$? P (? means relation poorly determined though somewhat unfavorable to P)

Infection after cardiac surgery (18/X–1519)
Innovation: prophylactic cephalothin in multiple doses
Standard: single prophylactic dose of cephalothin
Outcome: Using prophylactic antibiotics [cephalothin in multiple (I) vs single doses (S)] led to the conclusion that "There were no significant differences between the two groups in major and minor infections, deaths, or floral changes."
Gain: 5% reduction (not statistically significant)
R: $I = S$ (a disappointment for I)

Anesthesia for open-heart surgery (15/IV–1008)
Innovation: morphine in large doses as principal anesthetic agent
Standard: halothane anesthesia
Outcome: "There appeared to be hemodynamic differences between the agents, but neither mortality rates nor durations of hospital stay nor postoperative stay in the intensive care unit demonstrated a clear-cut advantage of either morphine or halothane for anesthesia during cardiac-valve operations."
Gains: hypertension percentages nearly equal; deaths unclear, but most (7 for 9) follow second-time operations.
R: $I = S$ (a success for I as a wider selection of anesthetic agents is now available)

Infection after appendectomy (24/II–503)
Innovation: prophylaxis with 0.5% chlorhexidine
Standard: no prophylaxis with chlorhexidine
Outcome: "In a controlled blind trial the instillation of 0.5 percent chlorhexidine (I) into the (contaminated) wound at gridiron appendicectomy has been found to be ineffective in preventing subsequent wound sepsis or in reducing hospital stay."
Gain: no gain
R: $I = S$ (a failure for I)

Infection after appendectomy (58/III–706)
Innovation 1: appendectomy plus surgical drainage
Innovation 2: appendectomy plus prophylactic antibiotics–ampicillin or tetracycline
Standard: appendectomy without drainage or antibiotics
Outcome: After appendectomy, "Drainage (I_1) *increased* the number of days of postoperative fever significantly ($p < .01$) in patients with turbid peritoneal fluid and interfered with wound healing in all groups of patients. . . . Antibiotics (I_2) ($p < 0.05$) significantly *reduced* the number of days of post-

operative fever in patients with perforated appendices without drainage." Antibiotics prevented intraperitoneal difficulties "but had no effect on wound healing."

Gain: almost 50% fewer days of postoperative fever in antibiotic group, 67% more days of fever in drainage group, than in a standard treatment group

R: $I_2 > S >> I_1$

Oxygen toxicity after open-heart surgery (88/IV-904)

Innovation: 100% oxygen after open-heart surgery

Standard: the minimal inspired oxygen concentration required to keep the arterial oxygen normal

Outcome: In cardiac patients (at least) "Fear of pulmonary oxygen toxicity should not prevent use of elevated inspired oxygen concentrations (*I*) in critically ill patients requiring artificial ventilation."

Gain: none

R: $I = S$ (a success for *I*)

Urine function after anesthesia (67/I-11)

Innovation: methoxyflurane anesthesia

Standard: halothane anesthesia

Outcome: "There was significant rise in the mean serum creatinine level and fall in the mean urine osmolality among patients who received methoxyflurane (*I*). No such changes were seen in those given halothane (*S*). These data suggest an effect of methoxyflurane on renal function, even when the severe symptomatic syndrome previously described does not occur."

Gain: serum creatinine: + 25% (*I*) +6% (*S*)
urine osmolality: - 24% (*I*) 0% (*S*)

R: $S > I$

Renal function after anesthesia (63/I-406)

Innovation: methoxyflurane anesthesia

Standard: halothane anesthesia

Outcome: ". . . methoxyflurane . . . must be considered a nephrotoxin. . . . Changes that were significant clinically . . . should be withheld [until better studies] from patients with known renal disease or . . . [until procedures] associated with a high incidence of postoperative renal complications [are carried out]."

Gain: Postoperatively, methoxyflurane (*I*) takes 24 days as compared with 6 for halothane (*S*) to reach maximum preoperative osmolality.

R: $S >> I$

Advanced cirrhosis of the liver with esophageal varices (16/XI-2001)

Innovation: surgery: prophylactic portacaval shunt

Standard: usual medical treatment

Outcome: When the medical control group (*S*) is compared with the prophylactic shunt group (*I*) in cirrhosis, the additional complications during treatment, such as portasystemic encephalopathy, hemosiderosis, and diabetes were at least as frequent and for some complications more frequent in the shunt group. Authors say that "appropriate control groups in evaluating the beneficial effects of a form of therapy must be extended to evaluations of its detrimental effect as well."

Gain: encephalopathy 50% (*I*) vs 33% (*S*)
R: $S > I$

Primary Therapies (Nonrandomized Controlled Trials)

Stab wounds of the abdomen (72/IX–1215)
Innovation: observation and selective management rather than routine laparotomy
Standard: routine surgery: laparotomy
Outcome: Instead of routine laparotomy (*S*) following stab wounds, "... it appears that clinical criteria ... *are* sufficient to differentiate seriously injured patients from those who can be managed non-operatively." This does increase the amount of observation required. "Observation and selective management (*I*) have a primary role in the care of patients with abdominal stab wounds."
Gain: reduced morbidity 27% (*S*) to 12% (*I*)
reduced hospitalization 7.9 days (*S*) to 5.4 days (*I*)
R: $I \gg S$

Cancer of the neck (94/V–1704)
Innovation: radiation treatment plus radical neck dissection
Standard: surgery: radical neck dissection alone
Outcome: In neck dissection, radiation treatment (*I*) reduces cervical recurrence substantially without increasing morbidity, but does not improve survival rate.
Gain: cervical recurrence rate 37% (*S*) vs 24% (*I*)
R: $I > S$

Advanced cirrhosis of the liver with hemorrhage from esophageal varices (76/V–1708)
Innovation: surgery: emergency therapeutic portacaval shunt
Standard: medical treatment
Outcome: "... early and definitive operative control of varix hemorrhage provides the cirrhotic patient with the greatest chance of surviving. ... emergency portacaval shunt (*I*) is the therapy of choice for most cirrhotic patients who bleed from esophageal varices."
Gain: 4 years' survival 43% (*I*) vs 3% (*S*)
R: $I \gg S$

Secondary Therapies (Nonrandomized Controlled Trials)

Renal failure after anesthesia (20/IV–1002)
Innovation: methoxyflurane anesthesia
Standard: halothane anesthesia
Outcome: "... methoxyflurane in clinical anesthesia ... restricted to situations where it offers specific advantages and where dosages less than 2.5 MAC hours can be attained." Overdose with inadequate equipment is a danger.
Gain: Dose-related abnormalities in renal function following methoxyflurane (*I*) occurred in 10/18 versus 0/8 in halothane (*S*) controls.
R: $S \gg I$

Renal function after anesthesia (62/XI–1015)
Innovation: methoxyflurane anesthesia
Standard: halothane anesthesia
Outcome: like other studies of methoxyflurane (*I*) on renal function plus search for toxic dosage levels.
Gain: less toxicity for halothane
R: $S > I$ (nearly $S = I$)

Thromboembolic complications following total hip surgery (21/VII–1908)
Innovation: anticoagulation with drug warfarin, starting on the fifth day after operation
Standard: no anticoagulation
Outcome: "The use of warfarin anticoagulation begun five days after surgery, according to our protocol, has been markedly successful in reducing fatal pulmonary embolism." Since increased wound infection has been observed following early anticoagulation in total hip arthroplasties, the authors "delayed" administration of warfarin (*I*). Because half the thrombo-embolic complications occur in the first 5 days, they now recommend a delay only to the 4th day.
Gain: reduced fatal pulmonary embolism 0.06% (*I*) vs 3.4% (*S*)
R: $I >> S$

Ileo-femoral venous thrombosis after hip surgery (26/VII–1901)
Innovation: prophylaxis with Dextran 70
Standard: no Dextran 70 treatment
Outcome: "This study does not therefore support the conclusion of other reports that Dextran 70 (*I*) is of value in preventing illo-femoral thrombosis after operations on the hip joint."
Gain: none
R: $I = S$ (a failure for the innovation)

Thoracic surgery (98/IX–1203)
Innovation: arterial blood-gas analysis during and after surgery
Standard: no arterial blood-gas studies
Outcome: The physician cannot readily tell from superficial symptoms that a patient being operated on for pulmonary problems is suffering from serious respiratory troubles either during or after the operation. In a quasi-experiment the authors appraise the value of arterial blood gases (*I*) during and after thoracotomy.
Gain: reduction in death from 16% (*S*) to 0% (*I*)
R: $I >> S$

Prostatectomy (43/XI–1020)
Innovation: prophylactic bactericidal antibiotics (two variants of the innovation are pooled here)
Standard: no use of prophylactic bactericidal antibiotics
Outcome: In prostatectomy ". . . prophylactic bactericidal antibiotics (*I*) reduced the incidence of postoperative sepsis, early and late urinary tract infection and overall morbidity in patients with preoperative bacteriuria and/or catheter drainage more than a week in duration."

Gain: reduction as stated
R: $I > S$

Urinary tract infections after prostatectomy
(36/IX–1119)
Innovation 1: chemotherapeutic treatment
Innovation 2: antibiotic treatment
Standard: untreated control group
Outcome: To prevent urinary tract infections after prostatectomy, "Routine administration of antibacterial medication . . . following transurethral resection of the prostate cannot be recommended." Use recommended only when urine is infected at time of operation and only according to sensitivity studies.
Gain: none
R: $S = I_1 = I_2$ (a failure for innovations)

Infection after appendectomy (40/II–504)
Innovation: delayed primary wound closure
Standard: initial wound closure
Outcome: "Delayed primary wound closure (I) in instances of perforated appendicitis has significantly reduced the incidence of superficial wound infection. . . ."
Gain: wound infection 2.3% (I) vs 34.1% (S)
R: $I >> S$

APPENDIX 9–II. ESTIMATING THE MEAN AND VARIANCE OF TRUE GAINS

The model of our process is that of a two-stage sampling operation. We regard an innovation and its standard as a pair drawn from a population of pairs of competing therapies. We think of their difference in performance as being obtained from the difference in their true performances, say $U - V \equiv Z$. In an experiment the investigator observes X as a measure of U for the innovation and Y as a measure of V for the standard, and so $X - Y \equiv W$ measures Z with error. We suppose X has mean U and standard deviation σ_X, Y has mean V and standard deviation σ_Y. In a moment we will consider sets of U, V pairs corresponding to randomized trials, but first let us look at properties of X and Y. Under our assumptions, the mean or expected value of W is

$$\text{Expected value } W = \text{Expected value } (X - Y) = U - V = Z$$

If we further assume that X and Y are independent as they are supposed to be in the randomized trials treated in this paper (though not in matched pair designs), then we can write for the expected value of the squared observed difference

$$\text{Expected value } W^2 = \sigma_X^2 + \sigma_Y^2 + (U - V)^2 = D + Z^2,$$

where $D = \sigma_X{}^2 + \sigma_Y{}^2$. Later we want to add up several $(U-V)^2$ to help us estimate the variance of the true differences. Consequently, we want to subtract D or an estimate of it from W^2 to isolate the part of the square dealing with the true difference Z.

When we have several experiments, we post the subscript i on all variables, with $i=1,2,\ldots,k$, where k is the number of experiments.

An estimate of the variance of the true differences Z_i would be, if we could compute it,

$$\text{Estimated Var } Z = \frac{\sum_{i=1}^{k} Z_i^2}{k} - \bar{Z}^2 \tag{1}$$

where $\bar{Z}$ is the average of the Z's. We cannot get expression (1) directly, but

$$\Sigma W_i^2 - \Sigma D_i$$

could estimate ΣZ_i^2 and $\bar{W}$, the average W, could estimate $\bar{Z}$, and so we might use

$$\frac{\Sigma W_i^2 - \Sigma D_i}{k} - \bar{W}^2 \tag{2}$$

to estimate expression (1). Next we must relate these quantities to our problem.

Our X's and Y's are observed binomial probabilities $\bar{p}_{Ii}$ and $\bar{p}_{Si}$, where I and S stand for innovation and standard, respectively. The $\bar{p}$'s are unbiased estimates of the corresponding true p's. The variances are

$$\text{Var } \bar{p}_{Ii} = \frac{p_{Ii}(1 - p_{Ii})}{n_{Ii}},$$

where n_{Ii} is the sample size for the innovation in the ith experiment. A similar formula holds for the standard. And so

$$\text{Var } \bar{p}_{Ii} + \text{Var } \bar{p}_{Si} = D_i.$$

The only trouble now is that we do not usually know the true p's and so we do not know the variance. But by replacing the p's in the variance formulas by their estimates, the corresponding $\bar{p}$'s, we can get at last an estimate of the D's.

$$\text{Estimated } D_i = \frac{\bar{p}_{Ii}(1 - \bar{p}_{Ii})}{n_{Ii}} + \frac{\bar{p}_{Si}(1 - \bar{p}_{Si})}{n_{Si}}. \tag{3}$$

This is what has been done in the calculations used for the simple estimates of the mean and variance of the differences in percentage success (survival or lack of complications) in Section IIIB–2. (For a few experiments we have treated a mixture of binomial distributions as if it were approximately binomial.)

App. 9–II Table 1 shows the details of the calculations for the primary therapies. Corresponding calculations give the quoted results for secondary therapies.

App. 9–II: Table 1. Primary Therapies: $\bar{p}_I - \bar{p}_S$

Sample Paper	*Gain* W_i	*(Gain)*^{2} W_i^2	*Est. of Variance** D_i	
68	.25	.0625	.0129	
17	−.18	.0324	.0170	
69	.16	.0256	.0067	
29	−.07	.0049	.0009	
93	−.09	.0081	.0064	
99 (a)	.19	.0361	.0172	
(b)	−.14	.0196	.0279	
19	.00	.0000	.0029	
9	−.04	.0016	.0106	
23	.02	.0004	.0014	
107 (a)	.07	.0049	.0083	
(b)	.06	.0036	.0084	
38	−.06	.0036	.0030	
		.2033	.1236	TOTAL

To estimate variance of true differences

$$\frac{.2033 - .1236}{13} = \frac{.0797}{13} = .0061$$

Average gain = .0131
The square of .0131 is .0002.
Estimated standard deviation of true scores
$= \sqrt{.0061 - (.0131)^2} = \sqrt{.0059} = .077$

*Computed from the data given in Appendix 9–IV using equation (3).

APPENDIX 9–III. ESTIMATING THE CUMULATIVE DISTRIBUTION

In using the approach of Appendix 9–II in the text, we assumed that the distribution of the true gains, the Z's, was approximately normally distributed. We have an alternative approach that puts less weight on this assumption. The general plan is Bayesian in outline but empirical in execution. The overall method is an application and slight generalization of Efron and Morris's empirical Bayes approach (Efron and Morris, 1974) based on a suggestion by Bradley Efron.

Let us assume, temporarily in the notation of Appendix 9–II, that Z's are drawn from a normal distribution with mean 0 and variance A. Further, for a given Z, W is distributed normally with mean Z and variance D, just as in Appendix 9–II, except that we impose the normality now. Since we deal with binomial differences, this should be a satisfactory approximation. When one observes a set of W's, the posterior distribution of Z_i is normal with

$$\text{Mean} = (1 - B_i)W_i \qquad \text{Variance} = (1 - B_i)D_i$$

where

$$B_i = \frac{D_i}{A + D_i}.$$

To estimate A, we estimate the D's as in Appendix 9–II, and we need to solve by iteration or otherwise the equations

$$A = \frac{\Sigma(W_j^2 - D_j)I_j(A)}{\Sigma I_j(A)}$$

where

$$I_j(A) = \frac{1}{2(A + D_j)^2}$$

The I's are weights, the inverse of the variance of the W^2's. The A corresponds to the variance we wound up estimating in Appendix 9–II.

To get at an empirical distribution function for the Z's, we use the following device. Pick a value of Z, say z. Compute

$$c_i = \frac{z - (1 - B_i)W_i}{\sqrt{(1 - B_i)D_i}},$$

This c_i is the estimated number of standard deviations z is to the right of the posterior mean of Z_i. If we compute the cumulative standard normal for c_i, $\phi(c_i)$, we have an estimate of the probability that the particular Z_i is less than z. To estimate the cumulative distribution for the Z's at z, we compute

$$\text{Estimate of } P(Z < z) = \frac{\sum_{i=1}^{k} \phi(c_i)}{k} \tag{4}$$

Now by picking a set of z's and making this calculation repeatedly we get an estimate for the cumulative of the Z's. Although the normality assumption is used at the beginning and in the smoothing, expression (4) is not normal.

To get a bird's eye view of these calculations, recall that if each comparison had been based on complete knowledge, we would represent it as a single point. To estimate the probability of a difference in percentages less than a given amount, z, we would use the proportion of comparisons whose points are to the left of z. Because the location of a percentage estimated from a limited sample is uncertain, we have replaced each point by a normal distribution, whose total density is 1—one point. Now instead of counting what proportion of points fall to the left of z, we can let each point offer an appropriate fraction of itself as falling to the left of z. Aside from the details of the Bayesian argument, this is what is going on.

In some statistical problems the assumption of 0 mean for the prior distribution is satisfactory because features of the situation either guarantee it, or a translation can handle it. We do not have such grounds in our problem and so we wish to allow the prior distribution to have a free mean M as well as a free variance A, both to be estimated by the data. Getting such estimates will require further iterations.

Let us use a superscript to designate the number of the iteration. Let us take A^0 to be the initial estimate of A. Then we can get an initial estimate of M, the mean of the prior distribution as

$$M^0 = \frac{\sum_i \frac{W_i}{A^0 + D_i}}{\sum_i \frac{1}{A^0 + D_i}}$$

where the W's are being weighted inversely as their variances.

Next we can form new W's

$$W_i^1 = W_i - M^0$$

and we can apply the method using a prior with 0 mean already described to get a new estimate of A, namely A^1. Next we re-estimate M to get

$$M^1 = \frac{\sum_i \frac{W_i}{A^1 + D_i}}{\sum_i \frac{1}{A^1 + D_i}}$$

Again subtract M^1 from W_i to get the second iterate of W_i:

$$W_i^2 = W_i - M^1,$$

and now use the original method to estimate A^2 and continue until the A's and M's converge numerically. Let us call these final values A^* and M^*. Then form

$$e_i = \frac{A^*}{A^* + D_i}$$

We estimate the true difference Z_i by

$$Z_i^* = M^* + e_i(W_i - M^*).$$

To estimate points on the cumulative we compute for any z

$$c_i = \frac{z - Z_i^*}{\sqrt{(1 - B_i)D_i}}$$

and then continue as before to get the average proportion to the left of Z.

An overview. The overall process does two things. First, it replaces each point by a distribution reflecting the uncertainty associated with the observed difference in the corresponding experiment. Then when we compute the fraction of experiments with values falling to the left of a point, each experiment contributes a portion of 1 rather than 0 or 1 as would be appropriate for infinite sample sizes in each experiment, or perfect knowledge of each true difference.

Second, the estimates, Z_i^*, of the true differences are pulled from W_i toward the center of the distribution of observed differences. Observed differences with larger associated variances are pulled more toward the center. With perfect knowledge, D_i is 0, then $e_i = 1$, implying that $Z_i^* = W_i$, thus no pulling toward the center. But when D_i is very large compared with A, then e_i is near 0, and Z_i^* is approximately M^*, essentially saying that the data are so weak that we pay much more attention to the average result for all experiments than to the observed difference. These are extremes; in the sampled studies, e_i is fairly large so that more weight is usually given to the specific experimental result than to the overall average.

APPENDIX 9-IV. BASIC DATA

The following materials give our code for the study: (1) the survival proportions used for the primary therapies and the sample sizes; (2) the survival proportions for the cancer of the prostate studies—part A comparing several direct therapies, and part B comparing dosages of estrogen; and (3) the proportions not having a given complication in the study of secondary therapies. Here the subscript I stands for innovation, S for standard. The text goes into more detail in the study of cancer of the prostate where the choices of I and S are rather arbitrary.

1. Primary Therapies*

Sample Paper		$\bar{p}_I$	X_I	N_I	$\bar{p}_S$	X_S	N_S
68	Therapeutic portacaval shunt**	.74	25	34	.49	17	35
17	Prophylactic portacaval shunt	.32	8	25	.50	15	30
69	Cancer of bronchus–radiotherapy (*I*)	.62	45	73	.45	32	71
29	TSPA (*I*) for cancer of colon and rectum	.45	212	469	.52	308	595
93	Breast cancer (implantation)**	.21	12	58	.29	17	58
99	HATG (*I*) aided transplant						
	related donor	.89	17	19	.71	12	17
	unrelated donor	.47	8	17	.61	11	18
19	Prednisone for cirrhosis	.59	99	169	.58	96	165
9	Prophylactic shunt	.54	26	48	.58	26	45
23	Chemotherapy in lung cancer	.079	8	101	.065	6	93
107	Breast cancer 5-year survival						
	internal mammary (I_1) vs radical mastectomy (*S*)	.69	37	54	.62	34	55
	chemotherapy (I_2) vs radical mastectomy (*S*)	.68	36	53	.62	34	55
38	Everting (*I*) vs inverting (*S*)	.91	32	35	.97	34	35

*$\bar{p}_I$ and $\bar{p}_S$ are survival proportions, X_I and X_S are numbers of survivors, and N_I and N_S are sample sizes for innovations (*I*) and standards (*S*), respectively; thus $\bar{p}_I = X_I/N_I$ and $\bar{p}_S = X_S/N_S$.

**These proportions are read from a graph. The closest $\bar{p}$ with an integer X is chosen.

2. Cancer of Prostate

Sample Paper		$\bar{p}_I$	X_I	N_I	$\bar{p}_S$	X_S	N_S
8	Cancer of Prostate						
	A. Comparing Therapies						
	Stage I S_3 vs S_2	.38	23	60	.50	30	60
	Stage II S_3 vs S_2	.51	48	94	.51	43	85
	Stage III S_5 vs *P*	.30	76	257	.32	85	262
	S_4 vs *P*	.31	82	266	.32	85	262
	S_1 vs *P*	.32	85	265	.32	85	262
	Stage IV S_5 vs *P*	.16	35	216	.15	34	223
	S_4 vs *P*	.10	21	203	.15	34	223
	S_1 vs *P*	.14	30	211	.15	34	223
	B. Comparing Dosages of Estrogen						
	Stage III 1 *DES* vs *P*	.52	38	73	.51	38	75
	Stage IV 1 *DES* vs *P*	.44	24	55	.25	13	53
	Stage III .2 *DES* vs *P*	.42	31	73	.51	38	75
	Stage IV .2 *DES* vs *P*	.31	16	52	.25	13	53
	Stage III *P* vs 5 *DES*	.51	38	75	.44	32	73
	.2 *DES* vs 5 *DES*	.42	31	73	.44	32	73
	1 *DES* vs 5 *DES*	.52	38	73	.44	32	73
	Stage IV *P* vs 5 *DES*	.25	13	53	.43	23	54
	.2 *DES* vs 5 *DES*	.31	16	52	.43	23	54
	1 *DES* vs 5 *DES*	.44	24	55	.43	23	54

For abbreviations consult Cancer of Prostate summary in Appendix 9–1.

3. Secondary Therapies*

Sample Paper		$\bar{p}_I$	X_I	N_I	$\bar{p}_S$	X_S	N_S
34	Heparin to prevent venous thrombosis						
	elective	.981	106	108	.84	99	118
	emergency	.87	20	23	.52	12	23
	medical	.974	37	38	.775	31	40
73	Ampicillin for colon surgery	.972	35	36	.59	20	34
70	Gastric decompression after vagotomy no tube (*I*) vs						
	nasogastrostomy (S_2)	.71	30	42	.49	23	47
	no tube (*I*) vs gastrostomy (S_1)	.71	30	42	.51	22	43
74	Neomycin-erythromycin in colon surgery	1.00	10	10	.70	7	10
57	Drainage in hepatic trauma						
	cholecystostomy (I_1) vs standard (*S*)	.66	23	35	.69	24	35
	choledochostomy (I_2) vs standard (*S*)	.41	15	37	.69	24	35
39	Antibiotics before heart surgery						
	pen + strep (I_1) vs placebo (*P*)	.73	22	30	.67	10	15
	oxacillin (I_2) vs placebo (*P*)	.74	20	27	.67	10	15
18	Antibiotic prophylaxis after cardiac surgery	.85	29	34	.80	24	30
3	Bowel preparation**	.78	39	50	.76	38	50
24	Chlorhexidine in contaminated wounds	.87	79	91	.87	152	175
58	Effects of drainage and of antibiotics after appendectomy***						
	drainage (I_1) vs no drainage (*S*)						
	normal	.52	13	25	.80	20	25
	acute	.36	35	96	.82	80	97
	gangrenous	.14	2	14	.74	14	19
	perforated	.15	4	26	.26	7	27
	antibiotic (I_2) vs none (*S*)						
	normal	.68	15	22	.64	18	28
	acute	.63	58	92	.56	57	101
	gangrenous	.53	10	19	.43	6	14
	perforated	.27	7	26	.15	4	27
38	Everting (*I*) vs inverting (*S*) in colon surgery						
	no wound infection	.49	17	35	.63	22	35
	no fecal fistulation	.57	20	35	.91	32	35

*The $\bar{p}$'s refer to proportions not getting a specific complication, the *X*'s to numbers not getting a specific complication.

**These proportions represent an average for the innovation and standard taken over the 12 local and general complications presented in the article.

***These proportions are read from graphs. The closest $\bar{p}$ with an integer *X* is chosen.

APPENDIX 9-V. REFERENCES FOR SAMPLE*

1. Andrews MJ: The incidence and pathogenesis of tracheal injury following tracheostomy with cuffed tube and assisted ventilation: Analysis of a 3-year prospective study. Br J Surg 58:749, 1971. (1–14)*
2. Andrews, MJ, Pearson FG: Incidence and pathogenesis of tracheal injury following cuffed tube tracheostomy with assisted ventilation: Analysis of a two-year prospective study. Ann Surg 173:249, 1971. (III–403)
3. Barker K, Graham NG, Mason MC, et al: The relative significance of preoperative oral antibiotics, mechanical bowel preparation, and preoperative peritoneal contamination in the avoidance of sepsis after radical surgery for ulcerative colitis and Crohn's Disease of the large bowel. Br J Surg 58:270, 1971. (I–407)
4. Blichert-Toft M, Jensen HK: Colles' fracture treated with modified Böhler technique. Acta Orthop Scand 42:45, 1971. (VI–1803)
5. Bonanno, PC: Swallowing dysfunction after tracheostomy. Ann Surg 174: 29, 1971. (III–410)
6. Böttiger LE: Prognosis in renal carcinoma. Cancer 26:780, 1970. (IV–901)
7. Bowen JC, Fleming WH: A prospective study of stress ulceration in Vietnam. South Med J 67:156, 1974. (XI–2005)
8. Byar, DP: The Veterans Administration cooperative urological research group's studies of cancer of the prostate. Cancer 32:1126, 1973. (I–6)
9. Callow AD, Resnick RH, Chalmers TC, et al: Conclusions from a controlled trial of the prophylactic portacaval shunt. Surgery 67:97, 1970. (II–511)
10. Campion BC, Frye RL, Pluth JR, et al: Arterial complications of retrograde brachial arterial catheterization: A prospective study. Mayo Clin Proc 46: 589, 1971. (VI–1806)
11. Caul EO, Clarke SKR, Mott MG, et al: Cytomegalovirus infections after open heart surgery: A prospective study. Lancet 1:777, 1971. (III–405)
12. Clark RE, Beasley WE III, Sode J, et al: Influence of hemodilution perfusion on total body and intracellular potassium: Critical prospective study. Surg Forum 20:40, 1969. (IX–1202)
13. Clarke RJ, McFarland JB, Williams JA: Gastric stasis and gastric ulcer after selective vagotomy without a drainge procedure. Br Med J 1:538, 1972. (V–1801)
14. Cohn LH, Powell MR, Seidlitz L, et al: Fluid requirements and shifts after reconstruction of the aorta. Am J Surg 120:182, 1970. (IX–1114)
15. Conahan TJ III, Ominsky AJ, Wollman H, et al: A prospective random comparison of halothane and morphine for open-heart anesthesia: One year's experience. Anesthesiology 38:528, 1973. (IV–1008)
16. Conn HO: Complications of portacaval anastomosis: By-products of a controlled investigation. Am J Gastroenterol 59:207, 1973. (XI–2001)
17. Conn HO, Lindenmuth WW: Prophylactic portacaval anastomosis in cirrhotic patients with esophageal varices. Interim results, with suggestions for subsequent investigations. N Engl J Med 279:725, 1968. (XI–2007)
18. Conte JE Jr., Cohen SN, Roe BB, et al: Antibiotic prophylaxis and cardiac surgery: A prospective double-blind comparison of single-dose versus multiple-dose regimens. Ann Intern Med 76:943, 1972. (X–1519)

*The number following the full reference is a special code useful in preparing materials for this study.

19. Copenhagen Study Group for Liver Diseases: Effect of prednisone on the survival of patients with cirrhosis of the liver. Lancet 2:119, 1969. (I-317)
20. Cousins MJ, Mazze RI: Methoxyflurane nephrotoxicity: A study of dose response in man. JAMA 225:1161, 1973. (IV-1002)
21. Coventry MB, Nolan DR, Beckenbaugh RD: "Delayed" prophylactic anticoagulation: A study of results and complications in 2,012 total hip arthroplasties. J Bone Joint Surg 55A:1487, 1973. (VII-1908)
22. Cox AG: Comparison of symptoms after vagotomy with gastrojejunostomy and partial gastrectomy. Br Med J 1:288, 1968. (II-506)
23. Coy P: A randomized study of irradiation and vinblastine in lung cancer. Cancer 26:803, 1970. (XI-505)
24. Crosfill M, Hall R, London D: The use of chlorhexidine antisepsis in contaminated surgical wounds. Br J Surg 56:906, 1969. (II-503)
25. Culp OS, Meyer, JJ: Radical prostatectomy in the treatment of prostatic cancer. Cancer 32:1113, 1973. (I-7)
26. Darke SG: Ilio-femoral venous thrombosis after operations on the hip: A prospective controlled trial using Dextran 70. J Bone Joint Surg 54B:615, 1972. (VII-1901)
27. DeHaven KE, Evarts CM, Wilde AH, et al: Early results of Charnley-Müller total hip reconstruction. Orthop Clin North Am 4:465, 1973. (VI-1808)
28. Drusin, LM, Engle, MA, Hagstrom, WC, et al: The postpericardiotomy syndrome: A six-year epidemiologic study. N Engl J Med 272:597, 1965. (VIII-801)
29. Dwight RW, Higgins GA, Keehn RJ: Factors influencing survival after resection in cancer of the colon and rectum. Am J Surg 117:512, 1969. (II-607)
30. Evarts CM, DeHaven KE, Nelson CL, et al: Interim results of Charnley-Müller total hip arthroplasty. Clin Orthop 95:193, 1973. (VII-1906)
31. Firat D, Olshin S: Treatment of metastatic carcinoma of the female breast with combination of hormones and other chemotherapy. Cancer Chemother Rep, 52:743, 1968. (I-110)
32. Fishman NH, Bogren HG, Carlsson ES: Angiographic estimation of the size of the aortic valve annulus. Arch Surg 101:717, 1970. (VIII-803).
33. Gaensler EA, Strieder JW: Pregnancy following pneumonectomy. Ann Thorac Surg 4:581, 1967. (V-1707)
34. Gallus AS, Hirsh J, Tuttle RJ, et al: Small subcutaneous doses of heparin in prevention of venous thrombosis. N Engl J Med 288:545, 1973. (X-1302)
35. Gaspard DJ, Cohen JL, Gaspar MR: Aortoiliofemoral thromboendarterectomy vs bypass graft. A randomized study. Arch Surg 105:898, 1972. (VI-1815)
36. Genster HG, Madsen PO: Urinary tract infections following transurethral prostatectomy: With special reference to the use of antimicrobials. J Urol 104:163, 1970. (IX-1119)
37. Gilbert JAL, Sartor VE: Regional enteritis: Disease patterns and medical management. Can Med Assoc J 91:23, 1964. (VIII-719)
38. Goligher JC, Morris C, McAdam WAF, et al: A controlled trial of inverting versus everting intestinal suture in clinical large-bowel surgery. Br J Surg 57:817, 1970. (II-507)
39. Goodman JS, Schaffner W, Collins HA, et al: Infection after cardiovascular surgery: Clinical study including examination of antimicrobial prophylaxis. N Engl J Med 278:117, 1968. (I-301)
40. Grosfeld JL, Solit RW: Prevention of wound infection in perforated ap-

pendicitis: Experience with delayed primary wound closure. Ann Surg 168: 891, 1968. (II–504)

41. Gunn A, Keddie NC, Fox H: Acalculous gall-bladder disease. Br J Surg 60: 213, 1973. (III–702)
42. Hedley AJ, Ross IP, Beck JS, et al: Recurrent thyrotoxicosis after subtotal thyroidectomy. Br Med J 4:258, 1971. (VI–1807)
43. Herr, HW: Use of prophylactic antibiotics in the high-risk patient undergoing prostatectomy: Effect on morbidity. J Urol 109:686, 1973. (XI–1020)
44. Howard PH Jr, Hardin WJ: The role of surgery in fever of unknown origin. Surg Clin North Am 52:397, 1972. (XI–913)
45. Howard RJ, Murphy WR, Humphrey EW: A prospective randomized study of the elective surgical treatment for duodenal ulcer: Two-to-ten-year follow-up study. Surgery 73:256, 1973. (VI–1814)
46. Hughes J, Lo Curcio SB, Edmunds R, et al: The common duct after cholecystectomy: Initial report of a ten-year study. JAMA 197:247, 1966. (IV–717)
47. Irani FA, Berkas E, Steiger Z: Evaluation of surgical treatment for duodenal ulcer: A prospective randomized study. Am J Surg 122:374, 1971. (IV–708)
48. Johnson WD, Grizzle JE, Postlethwait RW: Veterans Administration cooperative study of surgery for duodenal ulcer: I. Description and evaluation of method of randomization. Arch Surg 101:391, 1970. (III–602)
49. Jordan PH Jr, Condon RE: A prospective evaluation of vagotomy-pyloroplasty and vagotomy-antrectomy for treatment of duodenal ulcer. Ann Surg 172:547, 1970. (II–508)
50. Keighley MRB, Graham NG: The aetiology and prevention of pancreatitis following biliary-tract operations. Br J Surg 60:149, 1973. (III–703)
51. Kennedy T, Connell AM: Selective or truncal vagotomy? A double-blind randomized controlled trial. Lancet 1:899, 1969. (II–509)
52. Killingback MJ: Acute diverticulitis: Progress report, Australasian survey (1967–1969). Dis Colon Rectum 13:444, 1970. (V–1710)
53. Kimball CP: A predictive study of adjustment to cardiac surgery. J Thorac Cardiovasc Surg 58:891, 1969. (IX–1214)
54. Krishnamurthy GT, Blahd WH: Diagnostic and therapeutic implications of long-term radioisotope scanning in the management of thyroid cancer. J Nucl Med 13:924, 1972. (VI–1812)
55. Lawrence W Jr, Terz JJ, Rogers C, et al: Preoperative irradiation for head and neck cancer: A prospective study. Cancer 33:318, 1974. (VII–1904)
56. Lindbom G: Studies of the epidemiology of staphylococcal infections: II. Staphyloccoccal infections in a thoracic surgery unit. Acta Chir Scand 128: 421, 1964. (IV–805)
57. Lucas CE: Prospective clinical evaluation of biliary drainage in hepatic trauma: An interim report. Ann Surg 174:830, 1971. (III–704)
58. Magarey CJ, Chant ADB, Rickford CRK, et al: Peritoneal drainage and systemic antibiotics after appendicectomy: A prospective trial. Lancet 2:179, 1971. (III–706)
59. Malinow MR, Kremkau EL, Kloster FE, et al: Occlusion of arteries after vein bypass. Circulation 47:1211, 1973. (VIII–1010)
60. Mason MC, Clark CG: Psychiatric disorders after surgery for duodenal ulcer. Gut 11:258, 1970. (V–1709)
61. Mauney FM Jr, Ebert PA, Sabiston DC Jr: Postoperative myocardial infarction: A study of predisposing factors, diagnosis and mortality in a high risk group of surgical patients. Ann Surg 172:497, 1970. (IX–1116)

62. Mazze RI, Cousins MJ: Renal toxicity of anaesthetics: With specific reference to nephrotoxicity of methoxyflurane. Canad Anaesth Soc J 20:64, 1973. (XI–1015)
63. Mazze RI, Shue GL, Jackson SH: Renal dysfunction associated with methoxyflurane anesthesia: A randomized prospective clinical evaluation. JAMA 216:278, 1971. (I–406)
64. McCabe JC, Ebert PA, Engle MA, et al: Circulating heart-reactive antibodies in the postpericardiotomy syndrome. J Surg Res 14:158, 1973. (IV–1017)
65. McKeown KC: A prospective study of the immediate and long-term results of Polya gastrectomy for duodenal ulcer. Br J Surg 59:849, 1972. (VIII–711)
66. McMaster M: The natural history of the rheumatoid metacarpophalangeal joint. J Bone Joint Surg 54B:687, 1972. (VII–1902)
67. Merkle RB, McDonald FD, Waldman J, et al: Human renal function following methoxyflurane anesthesia. JAMA 218:841, 1971. (I–11)
68. Mikkelsen WP: Therapeutic portacaval shunt: Preliminary data on controlled trial and morbid effects of acute hyaline necrosis. Arch Surg 108:302, 1974. (XI–1910)
69. Miller AB, Fox W, Tall R: Five-year follow-up of the medical research council comparative trial of surgery and radiotherapy for the primary treatment of small-celled or oat-celled carcinoma of the bronchus. Lancet 2:501, 1969. (II–510)
70. Miller DF, Mason JR, McArthur J, et al: A randomized prospective trial comparing three established methods of gastric decompression after vagotomy. Br J Surg 59:605, 1972. (XI–2002)
71. Mills NL, Beaudet RL, Isom OW, et al: Hyperglycemia during cardiopulmonary bypass. Ann Surg 177:203, 1973. (VIII–1011)
72. Nance FC, Cohn I Jr: Surgical judgment in the management of stab wounds of the abdomen: A retrospective and prospective analysis based on a study of 600 stabbed patients. Ann Surg 170:569, 1969. (IX–1215)
73. Nash AG, Hugh TB: Topical ampicillin and wound infection in colon surgery. Br Med J 1:471, 1967. (II–606)
74. Nichols RL, Broido P, Condon RE, et al: Effect of preoperative neomycin-erythromycin intestinal preparation on the incidence of infectious complications following colon surgery. Ann Surg 178:453, 1973. (I–1)
75. Nissen ED, Goldstein AI: A prospective investigation of the etiology of febrile morbidity following abdominal hysterectomy. Am J Obstet Gynecol 113:111, 1972. (III–701)
76. Orloff, MJ: Emergency portacaval shunt: A comparative study of shunt, varix ligation and nonsurgical treatment of bleeding esophageal varices in unselected patients with cirrhosis. Ann Surg 166:456, 1967. (V–1708)
77. Orloff MJ, Chandler JG, Charters AC III, et al: Emergency portacaval shunt treatment for bleeding esophageal varices. Arch Surg 108:293, 1974. (VII–1909)
78. Pearson FG, Goldberg M, DaSilva AJ: A prospective study of tracheal injury complicating tracheostomy with a cuffed tube. Ann Otol Rhinol Laryngol 77:867, 1968. (VIII–806)
79. Pemberton PA: Pericapsular ostcotomy of the ilium for treatment of congenital subluxation and dislocation of the hip. J Bone Joint Surg 47–A:65, 1965. (X–1603)
80. Phillips, RS: Shiers' alloplasty of the knee. Clin Orthop 94:122, 1973. (VII–1903)
81. Piccone VA, LeVeen HH, Sawyer P, et al: Incidence and mechanisms of

myocardial infarction following coronary artery surgery. Angiology 24:590, 1973. (X–1311)

82. Resnick RH, Chalmers TC, Ishihara AM, et al: A controlled study of the prophylactic portacaval shunt. Ann Intern Med 70:675, 1969. (V–1705)
83. Rosen M, Mushin WW, Kilpatrick GS, et al: Study of myocardial ischaemia in surgical patients. Br Med J 2:1415, 1966. (X–1409)
84. Salmon JH: Senile and presenile dementia: Ventriculoatrial shunt for symptomatic treatment. Geriatrics 24:67, 1969. (V–1713)
85. Schowengerdt CG, Hunt JL: Respiratory acidosis during thoracotomy. Ohio State Med J, 68:358, 1972. (XI–2003)
86. Sevitt J: Fat embolism in patients with fractured hips. Br Med J 2:257, 1972. (VI–1804)
87. Silverstone JT, Tannahill MM, Ireland JA: Psychiatric aspects of profound hypothermia in open-heart surgery. J Thorac Cardiovasc Surg 59:193, 1970. (IX–1204)
88. Singer MM, Wright F, Stanley LK, et al: Oxygen toxicity in man: A prospective study in patients after open-heart surgery. N Engl J Med 283:1473, 1970. (IV–904)
89. Skyring A, Roberts R: Childhood ulcerative colitis: An epidemiological study in N.S.W. Med J Aust 1:955, 1965. (VIII–811)
90. Smith MD, Klebanoff G, Kemmerer WT: Exploratory laparotomy for staging in Hodgkin's disease: Diagnostic yield versus operative morbidity. Am J Surg 124:811, 1972. (X–1219)
91. Smith R, Grossman W, Johnson L, et al: Arrhythmias following cardiac valve replacement. Circulation 45:1018, 1972. (IV–915)
92. Smith RA, Nigam BK, Thompson JM: Influence of parental age on survival after resection for lung carcinoma. Lancet 1:843, 1973. (VI–1809)
93. Stewart HJ, Forrest APM, Roberts MM, et al: Early pituitary implantation with Yttrium-90 for advanced breast cancer. Lancet 2:816, 1969. (II–502)
94. Strong EW: Preoperative radiation and radical neck dissection. Surg Clin North Am 49:271, 1969. (V–1704)
95. Sweetnam R, Knowelden J, Seddon HS Sir: Bone sarcoma: Treatment by irradiation, amputation, or a combination of the two. Br Med J 2:363, 1971. (V–1711)
96. Takaro T, Pifarre R, Wuerflein RD, et al: Acute coronary occlusion following coronary arteriography: Mechanisms and surgical relief. Surgery 72: 1018, 1972. (X–1220)
97. Till AS: Carcinoma of the thyroid. Proc Roy Soc Med 58:309, 1965. (X–1605)
98. Tufo HM, Ostfeld AM, Shekelle R: Central nervous system dysfunction following open-heart surgery. JAMA 212:1333, 1970. (IX–1203)
99. Turcotte JG, Feduska NJ, Haines RF, et al: Antithymocyte globulin in renal transplant recipients: A clinical trial. Arch Surg 106:484, 1973. (VIII–1101)
100. Vilkki P, Tala E: Thyroid surgery in an area of low endemicity of goitre: A study based on 1456 thyroid patients treated in the surgical clinic, University of Turku, in 1947–1957. Acta Chir Scand Supplementum 313, 1963. (X–1607)
101. Vogelsang TM: The campaign against typhoid and paratyphoid B in western Norway: Results of cholecystectomy. J Hyg 62:443, 1964. (IV–718)
102. Wastell C, Colin JF, MacNaughton JI, et al: Selective proximal vagotomy with and without pyloroplasty. Br Med J 1:25, 1972. (VI–1802)

103. Whitaker RH: The fate of the prostatic cavity after retropubic prostatectomy. Br J Urol 43:722, 1971. (IX–1105)
104. Willerson JT, Moellering RC Jr, Buckley MJ, et al: Conjunctival petechiae after open-heart surgery. N Engl J Med 284:539, 1971. (III–402)
105. Wilson FC: Total replacement of the knee in rheumatoid arthritis: A prospective study of the results of treatment with the Walldius prosthesis. J Bone Joint Surg 54-A:1429, 1972.
106. Wilson FC: Total replacement of the knee in rheumatoid arthritis: Part II of a prospective study. Clin Orthop 94:58, 1973. (VII–1905)
107. Yonemoto RH, Barton DR, Byron RL, et al: Conservative mediastinal node dissection for the treatment of carcinoma of the breast. Surg Gynecol Obstet 136:417, 1973. (VIII–721)

APPENDIX 9-VI. SAMPLED PAPERS WITH REFERENCES TO ETHICAL ISSUES

Randomized Trial		*Controlled Trial*	*Series*
39	58	20	103
49	99		98
69	34		
9	18		
48*	16		

*This paper reports the design of a large study, but not its results.

10

The end result: quality of life

Bucknam McPeek
John P. Gilbert
Frederick Mosteller

In analyzing the 107 studies drawn through the MEDLARS search and presented in Chapter 9, quality of life following treatment frequently emerged as an important issue, as did long-run follow-up. We discuss these two related issues here, concentrating on those studies (about half the entire sample) that dealt with factors relating to quality of life or involving periods of follow-up greater than one year.

In many acute conditions a successful surgical procedure virtually restores the patient to his or her original state of health. The evaluation of such a therapy, appendectomy for example, does not generally require either long-term follow-up or a detailed assessment of the quality of the patient's life. On the other hand, many chronic conditions allow only a partial or temporary amelioration of symptoms. In addition, some treatments are themselves debilitating. In the latter two situations, therapies usually require a more thorough long-term follow-up for their ultimate evaluation.

Much of surgery is based upon the willingness of the patient to undergo the discomfort and risk of a surgical procedure in order to obtain an improved long-term result, even though the initial condition may not have been particularly life-threatening. Should the initial condition be life-threatening or potentially so, the choice between two procedures may depend upon the expected long-term result if both operations are equally effective in coping with the

Preparation of this paper has been facilitated by National Science Foundation Grant GS 32327X1; by the Miller Institute for Basic Research in Science, University of California-Berkeley; and by Grant #GM 15904 of the National Institute of General Medical Sciences.

threat to life. Although one would prefer to decrease short-term, nonlife-threatening morbidity, long-term results ordinarily have higher priority.

For a large proportion of both medical and surgical procedures, the patient's quality of life after the recovery phase matters most in choosing the treatment. To evaluate treatments properly and to select alternatives intelligently, those conducting medical research need to be able to explore the myriad factors that describe quality of life—the patient's residual symptoms, state of restored health, feeling of well-being, limitations, new or restored capabilities, and response to these advantages and disadvantages. A period of pain, discomfort, and limitation follows nearly all surgery—even a recovery unmarred by any complication. Following this period of recovery, the patient and physician can assess the results of treatment without the confusing aspects of temporary risk and disability specifically related to the treatment.

In many cases it is relatively easy to define particular types of morbidity associated with the original disease or with the surgical treatment. Thus, the various drainage procedures for ulcers with or without vagotomy all seem to have diarrhea and dumping as possible long-term sequelae. The rate of occurrence of each of these can be estimated by careful investigation, but their relative importance can be determined only by asking the patient how they affect his or her overall well-being. In practice, a surgeon probably learns from personal experience and that of teachers and colleagues what the implications of these various types of persistent symptoms are for the lives of patients. One of the problems in reporting large series and experimental comparisons of different treatments is how to communicate this knowledge and understanding of the subtle ways different symptoms affect the lives and quality of life for differing types of patients. How can a surgeon advise a patient who has never experienced any of the possible options which ones the patient would find least distressing?

What seems to be needed in investigations of quality of life following surgery are: (1) long-term follow-up, and (2) ability to appraise the patient's comfort and performance objectively and subjectively. The evidence from our sample is that modestly long-term follow-ups are frequently carried out. Some investigators repeat their examinations regularly and report each further follow-up. Nevertheless, mortality is more often reported than quality of life. Very long-term follow-up is rare, of course, but unfortunately may be needed. In discussing an operation for unstable hip in young children, Pemberton (79)* points out that the follow-up of two to eight years is not the issue since the hip is to last the patient a lifetime. "True end-result reports must await evaluation of these hips after twenty to forty years of walking and the time when the girls have borne children . . . " This operation illustrates both an extreme situation and the appreciation of the surgeon for the need for long-term follow-up of quality of life.

Because quality of outcome depends on the condition of the patients and on how well they adapt to the condition, both objective and subjective measures

*Refers to a sampled paper, a list of which appears in Appendix 9-V of Chapter 9. Reference articles not included in the sample papers are referred to by author and date. These articles are listed under References at the conclusion of this chapter.

will be required. The further development of such measures should benefit from close cooperation between surgeons and social scientists. Unless surgeons provide the leadership for such cooperation, it seems unlikely that measures that are both relevant and reliable will be developed.

TREATMENT OF CANCER

Among the papers in our sample, sixteen (6, 8, 23, 25, 29, 31, 54, 55, 69, 90, 92, 93, 94, 95, 97, 107) dealt with the treatment of cancer. The authors of the papers followed the patients involved for periods ranging from six months to twenty years. Almost all reported on the survival and the recurrence rates of their patients. With a few exceptions, most of these studies were unable to document any striking difference in either survival or the rate and time of recurrence among the different treatments tried. Once we note this general lack of marked differences in effectiveness of the treatments, we see that it might be fruitful to have been able to investigate and report in a reliable and reproducible way contrasts among these treatments in the quality of life, or of the death, experienced by patients with the same disease but having different treatments (see Chapter 19 on breast cancer). Such an inquiry might be particularly relevant because the therapies involved such varied elements as castration, hormones, irradiation, chemotherapy, and surgery of greater or lesser extent.

The continuing experimentation necessary for the development of new and better methods for treating cancer is of primary importance, but should we not also document effects of these therapies on the quality of life well before death and note the particular difficulties of the final months of life so that the experience of all physicians can be broadened and their wisdom and compassion strengthened? (See Chapter 3 on social costs due to disease.)

One of the difficulties that lie in the way of such evaluations of the impact of medical therapies upon the quality of the lives of patients is the difficulty of measuring this effect in a way that is informative and relevant, yet reliable. In order to do this, surgeons will have to rely not only upon objective criteria of presence or absence of disease or disability, but also on less objective measures that indicate how much improvement or how much disability the patient thinks he or she has as a result of the therapy. It is likely that much more development will be required for such interviews to become reasonably informative (Grogono and Woodgate, 1971).

TREATMENT OF ULCERS

Ten (13, 22, 45, 47, 48, 49, 51, 65, 70, 102) papers we reviewed reported studies of the surgical treatment of peptic ulcer. Of these, five reported a long-term follow-up—more than a year—in some detail. Overall, they reported similar findings: a generally low mortality and morbidity, and indicated the need for a careful analysis of the patient's residual symptoms, gastrointestinal function, and the patient's own view of his or her state of health in evaluating a treatment for peptic ulcer. This requires a long follow-up—certainly in excess of a year or

Table 10-1. Visick Classification

Category	*Definition*
I. Excellent	Absolutely no symptoms; perfect result.
II. Very Good	Patient considers result perfect, but interrogation elicits mild occasional symptoms easily controlled by minor adjustment to diet.
III. Satisfactory	Mild or moderate symptoms not controlled by care and which cause some discomfort; however, patient and surgeon are satisfied with result, which does not interfere seriously with life or work.
IV. Unsatisfactory	Moderate or severe symptoms or complications which interfere considerably with work or enjoyment of life; patient or doctor dissatisfied with result. Includes all cases with proved recurrent ulcer and those submitted to further operation, even though the latter may have been followed by considerable symptomatic improvement.

two. It requires an assessment by both a medically trained observer and the patient, together with some sort of scaling of the information obtained. We were particularly impressed with the ideas behind the Visick classification (Visick, 1948), modifications of which were used in several papers in the sample (see also Chapter 11 on ulcer surgery).

An instructive example is the randomized clinical trial of several operations for duodenal ulcer from a Veterans Hospital in Michigan (47). Three separate operations were studied (vagotomy and pyloroplasty, segmental gastric resection with pyloroplasty, and vagotomy and hemigastrectomy) in patients coming to elective surgery for proven duodenal ulcer. If at operation any one of the procedures could be done safely, the patient was admitted to the study and a sealed envelope opened to select the operation randomly. Evaluation of the procedure included mortality as well as a variety of short-term morbidity measures. Follow-up studies from three to six years after surgery reached 80% of the 131 patients. Most patients were followed at regular intervals at a special clinic where signs and symptoms of alimentary dysfunctions were sought, and a questionnaire was sent to evaluate the present status of patients. The modified Visick classification was used to grade patients into four categories as shown in Table 10-1.

TREATMENT OF ORTHOPEDIC DISABILITIES

Twelve papers in our sample reported evaluation of orthopedic surgery. Four of these (21, 26, 66, 86) dealt exclusively with operative or immediate post-operative findings. The remaining eight (4, 27, 30, 79, 80, 95, 105, 106) reported follow-up of patients over a longer interval (in some cases up to four years or eight years after operation). Anatomic structure, physiologic function, and the end-result are nowhere related more directly than in orthopedic surgery.

It is not surprising that careful long-term assessment of function and results has been of traditional concern to orthopedic surgeons. The wide use of x-rays in orthopedic diagnosis and the ease of clearly detecting the structural result of orthopedic surgery, has, in most cases, made repeated noninvasive examination of postoperative orthopedic patients possible. While some results in the evaluation of orthopedic surgery are subjective (such as pain), many are amenable to objective study (for example, range of motion, gait, deformity, instability, and strength). It is on these results, both subjective and objective, that the quality of life achieved by the patient and the degree of improvement depends. A variety of instruments has been developed to enable the systematic recording of the functional results of orthopedic surgery. Among these is the Iowa Hip Score (Larson, 1963), which several authors (29, 30) suggest as an objective and reliable means of evaluating patients for surgery as well as for recording the changes following operation.

TREATMENT OF ESOPHOGEAL VARICES

Seven papers evaluated the portacaval shunt operation in treating esophogeal varices in cirrhotic patients. Four dealt with portacaval shunt in patients with known varices but not actually bleeding (9, 17, 68, 82). Two concerned its use as a form of emergency therapy in patients with active variceal hemorrhage (76, 77), and one reported the incidence of symptoms in a combined group of both prophylactic and emergency operations (16). Most of these studies followed surviving patients for two or more years. The results of the studies of prophylactic shunts are mixed when survival effectiveness of this operation is compared with a conventional nonsurgical approach. These mixed results may be caused by differences in the pool of patients treated, either medical or socioeconomic, or by differences in the treatment.

In this very high-risk group of patients, their physicians understandably have focused on issues of survival and on the incidence of specific complications. So far we seem to have little or no data to help us evaluate these differences on the lives of the patients surviving. In addition to their rate of survival, should we not also discover how well the survivors of this procedure are managing and enjoying their lives? Some papers discuss whether or not the patients were still drinking, whether they were employed, able to do housework or other appropriate activities for their age. But often these matters were touched on only in passing, and few reported information systematically. The meaning of such comparisons between groups treated differently is unclear, and valuable information might well be obtained by gathering more data on quality of life factors in the lives of the surviving patients.

SUMMARY AND CONCLUSIONS

The studies in the four areas cited above suggest that we need further methods to appraise quality of life and that fresh research is required to determine how patients can report more accurately on their situation. With surgical leadership, methods used by social scientists for subjective measurement might be profitably adapted.

These four areas of surgery show us that the degree of long-term follow-up varies considerably from one area to another. Although physicians seem to be willing to follow their patients for a period longer than therapy requires, some obvious problems arise. Patients who return to provide this information do not always benefit individually from their visits, and the physician may question whether, on balance, such visits use professional time well and whether it is ethical to so use the patient's time. These problems might be solved in part by compensation for both the patient and the physician.

Less intensive use of physicians is an alternative suggested by several people, including Charles Sanders, M.D. (personal communication). Paramedical personnel could be recruited to assist in doing these long-term follow-up studies. Reasons for such an approach would be that follow-up studies do not require the full range of training of physicians. Developing questionnaires, administering them, and carrying out the detective work necessary to find missing patients, or at least their outcomes, are specialized time-consuming tasks. Their general supervision might be carried out by physicians who need not deal with the details.

The problems just described require substantial long-term funds if suitable follow-up and evaluation of quality of life are to be carried out. Too, they require mechanisms for institutional follow-up similar to our present tumor registries, tuberculosis and venereal disease programs, or large longitudinal studies like the Framingham Heart Study. This mechanism will be most important where the experience of many physicians is to be pooled or where the length of follow-up is a lifetime, as may be appropriate in some surgery for children.

Often the patient accepts the risks and discomfort inherent in surgery with the expectation that the quality of his or her life will be improved. Thus, the ultimate goal of much of surgery is to increase the patient's productive and enjoyable life. That many papers in our sample touched upon this aspect of surgical outcome indicates that surgeons are well aware of this point. Without well-designed and carefully executed clinical trials, we cannot expect to demonstrate on the basis of experience the long-run effectiveness of therapies.

Acknowledgment

George Zuidema, M.D., and Charles G. Child, II, M.D., have given us permission to revise our paper "On Quality of Life" prepared for the Study on Surgical Services for the United States currently in press and to present it here.

References

Grogono AW, Woodgate DJ: Index for measuring health. Lancet 2:1024, 1971

Larson CB: Rating scale for hip disabilities. Clin Orthop 31:85, 1963

Visick AH: A study of the failures after gastrectomy. Ann R Coll Surg Engl 3:266, 1948

11

Experiments in surgical treatment of duodenal ulcer

William G. Cochran
Persi Diaconis
Allan P. Donner
David C. Hoaglin
Nicholas E. O'Connor
Osler L. Peterson
Victor M. Rosenoer

1. INTRODUCTION

This chapter presents a critical survey of randomized clinical trials comparing vagotomy and pyloroplasty with vagotomy and antrectomy as elective treatments for duodenal ulcer.

The second section describes the study group and the iterative process which led to this report. Section 3 sketches the health impact of peptic ulcer disease. Section 4 summarizes the natural history of the disease and briefly describes the two operative treatments.

The study group drafted lists of medical and statistical criteria to be used in comparing the selected studies. These criteria appear in Sections 5 and 6. For the four published studies a detailed consideration (in Section 7) includes tabulations of their critical features, a discussion of the overall findings, and a discussion of their major medical and statistical problems.

Section 8 contains a detailed discussion of principal problem areas common to all studies. The statistical problems are sample size, the need in these investigations for nonoperated controls, and problems of loss to follow-up and of ran-

•Supported in part by grants from the Robert Wood Johnson Foundation through the Harvard Faculty Seminar on Human Experimentation in Health and Medicine during 1973–74.
•Supported in part by Division of Research, Lahey Clinic Foundation, Grant# 0683.
•Dr. Peterson was a fellow at the Center for Advanced Study in the Behavioral Sciences (1974–75) under a program of senior medical fellowships supported by the Kaiser Family Foundation when this report was being written and revised.

domization. Medical problems include tests for completeness of vagotomy (the Hollander test) and evaluation of outcome and side effects according to the Visick scale.

Section 9 contains a summary of the group's findings and general recommendations.

2. BACKGROUND TO THE PRESENT STUDY

The Working Group on Protocol Issues prepared this report as part of the Faculty Seminar on Human Experimentation in Health and Medicine held at Harvard University during the 1973-74 academic year and continued as the Faculty Seminar on Analysis of Health and Medical Practices during 1974-75. Focusing on surgical treatment of duodenal ulcer gave the group many concrete examples of problems in preparation, implementation, and assessment of protocols for clinical trials; but attention was not confined to this one area, and many of the findings reported here should be useful in other areas as well.

The decision to study surgical treatment of duodenal ulcer disease was taken at the urging of a physician member of the group, who reported sharp disagreement among surgeons about the relative merits of the several operations used. Surgical treatment at present includes three or four operations which could be reliably characterized by risk. The most common symptom, pain, is subjective and variable, thus posing measurement problems in defining disease severity. The smaller group of patients who suffer severe hemorrhage, perforation, or gastric outflow obstruction provides more objective evidence of disease severity. Following patients over several years to determine early, intermediate, and late results raises interesting practical problems. These complex problems made the subject attractive for critical review.

A major goal of the review was to find possible solutions for some of these problems. Such a review, it was foreseen, might raise a number of policy issues. Was there as much uncertainty about the effectiveness of the several operations as the reported discussion by surgeons suggested? Could an independent review contribute to the resolution of any problems that might be found? In part the group was also testing the utility of a rigorous review using defined standards as a scientific tool in examining policy questions.

To assess the relative merits of operations used in elective surgical treatment of peptic ulcer disease, one turns first to randomized comparative studies because they are substantially more reliable in eliminating biases than are nonrandomized studies. While this position is not universally accepted, the evidence is decidedly in its favor. (Section 8.7 discusses some aspects of randomization.) To narrow and simplify the study, the group limited it to elective gastric surgery, thus eliminating operations for bleeding, perforation, and obstruction. We further decided to concentrate on two operations, vagotomy with antrectomy and vagotomy with drainage. The small number of randomized studies involving comparison of these two widely used operations made it possible to examine each study in considerable detail.

The group drafted sets of medical and statistical criteria to apply to such studies. We had also examined a number of clinical trials in which partial gastrectomy was compared with drainage operations. The clear preference in recent years for vagotomy in combination with less extensive gastric surgery led to the later restriction. The criteria used in the final study were developed during the early exploratory period. A search (based on the Index Medicus) of the English-language literature published since 1948 produced a list of about 75 trials in the problem area. Closer examination (by teams pairing a statistician and an M.D.) eliminated those which did not report randomized comparisons of the two surgical procedures and left a total of four studies: Price et al. (1970), supplemented by Johnson et al. (1970) and Postlethwait (1973), Jordan and Condon (1970), Sawyers and Scott (1971), and Howard et al. (1973). The careful work underlying these four extensive studies proved very valuable as a basis for our work. Without the substantial progress which their authors had already made, we would have been able to learn far less about comparative studies in this problem area.

The full group then read, discussed, and evaluated the published reports of the four studies, applying the medical and statistical criteria. This allowed elaboration of the various criteria as particular features of individual studies and reports were considered. The results of these deliberations are given in the remainder of the present report.

3. IMPACT ON HEALTH

Peptic ulcer disease* is a common and recurring cause of morbidity. Its prevalence rate is 22.0 per thousand among males and 12.6 per thousand among females (Wilson, 1974). The highest prevalence rate is found in the age group 45 to 64, where the rates per thousand population are 45 for males and 22.8 for females. Prevalence varies with income, from 22 per thousand among persons with incomes under \$5,000 per annum to 14.6 per thousand among persons with incomes above \$10,000 (in 1968).

Though peptic ulcer is not one of the most common causes of disability, it is nevertheless significant (Namey and Wilson, 1973). Among the approximately 22 million persons with some activity limitation due to health, approximately 550,000 (or 2.5%) suffer some limitation on their normal activities because of peptic ulcer disease.

A 1969-70 study of hospitalizations in New England (exclusive of Connecticut) found that the average charge per hospital stay was \$772 (Jones et al., 1976). Peptic ulcer patients, whose admission rate was 1.9 per thousand population (1.2% of all admissions), incurred substantially higher bills per stay (\$1,153 on the average). A calculation based on these data indicates that more than \$16 million in charges for hospitalization are incurred by peptic ulcer patients annually, representing 1.85% of the estimated charges for all hospitalization, or nearly \$2 per New England resident.

Finally, peptic ulcer, though not among the most common causes of death, is nevertheless a significant one (Namey and Wilson, 1973). In 1968 there were

*The term "peptic ulcer" includes esophageal, gastric, duodenal, and anastomotic ulcers. Among these, duodenal ulcers are by far the most common.

about 10,000 deaths in the United States from peptic ulcer disease. This represents about 0.53% of all deaths.

4. NATURAL HISTORY AND SURGICAL THERAPY

Most studies and descriptions of duodenal ulcer disease are based upon patients treated in medical centers for particularly complex and intractable problems. It is often difficult, therefore, to use such studies as a basis for describing the natural history of duodenal ulcer disease for the population as a whole. From the more careful clinical studies we judge that the average healing time of a duodenal ulcer is about 6 weeks. A high percentage of patients will have recurrences. However, a large percentage will recover and be completely free of recurrences within five years (45-90%). The probability that patients will be cured and become symptom-free apparently diminishes with disease duration. A substantial number of ulcer patients will require hospitalization (40%), though this is likely to be influenced by health insurance coverage as well as by the disease. A minority of patients with duodenal ulcers will have bleeding complications with their disease (15-20%). A smaller proportion (7-10%) will experience a perforation of their ulcer.

The surgical therapy of duodenal ulcer disease is directed at reducing the amount of acid secreted by the stomach. This plan makes the basic assumption that an increase in acid secretion by the stomach is associated with an increased incidence of duodenal ulcer disease. The vagus nerves, which run alongside the esophagus and innervate the stomach, control the cephalic phase of gastric acid secretion and provide a stimulus to motility. Cutting these nerves thus decreases secretion of acid by the parietal cells in the upper half of the stomach, but it also decreases motility so that emptying of the stomach is impaired. By widening the outlet of the stomach, a pyloroplasty provides adequate emptying or drainage. An antrectomy achieves better drainage by removing the lower portion of the stomach. Since that portion of the stomach contains the cells which secrete the hormone gastrin, a powerful stimulator of acid secretion by the parietal cells, the combination of vagotomy and antrectomy reduces acid secretion in two ways.

5. MEDICAL CRITERIA

Initially, the group had an extensive list of medical criteria for evaluating surgical studies. However, the discovery in reviewing the papers that many of the relevant details were not included led to a narrowing of the list.

The basic preoperative information is the patient's age and sex and the history and presence of ulcer and other diseases which may influence risk or outcome. Details of the patient's history should include the length of time the patient has had ulcer symptoms and the duration and severity of those symptoms (if possible, in terms of the amount of work lost, frequency and duration of dieting, medication, adherence to treatment, and number and duration of hospitalizations required).

In establishing the diagnosis of an ulcer, one or more of the following criteria would be acceptable:

1. Ulcer seen on an upper gastrointestinal barium x-ray.
2. Ulcer seen by endoscopy.
3. Confirmation of the ulcer either at surgery or by the pathologist.

Postoperatively, the study should yield the following information:

1. Operative mortality, which includes death up to 30 days following the operation.
2. Length of stay in the hospital following operation.
3. Length of time it takes to return to the patient's usual activity.
4. Length of time the patient was followed-up.
5. Incidence of ulcer symptom recurrence.
6. Recurrence of a proven ulcer (proven by one of the above criteria).
7. Incidence and severity of dumping following the operation.
8. Incidence and severity of diarrhea (consisting of three or more bowel movements per day).
9. Amount of weight loss following surgery.
10. Permanent change in meal frequency and amounts.

6. STATISTICAL CRITERIA

The statistical criteria used in this study are as follows:

(1) The specific aims of the study should be clearly stated, and the total sample size should be consistent with these aims.

(2) The patients selected for the trial should be representative of a larger population of patients at risk of having the operation(s) under study. The requirements for eligibility should be listed. If certain kinds of patients were excluded from the trial, this should be stated, along with the reason for exclusion and the number of patients excluded. On the other hand, if there is a bias toward *including* certain kinds of patients, this should also be stated.

(3) Factors affecting the randomization procedure should be specified in detail. If patients were withdrawn or not given the randomly selected operation or omitted from the study after randomization, there should be sufficient information presented to judge the effect this may have had on the comparison of the treatments. Ideally, there should be a control group consisting of patients with characteristics as similar as possible to those in the treatment groups. For a disease as poorly understood and as unpredictable as duodenal ulcer, this is particularly important.

(4) The treatment (surgical) procedures should be described, together with the range of modifications permitted.

(5) The measurements recorded for the patients must be clearly defined and should be objective whenever possible. The processes by which the measurements are taken should be described in detail and should be consistent from patient to patient for all treatments. Follow-up should be "blind" whenever possible.

(6) Frequency distributions of important clinical characteristics such as age, sex, disease severity, complications, and other diseases in the study population

should be given. The treatment groups should be compared with regard to the most important of these so that comparability or its lack can be assessed.

(7) Frequency distributions of modifications in the surgical procedure for each treatment group should be given, as well as distributions for surgical and pathological findings, if any.

(8) Follow-up procedure should be carefully described. If there is substantial loss to follow-up, the authors should indicate how they dealt with the resulting possibility of bias. All missing cases must be accounted for.

(9) The authors should indicate clearly which statistical procedures were used in addition to reporting a *P* value. Wherever they may be of value in judging the size of differences between treatment effects, estimates of variability (such as standard errors) should be given.

(10) The conclusions from the study should be clearly stated. It should be possible to assess the seriousness of any deficiencies in design or execution of the study from the material presented.

With a few modifications these criteria can readily be applied to randomized clinical trials on other problems.

We discuss several general points here and return in Section 8 to sample size, randomization, follow-up, and the possibility of a control group, giving particular attention to how these arise in studying surgical treatment of duodenal ulcer.

From experience we appreciate the difficulties which may arise in the sampling phase of an ideal study (Cochran, Mosteller, and Tukey, 1954). It is seldom feasible to proceed by first defining the target population to which we wish the results of the study to apply and then selecting for the experiment a study group which is a random sample from this population. It remains true, however, that the most useful studies are those in which the study group is evidently representative of a population which presents itself to others who can use the results. If several target populations may be distinguished, the report should identify them and indicate how broadly the results may apply. Overall, clear statements of the criteria for inclusion in the study and information about relevant characteristics of the patients are valuable in documenting the relationship between study group and target population.

Naturally enough, not all measurements can be objective. A common example in the treatment of duodenal ulcer is "patient satisfaction." When asked about satisfaction with the outcome, a patient may feel that some sort of positive answer is expected. Such a subtle bias could be very difficult to assess.

As a general rule, the papers we have examined could well give substantially more detail on characteristics of the study populations. Simple frequency distributions for single characteristics are not commonplace, and such counts for important *combinations* of characteristics seldom appear.

7. DISCUSSION OF PAPERS STUDIED

In examining and comparing the four surgical studies, the group applied the medical and statistical criteria presented in Sections 5 and 6. Since these criteria were sharpened during preliminary comparisons of various studies, they cannot be expected to show any one paper in the most favorable light. Thus the discussions of the individual studies often point out possibilities for improvement, and space limitations do not permit us to emphasize their numerous strengths.

To aid the reader in comparing the four papers studied, we use tabular form to present information on attributes, follow-up, and outcomes of each one. Since some entries in the three tables are abbreviated, we explain them before proceeding to the discussion of each paper. ("N.R.," which appears in all three parts, indicates that the information was not reported or was inadequate.)

Attributes of Study (Table 11-1)

Most of this information is self-explanatory. "Typical age" is used instead of "average age" because some studies reported median age or some other summary value. The information on "surgeons" gives a rough indication of the level of training and experience of those who performed the operations. "Timing of randomization" is discussed further in Section 8.7. In characterizing "diagnosis" we sought to determine how the presence of an ulcer was established; this is particularly important in analyzing recurrence. One of the critical attributes of a randomized clinical trial is definition of the patients accepted as eligible for randomization. The treatment of this study measure was disappointing in these four generally good studies. Only one (Howard et al., 1973) gave a quantitative description of severity of the disease.

Follow-up (Table 11-2)

A reference to a numbered table (for example, "(Table I)" under Postlethwait) indicates that the information is given in some detail by that table of the particular paper and could not adequately be summarized. Under "timing" the shorthand "1,3,6(6)36(12)" means that patients were seen at 1 month, 3 months, from 6 months to 36 months at intervals of 6 months, and thereafter at intervals of 12 months (the number in parentheses gives the interval length). The entry "blind?" indicates whether the interviewer knew what operation that patient had had, while "independent?" reflects whether the interviewer was someone other than the surgeon(s) involved.

Outcomes (Table 11-3)

The three major treatment outcomes are early and late deaths and improvement of symptoms. As is customary, "operative mortality" counts deaths up to 30 days after operation. "Total mortality" includes later deaths from causes unrelated to the operation. "Success" gives the percentage of patients whose overall result was judged excellent or good on a Visick-type scale (described in Section 8.6).

Table 11-1. Attributes of four randomized surgical studies of duodenal ulcer. (P = vagotomy/pyloroplasty; A = vagotomy/antrectomy)

		Jordan/Condon	*Sawyers/Scott*	*Howard et al.*	*Postlethwait*
Number of patients	P	108[a]	40	100	337
	A	92	39	73	331[b]
Percent male	P	100%	(72.2%)	100%	100%
	A	100%		100%	100%
Typical age (years)	P	49	(range = 16 to 76)	54	46
	A	46		53	47
Hospital(s)		V.A.*	university	V.A.	V.A.
Surgeons		95% residents	authors	90% residents	residents and attending staff
Timing of randomization		before operation	N.R.	during operation	during operation
Diagnosis		X-ray	N.R.	X-ray, acid	N.R.
Indication for surgery		based on "clinical history"	N.R.	duration of pain in years (mostly 5 to 10)	intractability, not defined beyond "usual symptoms"

*Veterans Administration

[a]The original randomization assigned 98 patients to pyloroplasty and 102 to antrectomy, but the protocol was violated in 10 cases because resection was considered too hazardous.

[b]This study also involved hemigastrectomy and gastric resection. An alternative analysis could combine the results for antrectomy and hemigastrectomy.

Table 11-2. Comparison of follow-up in four surgical studies of duodenal ulcer.

	Jordan/Condon	*Sawyers/Scott*	*Howard et al.*	*Postlethwait*
length (mo.) min, mean, max	24,NR,60	12,30,45	24,NR,120	(Table I)
timing (mo.)	1,3,6(6)36(12)	N.R.	N.R.	6,24,60
% loss	14.4 (3 yrs.)[c]	N.R.	N.R.	15.3 (5 yrs.)
blind?	no	N.R.	N.R.	yes
independent?	at 3 yrs.	N.R.	N.R.	yes

[c]Table 1 in the paper gives the number of patients expected and those actually studied at yearly intervals up to five years. Because of an unexplained sharp drop from the number studied during the third year to the number expected during the fourth year, we give the loss after three years.

Table 11-3. Comparison of selected outcomes in four surgical studies of duodenal ulcer. (All values in %)

		Jordan/Condon	*Sawyers/Scott*	*Howard et al.*	*Postlethwait*
operative mortality	P	1.9	0	0	0.6[d]
	A	0	0	0	0.9
total mortality	P	8.3	0	0	N.R.
	A	4.3	0	0	
recurrence					
rate	P	7.4	0	10.0	6.6
	A	0	2.6[e]	3.9	1.7
delay		(Table 9a)	17 mo.[e]	(Table VI)	(Table I)
proof		N.R.	x-ray	x-ray, surgery	surgery
diarrhea	P	(Table 8)	17.5	14.0	20.7
	A		5.1	22.0	21.5
dumping	P	(Table 6)	25.0	8.5	N.R.
	A		20.5	27.0	
weight loss		(Table 7)	N.R.	(Table V)	N.R.
success (V-scale)	P	(Table 13)	95.0	N.R.	83.0
	A		97.4		89.2

[d]If we included related deaths which occurred at 31, 35, 37, and 37 days after operation, these rates would rise to 0.9 and 1.5, respectively.
[e]One patient developed a recurrent ulcer at 17 months.

Jordan and Condon (1970)

Among the patients in this study initially randomized to vagotomy and resection, ten were judged to be in too hazardous a condition for a resection, and hence those 10 patients had a vagotomy and pyloroplasty and were left in the study. The patients having vagotomy and pyloroplasty had the only operative mortality (2 patients) and the only ulcer recurrences (8 patients). The paper does not state whether any of the deaths or recurrences came in those 10 patients who were initially randomized for resection, so it is not possible to determine whether this departure from the protocol may account for the increased incidence of postoperative mortality and ulcer recurrence in the vagotomy and drainage group. The noticeable age difference between the two groups leaves a similar unanswered question. It is worth mentioning that this study is the only one of the four in which the operative mortality was higher for vagotomy/pyloroplasty than for vagotomy/antrectomy.

A second problem is that patients with emergency indications for ulcer surgery were included in the study, and it is not clear which cases of ulcer recurrence or mortality were patients operated on for emergency indications.

A third difficulty is that the percentage of follow-up, though initially high, declined rapidly: 81% of the patients were followed for 3 years, but only 20%

were followed for a full 5 years. This is too short a period of time to determine the true ulcer recurrence rate for either procedure.

Sawyers and Scott (1971)

This brief paper has several deficiencies. First, the study sample, with only 40 patients per treatment, is too small to establish statistically significant differences in rates of operative mortality or ulcer recurrence between the two groups. (Section 8.2 discusses this in more detail.) Second, the sample may not have been typical of the larger group of patients with ulcer disease in that the male-to-female ratio in this series was three to one. Furthermore, there was no breakdown of sex distribution by operation. Third, follow-up time was short: the minimum was 12 months, and the mean was 30 months. This is too short a time to make an accurate statement about ulcer recurrence. Fourth, the authors did not clearly outline their criteria for diagnosis of a duodenal ulcer either preoperatively or as a recurrence. (Only one patient seemingly had a recurrence.) Fifth, no data were given on the incidence of recurrent ulcer symptoms following operation. The conclusions reached by the authors are based not only on their own data, but also on data from other published studies.

Howard, Murphy, and Humphrey (1973)

This is a brief but informative paper. The groups are well outlined and described prior to surgery as well as following surgery. This study demonstrated no important difference in mortality rate or ulcer recurrence for the two groups. One criticism is that the paper does not give the number of patients lost to follow-up. Also, although the maximum length is much better than in the other series, the follow-up is still a bit short to determine the true ulcer recurrence rate. One table (Table VI) shows that patients were still suffering recurrent ulcers as late as 4 and 5 years after their operation. There was a high incidence of recurrence after vagotomy and drainage; however, the numbers of patients in the study were not large enough to make this difference significant.

Postlethwait (1973)

This paper has to be considered together with earlier reports on this group of patients (Price et al., 1970; Johnson et al., 1970); we emphasize it because it is the most recent in the series. It is, in general, an excellent paper and the only one which describes the patients lost to follow-up and attempts to assess the effects of the losses. There is some confusion, however, in indications for operation on patients in the study. In the 5-year follow-up paper, the patients were described as those undergoing elective surgery, and patients needing emergency surgery were excluded. However, the earlier paper (Price et al., 1970) states clearly that half the patients were operated on for perforation, hemorrhage, or obstruction. Thus it is not clear how directly the results apply to elective operations for duodenal ulcer disease. The length of follow-up, however, is admirable, and the system of randomization (Johnson et al., 1970) is also very good.

Finally this is the only one of the four studies with sample sizes which are large enough to provide a good chance of detecting the small differences in rates of mortality and recurrence which are associated with the two operations (see Section 8.2).

8. PROBLEM CONSIDERATIONS

In this section we return to several important considerations and discuss them in more detail. Some, such as the Visick scale and tests for completeness of vagotomy, are particular to treatment of duodenal ulcer but typical of problems which can arise in other surgical studies. Others–randomization, follow-up, aggregation, and sample size–must generally be faced in any study.

8.1 Combining the Evidence from Various Studies

For the operations studied, the four papers selected for review tend to show differences in outcomes that are consistent with those reported from a number of nonrandomized series. In general, vagotomy and pyloroplasty was a safer operation than vagotomy and antrectomy. Vagotomy and pyloroplasty, however, was not quite as good an operation as vagotomy and antrectomy when measured by relief of ulcer symptoms. These differences were small and not always consistent; none reached statistical significance. It would be useful if the results of the four studies could be combined. Then small one-sided effects which are not significant individually might yield an overall significant finding. Such a combination seems initially sensible in view of the similarity of the patients and clinics involved, but a closer look shows that any combination without more specific data than are currently available would be unwise.

What if the comparison were limited to recurrence rates following operations on elective patients only? One problem is that three of the studies have apparently pooled emergency and elective patients. While the overall breakdown into emergency and elective is described, no breakdown by operation is given. A second problem arises when we ask which recurrence rate should be studied. Two clear candidates are

$$R_1 = \frac{\text{number of recurrences}}{\text{total in study from start}}$$

and

$$R_2 = \frac{\text{number of recurrences}}{\text{number remaining alive in study}}$$

A potential problem with R_1 is that one of the operations might have a higher death rate and higher recurrence rate, but the higher recurrence rate would not be evident because too few patients were exposed to the possibility of recurrence. Similar comments apply to follow-up losses. The second rate R_2 represents the fraction of those remaining in the study for a fixed period who developed a recurrent ulcer. Unfortunately, it is not possible to estimate R_2 for elective patients from the data currently available. A further difficulty is that the studies have far from uniform lengths of follow-up. Postlethwait (1973) reports a uniform follow-up of 5 years, but the other papers have various mixtures of length of follow-up which are not always well reported. We discuss the special problems of follow-up further in Section 8.5. Our overall conclusion is that, given the variation of reporting, there is no reliable way of combining the findings from the four studies.

We have become aware that peptic ulcer disease presents an unusual problem for the clinical investigator. The difficulty of making accurate and reliable measurements and the requirement for lengthy follow-up may explain why the many clinical studies published have left the value of the various operations used unproven. Occasionally the conclusions of different studies have been contradictory. It would be desirable if one of the professional organizations concerned with gastroenterology were to publish standards to guide investigation and reporting. Standard descriptions of symptoms (such as duration, severity, dieting, medications, and hospitalization), treatment, and follow-up (including intervals, duration, methods of reassessment, and details of losses), if used by all investigators, would provide a basis for combining different studies, much as in multicenter trials.

8.2. Sample Size

In the statistical analysis of the results of an experiment that compares two operations, the two groups of patients in the experiment are regarded as samples drawn from the much larger aggregate or population of patients about whom we are trying to learn. For any postulated percentages P_1, P_2 of occurrence in this population of some outcome of the operations, formulas are available (Cochran and Cox, 1957, pp. 23-27) for calculating the probability of finding a statistically significant difference in the experiment, at any chosen level of significance, for any specified sample sizes n_1, n_2. These formulas can help the investigator in planning an experiment. In the randomized experiment on the Salk polio vaccine trial (Francis et al., 1957), for instance, the calculations suggested that at least 200,000 children in each group (vaccine and placebo) would be necessary to guarantee a high probability of finding a significant difference if, in fact, the vaccine reduced the risk of paralytic polio by 50% in the population of children in grades 1-3.

Most medical or surgical experiments have numerous outcomes that are measured and compared for the two procedures. Usually the investigator selects from one to three of these outcomes that he regards as most important and makes the calculation of n_1, n_2 separately for each one. The next problem is to decide on outcome values P_1 and P_2 that are realistic. This problem is simplified if operation 1 is a standard method on which past data about P_1 values have accumulated. The investigator can then name a value P_2 such that he regards the difference $(P_2 - P_1)$ as of scientific or practical importance. He can then find the sample size required in the experiment in order to have only a small probability of finding an inconclusive, nonsignificant result if the "true" difference is

$(P_2 - P_1)$ or greater. When there are little past data on the performance of either operation, selection of P_1, P_2 values may be very difficult and the sample size calculation of limited help.

In comparing vagotomy/pyloroplasty (VP) and vagotomy/antrectomy (VA), the deaths (during the operation and first month post-op) are important outcomes. For these deaths the average death rate $(P_1 + P_2)/2$ in the four studies was about 1%. With these low P values, sample sizes needed to "discriminate" in this sense between P_1 and P_2 are very high, e.g., $n = 850$ in each group for $P_1 = 0.5\%$ and $P_2 = 2\%$ in order to have an 80% chance of detecting this difference at the 5% level.

The three studies that reported on ulcer recurrences within 5 years showed rates of about 8% for VP and 3% for VA. Some questions remain since the follow-up period was not always fully reported. If, for instance, these values held in the population of patients sampled by these experiments, the probability of finding a significant difference at the 5% level (two-tailed test using inverse sine transformation) is:

Sample Size $(n_1 = n_2 = n)$	Probability
100	0.34
200	0.60
300	0.78

Thus, sample sizes of somewhat over 300 would be needed to confidently distinguish between $P_1 = 8\%$ for VP and $P_2 = 3\%$ for VA, while this sample size can expect to detect only a marked difference in the death rates.

Analogous sample size calculations are available (Cochran and Cox, 1957) when the outcome is a discrete or continuous variable or when the primary interest is in a good estimate of the difference $(P_1 - P_2)$. (See Chapter 12 for further discussion of sample size and power of tests.)

8.3 Nonoperated Controls

In this section we return to the possibility of a control group (Statistical Criterion 3) in which patients would receive further medical therapy instead of a surgical treatment. This can be justified ethically when intractability is the only indication for surgery, because patients may recover, or their disease may become inactive (the more modest description used by gastroenterologists) many years after onset. In some cases it should provide a more accurate basis of information in choosing a therapy for duodenal ulcer disease. For example, when the natural history of the disease may be changing, such a control group would be an important reference point. If, by contrast, medical therapy had been thoroughly demonstrated to be inferior, then the study would focus on comparing surgical treatments, and a nonoperated control group would be of little benefit.

Our search of the literature did not locate any mention of nonoperated control groups. This may be the consequence of surgery being restricted to patients who have had a reasonable trial of medical therapy and who continue to experience disabling symptoms. It would be difficult under these circumstances to randomize such patients into a nonoperated control group to continue ineffective (for them) medical therapy. Nonetheless, in light of the possible strengthened inferences that a control group permits, we feel that this possibility deserves further comment.

8.4 Tests for Completeness of Vagotomy

The insulin test introduced in 1946 by Hollander has been extensively used to determine the completeness of vagotomy. Hypoglycemia is a potent cause of gastric acid secretion, the stimulus being mediated through the vagus nerves. In 1942, Jemerin, Hollander, and Weinstein reported that the insulin test was reliable in differentiating innervated (positive result) from denervated (negative result) gastric pouches in dogs. In the clinic, the result was less clear: 48% of the vagotomized patients had positive insulin test 10–14 days postoperatively. Lewis (1951) stressed the contrast between the ease with which complete insulin negativity is produced by vagotomy in the dog, and the frequency with which a positive response to insulin is found in man after a presumably complete operation.

On theoretical grounds we must question the validity of the insulin test. The notion that stimulation of acid secretion by insulin is mediated solely by the vagus in man is an unproven assumption. Even more suspect is the corollary that any response to insulin after vagotomy indicates an incomplete vagotomy, as there is no independent test for completeness of the vagotomy. Certainly, incomplete vagotomy or the recovery or regeneration of injured fibers may contribute to a positive insulin response after vagotomy. However, nonvagal neural mechanisms may become operative after vagotomy as suggested by Kronborg (1973), and nonneural mechanisms such as the hypoglycemic release of epinephrine, which in turn releases gastrin and stimulates acid gastric secretions (Stadil and Rehfeld, 1973), may play an important role.

Re-exploration studies by Fawcett et al. (1969) and Kronborg (1973) indicate that a positive insulin test can occur in the presence of a surgically complete vagotomy. The percentage of patients with a positive Hollander test in whom intact vagi were found was not greater than the percentage with negative insulin tests.

Does the insulin test, then, have any place in assessing the clinical results of vagotomy? With the evidence before us, no definite conclusion can be drawn. Many surgeons feel that it is important for them to have some objective evidence that they have indeed cut the vagi. In this situation the insulin test provides uncertain supportive evidence.

8.5. Follow-up

In this section we discuss length, causes of missing information, techniques for reducing losses, and treatment of the resulting data.

The duration of follow-up necessary to encompass all cases of ulcer recurrence following ulcer surgery is not really well established. It appears that, both for vagotomy/pyloroplasty and for vagotomy/hemigastrectomy, the length of follow-up should be at least 8 years. In several published studies (Howard et al., 1973; Goligher et al., 1964 and 1968; Brooks et al., 1975) ulcer recurrences, plotted against time, seem to follow a roughly bimodal distribution with early recurrences coming within the first 3 years and then late recurrences occurring between 5 and 8 years.

Detailed analysis of the follow-up data should include life-table applications to provide estimates of the mean length of time until recurrence or death, as well as the distributions of these events. If the number of patients permits, it is useful to see the effects of factors like age and disease severity on these distributions.

Thorough analysis of follow-up data becomes more difficult when patients are lost to follow-up. There are four principal causes of missing follow-up information: (1) Experiments must be evaluated after a finite length of time. (2) Patients enter the experiment at different times. (3) Patients die from unrelated causes. (4) Patients are lost to follow-up for other causes.

We briefly discuss each of these four problems.

1. Length of follow-up has been mentioned above and in Section 8.1. Studies must continue long enough to allow recurrences to take place. We recommend a minimum length of 8 years. Whatever the length of the study, reports must be completed, and the classical problem of using censored data (that is, data from which a known number of potential observations are missing at one or both extremes) to assess survival curves arises (see the references cited below).

2. Most clinical studies continue for several years during which patients enter the study continuously until an adequate number of subjects has been treated. This seems inevitable in large-scale comparisons of surgical treatments. Among the papers, the study by Howard et al. had follow-up varying from 2 to 10 years for this reason. Jordan and Condon are less definite about the length of follow-up, but their Table 1 (p. 548) indicates new patient entries throughout the 5-year trial. Life-table procedures are designed to handle these types of data.

3. Postoperative death rates have immediate utility in comparing safety of two treatments, and all the studies considered have separate accounting for patients who died postoperatively or died later from "unrelated causes." None, however, makes use of the total mortality in the comparison of the two operations. While it is clear that gastric surgery can be performed with considerable safety, the amount of diarrhea and dumping after operation indicates physiological derangements of sufficient severity to make some excess of deaths among surviving patients quite possible. Careful follow-up of sufficient patients to provide assurance on this point is certainly justified. Deaths from "unrelated causes" therefore cannot be lightly ignored; they may prove in time to be "related causes." Neglecting these patients and analyzing the data as if they were never in the study also bias mean recurrence rates upward since patients who were known to be free of recurrences for some time are omitted from the computation.

4. Patients may be lost to a study for reasons like emigration or lack of cooperation. Price et al., the only one of the four studies to clearly describe losses,

lost over 15% of the patients under study. With recurrence rates as similar as they are for the two operations under study, even a slight difference in losses from each group could render comparisons of observed recurrence rates meaningless. Price et al. performed the useful check of reviewing the records of lost patients to see if there were significant differences in operation, age, condition, or other characteristics and found no differences.

A search produced few references to available techniques for guarding against follow-up losses. There seems to be no substitute for determination. Several Ph.D. dissertations were found at the Harvard School of Public Health in which graduate students taking up a problem 10 to 15 years after a study managed to locate about 95% of the patients previously studied. William Taylor* of the Mayo Clinic writes that they frequently have losses under 5% in studies involving very long-term follow-up. This is achieved by writing letters directly to patients and not going through their doctors; if no reply is forthcoming, the telephone is used. If the patient is not found, a vigorous search is undertaken, including use of bill-collecting agencies, who apparently have experience with similar problems. A loss as high as 15% in a population as well documented as veterans appears unnecessary and wasteful.

There are two extreme approaches to treatment of missing patients, each with its biases. First, it may be argued that if a patient had a recurrence, he would be likely to rejoin the study, so it is assumed that all lost patients are disease-free. This approach clearly results in a bias toward lower estimated recurrence rates. Second, some studies eliminate all data pertaining to patients lost to follow-up. Since such patients were known to be disease-free for a certain length of time, this procedure will result in a bias toward higher recurrence rates. Discussion of similar problems and techniques for handling them will be found in the references below.

A battery of statistical techniques has been developed to try to deal with problems of follow-up (1 through 4 above). Koch et al. (1972) describe methods using techniques developed for contingency tables. The method of Kaplan and Meier (1958) is widely used for estimating survival curves in the face of various types of missing data. Efron (1967) discusses the comparison of two treatments under the conditions discussed in 1 to 4 above. All three papers contain many references to the statistical and medical literature.

8.6 Visick Scale

The Visick scale (1948) has been used by Goligher (1970) and others to evaluate the overall symptomatic state of the patient. It is a four-point scale on which the patient is rated from unsatisfactory to excellent following an assessment made by one or more judges. The assessment may take place once (Visick recommends 6 months to 12 years after the operation) or periodically. The purpose in any case is to gauge the severity of the operation's side effects in a manner which is both standardized and objective. However, the reproducibility of the clinical assessment by different physicians is unknown at present, and the Visick scale's

*Personal communication to Osler Peterson.

true worth is undocumented. (For further discussion of Visick scale see Chapter 10.)

8.7 Randomization

In view of the emphasis given to randomized studies throughout this chapter, some further discussion of randomization and of particular features of the present problem is desirable. This section reviews the concept and implications of randomization, describes its application to ulcer surgery, and examines some implications of a randomization scheme in one of the published studies.

The basic notion of randomization is simple: patients or experimental subjects are assigned to treatments by chance in such a way that each patient has an equal chance of receiving any of the treatments under study. Such familiar chance mechanisms as tossing a coin or drawing a card from a well-shuffled pack could provide the random element, but it is generally preferable to use a table of random digits or some other device whose randomness is reliable and thoroughly understood.

The purpose of randomization is almost equally simple. In any substantial experiment a great many factors may affect the outcome, and differences between the results of treatments are seldom overwhelmingly clear, even after careful analysis. Randomization makes it possible to avoid biases (from expected as well as unexpected sources) which could cause difficulty in deciding whether an apparent difference between treatments is a consequence of real differences between the treatments or is simply an artifact of the way patients were assigned to treatments. Without randomization, conclusions from the comparison are in doubt. It is important to realize that one cannot expect the same benefits from a scheme of haphazard assignment, performed without any *intentional* biases, because the underlying "random" mechanism cannot be well understood, and subtle biases may, in fact, be present. Overall, the role of randomization in evaluating social, medical, and sociomedical programs has been nicely stated by Gilbert, Light, and Mosteller (1975): "randomization, together with careful control and implementation, gives strength and persuasiveness to an evaluation that cannot ordinarily be obtained by other means." (Gilbert, McPeek, and Mosteller elaborate on these questions in Chapter 9.)

In planning and carrying out a randomized controlled trial of (elective) surgical treatments for duodenal ulcer, the basic randomization procedure should be straightforward, but practical problems can arise. Chief among these are the specification of the target population and the timing of the actual randomization. When several surgical procedures are to be compared, it may be that not all patients are suitable candidates for all the operations. In this case, the decision on whether to include the "nonoperable" patients in the population of experimental subjects has considerable impact on the inferences ultimately formulated. Since a patient might often be "nonoperable" because of poorer health, a decision to exclude such patients would naturally reduce the scope of justifiable inferences; conclusions would then apply only to a subpopulation healthier than the general population.

If "nonoperable" patients are not automatically excluded, the timing of the randomization becomes important, and some sort of "escape mechanism" may be required. Three possibilities and their consequences are:

1. *Randomize before the operation begins.* A patient assigned to an unacceptable treatment is then removed from the study. The more severe operations would receive healthier patients, and a bias could favor such operations.

2. *Randomize before the operation begins.* A patient assigned to an unacceptable operation would be treated with a specified "default" operation. As in alternative 1, bias would tend to favor the more severe operations. In the present case, however, it is possible to estimate this bias by comparing patients originally assigned to the default operation with those assigned to it for reasons of poorer health.

3. *Randomize either before the operation or during it* (when complications have just become evident). A patient assigned to an unacceptable operation is rerandomized among the acceptable operations. An unbiased comparison is possible within each subset of operations over which randomization or rerandomization is performed. Further discussion at the end of the section deals with an example.

The central issue in this discussion of timing is the role a patient's condition may play in selecting the operation. It is important to have a clear understanding of the relation between the experimental population and the general population of patients who might be candidates for treatment by one or more of the operations compared in the experiment.

The extensive study reported on by Price et al. (1970) and Postlethwait (1973) provides an interesting example.

> "Briefly, the operations selected for application on a random basis were vagotomy and drainage, vagotomy and antrectomy, vagotomy and hemigastrectomy, and gastric resection. . . . After abdominal exploration, the surgeon determined whether or not the condition of the patient and the pathologic changes in the duodenum would permit any one of the four operations to be performed without endangering the welfare of the patient or compromising the outcome. The suitable patients were randomly assigned by opening the next numbered sealed envelope, and the indicated operation was performed [Postlethwait, p. 387]."

Here the randomization is a variant of possibility 3 above. While the procedure used in this study is certainly a very good one, it is important to realize that comparisons between some operations must be interpreted with care. For example, in using the results for vagotomy/drainage and vagotomy/antrectomy one must keep firmly in mind the selectivity imposed by requiring that the condition of the patient permit the more severe operation of gastric resection. In this important respect the study group is not necessarily representative of the general population of patients who would be suitable candidates for either vagotomy/drainage or vagotomy/antrectomy if those two were the only operations considered.

In this experiment a slightly more elaborate randomization scheme might have provided a basis for broader conclusions. Such an alternative may be valuable when, as may have been the case here, many patients are not eligible for randomization over the full set of operations. Price et al. report that "1,358 patients who met certain criteria were randomly assigned one of [the] four operations. During the same period, 1,630 patients had definitive operations for duodenal ulcer but the type of operation was not randomly assigned" (p. 233). It seems likely that many of the "rejected" patients might have been eligible for randomization over a subset of the four operations. Since the four operations are ordered by extent of resection (and, most likely, by severity), only two such subsets are likely to be sensible: (vagotomy/drainage, vagotomy/antrectomy, vagotomy/hemigastrectomy) and (vagotomy/drainage, vagotomy/antrectomy). One might hope that this approach would yield considerably more information without seriously complicating the administration of the study.

9. SUMMARY AND CONCLUSIONS

Elective surgery for intractable duodenal ulcer offers a substantial focus for a broad critical examination of protocol issues. By systematically studying published reports on four randomized studies which compare vagotomy/pyloroplasty with vagotomy/antrectomy, our group of physicians and statisticians has been able to consolidate some quantitative results on the outcomes of these two operations and to identify several possibilities for improvement in reporting and analysis of results from surgical experiments.

While the relation between gastric acid and duodenal ulcer is not well understood, the prevalence of the two treatments described in this chapter makes consideration of their risks and effects mandatory. The exercise of summarizing the four studies (Jordan and Condon, 1970; Sawyers and Scott, 1971; Howard et al., 1973; and Postlethwait, 1973) in a single comparative table (see Section 7) was beneficial because it facilitated evaluations and at the same time emphasized the difficulties of putting studies on a common basis. This was especially true for follow-up because few of the necessary details were available.

In view of this it is not easy to make definite statements about the overall picture of outcome on the basis of these four studies. Since the results would obviously be useful, however, we attempted to do so for five major outcomes: operative mortality, recurrence, weight loss, dumping, and diarrhea. *Operative mortality* is the easiest outcome to assess; for both vagotomy/pyloroplasty and vagotomy/antrectomy it is acceptably low, and none of the four studies shows a significant difference between the two procedures. *Recurrence* rate is higher for vagotomy/pyloroplasty than for vagotomy/antrectomy, and the difference was statistically significant in the Postlethwait study. For this outcome, as well as for others, we must be cautious: loss to follow-up is substantial, and it may affect these comparisons. Length of follow-up may also be too short. We wish the evidence were stronger. *Weight loss* shows no real difference between the two procedures, but only two of the papers include any numerical evidence. The evidence on *dumping* is mixed, and it seems wisest not to attempt a conclusion. Jordan and Condon report year-by-year data on sweating, palpitation, and weakness and find no difference. The difference for Sawyers and Scott is not significant, but Howard et al. found vagotomy/antrectomy significantly worse (at the 5% level). Postlethwait reports finding a significant "linear trend of less dumping in direct relationship to the amount of stomach removed" but gives no data which would permit direct comparison of vagotomy/pyloroplasty and vagotomy/antrectomy. On *diarrhea* the findings are generally in agreement, and we can suggest a conclusion: no difference between the two procedures.

While these conclusions are a natural product of our study, the difficulties encountered in reaching them are more important and more general. It is quite reasonable to try to reach firmer conclusions and a more comprehensive view by combining the results from available studies. This is, at least implicitly, what anyone reviewing the literature would do; one expects evidence to accumulate as research proceeds. Our attempt to do this systematically and quantitatively, however, leads us to emphasize the problems in reaching a satisfactory and defensible synthesis of evidence from several studies. Often, we have found, the published reports make this process unnecessarily difficult.

A prominent example is the definition of intractability. None of the four studies we examined gave a clear and precise description of criteria for intractability. This one reporting flaw is typical of a number of others, but none of them is difficult to remedy. We conclude that much more attention should be given to establishing uniform definitions and methods of reporting and analysis.

Another serious problem is the very considerable percentage of patients lost to follow-up. If these losses are not drastically reduced, there may be biases of unknown size and direction, and the effective number of patients in the study will be substantially reduced.

In making effective use of the patients in a study, careful attention must also be paid to the method of randomization, especially when three or more surgical treatments are being compared (see Section 8.7).

The question of adequate sample size is intimately related to the problems of comparing and combining results from several studies. If results on key outcomes cannot be combined across studies, then it may be quite difficult to justify a trial in which the number of patients is too small to give a high probability of reaching a definitive conclusion.

Overall, these steps would help a number of surgical experiments to produce stronger and more useful results. We look forward to opportunities to put many of them into effect.

Acknowledgments

The authors are grateful to Paul A. Blake, Pierce Gardner, Bernard Rosner, and James H. Warram, Jr., for valuable discussion at various stages and to John P. Gilbert and Frederick Mosteller for critical reading of earlier drafts.

References

Brooks JR, Kia D, Membrano AA: Truncal vagotomy and pyloroplasty for duodenal ulcer. Arch Surg 110:822, 1975

Cochran WG, Cox GM: Experimental Designs. Second edition. New York, John Wiley and Sons, 1957

Cochran WG, Mosteller F, Tukey JW: Principles of sampling. J Am Stat Assoc 49: 13, 1954

Efron B: The two sample problem with censored data, Proceedings of the Fifth Berkeley Symposium on Mathematical Statistics and Probability. Vol. 4. Edited by LM LeCam, J Neyman. Berkeley, California, University of California Press, 1967, p 831

Fawcett AN, Johnston D, Duthie HL: Revagotomy for recurrent ulcer after vagotomy and drainage for duodenal ulcer. Br J Surg 56: 111, 1969

Flood CA: The results of medical treatment of peptic ulcer. J Chronic Dis 1: 43, 1955

Francis T, Napier JA, Voight RB, et al: Evaluation of the 1954 Field Trial of Poliomyelitis Vaccine, Final Report. Ann Arbor, Michigan, Edwards Brothers, Inc., 1957

Fry J: Peptic ulcer: a profile. Br Med J 2:809, 1964

Gilbert JP, Light RJ, Mosteller F: Assessing social innovations: An empirical base for policy. Evaluation and Experiment: Some Critical Issues in Assessing Social Programs. Edited by CA Bennett and AA Lumsdaine. New York, Academic Press, 1975

Goligher JC: The comparative results of different operations in the elective treatment of duodenal ulcer. Br J Surg 57: 780, 1970

Goligher JC, Pulvertaft CN, Watkinson G: Controlled trial of vagotomy and gastro-enterostomy, vagotomy and antrectomy, and subtotal gastrectomy in elective treatment of duodenal ulcer: Interim report. Br Med J 1: 455, 1964

Goligher JC, Pulvertaft CN, de Dombal FT, et al: Five- to eight-year results of Leeds/York controlled trial of elective surgery for duodenal ulcer. Br Med J 2:781, 1968

Hogan MD: A Study of Postoperative Complications Following Surgery for Duodenal Ulcer. Ph.D. thesis. Chapel Hill, North Carolina, Department of Biostatistics, University of North Carolina, 1969

Howard RJ, Murphy WR, Humphrey EW: A prospective randomized study of the elective surgical treatment for duodenal ulcer: Two- to ten-year follow-up study. Surgery 73:256, 1973

Johnson WD, Grizzle JE, Postlethwait RW: Veterans Administration cooperative study of surgery for duodenal ulcer–I: description and evaluation of method of randomization. Arch Surg 101:391, 1970

Jones SH, Carr J, Peterson OL: A comparison of hospitalizations in New England before and after Medicare. Social Security Bulletin (in press), 1976

Jordan PH, Condon RE: A prospective evaluation of vagotomy-pyloroplasty and vagotomy-antrectomy for treatment of duodenal ulcer. Ann Surg 172: 547, 1970

Kaplan EL, Meier P: Nonparametric estimation from incomplete observations. J Am Stat Assoc 53:457, 1958

Kennedy T: Which vagotomy? Which drainage? Proc R Soc Med 67:3, 1974

Koch GG, Johnson WD, Tolley HD: A linear models approach to the analysis of survival and extent of disease in multidimensional contingency tables. J Am Stat Assoc 67:783, 1972

Kronborg O: The discriminatory ability of gastric acid secretion tests in the diagnosis of recurrence after truncal vagotomy and drainage for duodenal ulcer. Scand J Gastroenterol 8:483, 1973

Lewis FJ: The effect of parasympathetic or sympathetic denervation on total stomach pouch secretion in dogs. Surgery 30:578, 1951

Lipetz S: Gastro-intestinal ulceration and non-ulcerative dyspepsia in an urban practice. Br Med J 2:172,1955

Namey C, Wilson RW: Age patterns in medical care, illness and disability, U.S. 1968–69. Data from the National Health Survey, Series 10, No 70 (DHEW Publication No [HSM] 73-1026). Washington, DC, Government Printing Office, 1973

Postlethwait RW: Five year follow-up results of operations for duodenal ulcer. Surg Gynecol Obstet 137:387, 1973

Price WE, Grizzle JE, Postlethwait RW, et al: Results of operation for duodenal ulcer. Surg Gynecol Obstet 131:233, 1970

Sawyers JL, Scott WH: Selective gastric vagotomy with antrectomy or pyloroplasty. Ann Surg 174:541, 1971

Stadil F, Rehfeld JF: Release of gastrin by epinephrine in man. Gastroenterology 65:210, 1973

Visick AH: A study of the failures after gastrectomy. Ann R Coll Surg Engl 3: 266, 1948

Vital Statistics of the United States, 1968. Vol. 2, part A. DHEW, Public Health Service, National Center for Health Statistics

Wilder CS: Limitation of Activity and Mobility due to Chronic Conditions, U.S., 1972. Data from the National Health Survey, Series 10, No 96 (DHEW Publication No [HRA] 75-1523). Washington, DC, Government Printing Office, 1975

Wilson RW: Prevalence of Selected Chronic Digestive Conditions, U.S., July-December 1968. Data from the National Health Survey, Series 10, No 83 (DHEW Publication No [HRA] 75-1510). Washington, DC, Government Printing Office, 1974

12

Gastric freezing: an example of the evaluation of medical therapy by randomized clinical trials

Lillian Lin Miao

Over the span of seven years, 1962-69, the medical field successively witnessed the discovery, the adoption and finally the abandonment of gastric freezing as a treatment of duodenal ulcer. This experience demonstrates one way the medical profession has monitored and evaluated its own procedures.

Dr. Owen Wangensteen, a leading surgeon at the University of Minnesota Hospital, and President of the American College of Surgeons in 1959-60, first introduced gastric freezing to his colleagues in 1962. The gastric freezing treatment may be described as follows: A patient is asked to sit on a hospital bed. He or she is then asked to swallow an empty ballon which has tubes attached. After the balloon has been positioned in the stomach, it is continually irrigated with coolant for about an hour. During the freezing, the temperature of the coolant entering the patient is maintained at -10°C by attaching the inflow and outflow coolant to a hypothermia machine. This is simply a refrigeration unit which keeps a uniform temperature during the freezing. At the conclusion of the procedure, the machine is turned off but the balloon is left inside for an additional 10 minutes until its flexibility has been restored by warming. Then the balloon is removed.

The physiological principle employed in gastric freezing is a sound one. Lowering of the stomach temperature temporarily reduced secretion of acid. In fact, the freezing is an outgrowth of the gastric *cooling* technique (coolant at 5-10°C)

This work was facilitated by grant GS-32327X2 from the National Science Foundation.

which has been successful in the emergency treatment of massive upper gastrointestinal hemorrhage (Wangensteen et al., 1958).

The Wangensteen et al. report, published in the *Journal of American Medical Association* (1962), convinced many practitioners that the new procedure was a better treatment of ulcer, especially for those patients who would otherwise require surgery. Wangensteen reported: (a) gastric freezing "significantly decrease[d]" gastric secretions; (b) it relieved pain; (c) it was safe; (d) the treatment was simple; employing a specially designed $1,800 apparatus, it could be done on an outpatient basis.

In order to understand the excitement of the medical profession over this innovation, we recall some salient features of duodenal ulcer and its management. "Physiologically, peptic ulcer represents the failure of localized areas of the gastroduodenal mucosa to withstand the destructive effects of acid and pepsin in the gastric content" (Kirsner, 1964). Duodenal ulcer, peptic ulcer of the duodenum, is a chronic disease with a great tendency to relapse and/or to heal spontaneously. Its main symptoms are rhythmic pain, vomiting, and weight loss. From the basis of the symptoms alone, it is almost impossible to differentiate a patient with duodenal ulcer from one with gastric ulcer. However, there are a few differences in the natural history of the ulcers, and it is believed that duodenal ulcer is more prevalent by a factor of 4 to 1 over gastric ulcer (Kukral, 1968). Until 1962, the usual medical therapy, directed only at relieving symptoms, but with no curative effects, was by antacid drugs, sedatives, diet change, bedrest, and/or modification of the patient's living routine. In the case of severe, recurrent hemorrhaging, the only known treatment of duodenal ulcer was surgery. The surgical treatment had an associated mortality rate of 5-10%, and among survivors ulcer recurs in at least 5-10% of the patients, with a minority of these suffering from troublesome side effects as well (Walker, 1973). Therefore, the highly positive initial reaction by the profession to the new therapy was not surprising. Subsequent feature articles and reports in both medical bulletins as well as lay publications further publicized gastric freezing to the medical profession, the patients, and the public at large. Many small clinics across the country immediately adopted the procedure as the standard treatment of duodenal ulcer (Nichols, 1963).

DOUBTS

However, some physicians were troubled by the lack of long-term evaluations of gastric freezing in the first report. One year after the introduction of the procedure, cautionary notes and skepticism appeared in well-regarded medical journals (Brown and Taylor, 1963; Holland and Morkovin, 1963). An editorial in *New England Journal of Medicine* (1963) perhaps best summarizes the view of these physicians:

"One must realize, however, that because of enthusiasm or in response to various pressures, information regarding a new test or therapeutic regimen may be provided to physicians before complete or confirmatory tests have been achieved. This creates a situation in which the physician is in a dilemma. He must decide whether to assume a critical and conservative role in the best interests of his patients or to yield to the urging of the same patients and his medical colleagues to employ the new technique without complete knowledge of risk, complications, and ultimate value."

Further doubt was expressed by a panel symposium on gastric freezing (Hightower and Bernstein, 1963) during the sixty-fourth annual meeting of the American Gastroenterological Association in San Francisco in May 1963. It was recommended that the treatment not be accepted as an approved technique for large-scale use before carefully conducted studies could ascertain its value. As a consequence, a multiclinic, cooperative, double-blind, randomized clinical trial was initiated. This study was to play an important role in the evaluation of gastric freezing.

REPORTS OF STUDIES

Meanwhile, a large number of gastric freezing reports with conflicting results, some encouraging and others discouraging, appeared in the literature. These studies were aimed at: (a) testing the claims made earlier; (b) investigating the duration of the benefits attributed to the procedure; and (c) postulating possible adverse effects associated with the freezing of the stomach. Table12-1 lists studies of gastric freezing published between 1962 and 1969 together with a few of their properties.

Among the studies in Table 12-1, 14 are observational, 2 are controlled, and 6 are randomized double-blind studies.

For the observational studies, the sample sizes ranged between 10 and 185 with 6 of the 14 studies having sample sizes less than 35 (Wangensteen et al., 1962; Berg et al., 1964; Hitchcock et al., 1964; Karacadag et al., 1964; Heineken et al., 1963; Bernstein et al., 1963). The follow-up period for the 14 studies varied between 2 weeks and 31 months. Apart from the finding that gastric freezing produced no long-term suppression of acid secretion, the conclusions about its efficacy were varied. The percentage of patients reporting with complete relief was used as a measure of efficacy. Here results ranged from 13% to 100%, with 6 studies indicating 13-36% relief (Berg et al., Hitchcock et al., Karacadag et al., 1964; Scott et al., 1965; Barner et al., 1966; McIntyre et al., 1969), and another 5 of the 14 studies indicating 65-78% relief (Artz et al., 1964; Bernstein et al., 1964; Manlove, 1965; Bernstein et al., 1963; Peter et al., 1962). In two studies (Wangensteen et al., 1962; Heineken et al., 1963) (including the original Wangensteen study), 100% of patients reported complete relief.

The evidence from the controlled studies (McIntyre et al., 1966; Lubos et al., 1966) (respectively of sample sizes 19, 17 in control groups and 89, 171 in the freezing groups) suggested that gastric freezing is no more effective than the medical therapy. However, one of the studies (McIntyre et al., 1966), was on gastric secretory changes alone, and the only comment relating to the patient's recovery from the illness was "a small proportion of patients [has been] completely relieved of symptoms for over 3 years."

Unlike randomized double-blind studies initiated by the American Gastroenterological Association (Ruffin et al., 1969), which has approximately 80

Table 12–1. Studies on gastric freezing, 1962–69.

Study	*Type of study*[1]	*Length of follow-up*	*Sample size*	*Average age*	*% with*[2] *complete relief & definite improvement*	*Acid*[3] *secretin (compared to pre-freezing level)*	*% developed gastric ulcer*	*% gastro-intestinal hemorrhage*	*Deaths*[4]
Wangensteen (1962)	Observ.	2–6 weeks	19	–	100	100% decrease overnight for all patients	–	–	–
Peter (1962)	Observ.	2–6 weeks	86	–	majority	significant depression over night	–	–	–
Artz (1964)	Observ.	3 months	150	40	72	54% returned in 3 months	1	–	2
Bernstein (1964)	Observ.	18 months	185	40	69	–	2	–	2
Berg (1964)	Observ.	6 months	13	44	13	80% returned in 3 months	–	–	0
Hitchcock (1964)	Observ.	9 months	29	–	14	majority returned in 6 weeks	2	14	1
Karacadag (1964)	Observ.	9 months	22	–	18	100% returned in 3 weeks	–	–	0
Scott (1965)	Observ.	12 months	60	–	21	71% returned at end of 1 year	12	–	1
Manlove (1965)	Observ.	6 months	53	–	78	–	–	9	0
Barner (1966)	Observ.	31 months	91	–	31	26% had an increase in acid secretin	3	–	3
White (1964)	Observ.	10 months	120	–	–	–	3	10	0

(Continued)

Table 12–1 continued

Study	*Type of study*[1]	*Length of follow-up*	*Sample size*	*Average Age*	*% with*[2] *complete relief & definite improvement*	*Acid*[3] *secretin (compared to pre-freezing level)*	*% developed gastric ulcer*	*% gastro-intestinal hemorrhage*	*Deaths*[4]
McIntyre (1969)	Observ.	3.8–4.9 years	85	–	20	–	3.5	5.9	–
Heineken (1963)	Observ.	4 weeks	10	–	100	60% patients had 50% reduction, 10% patients had 25% red., 10% patients had 35% red., 20% patients had no red.	–	–	–
Bernstein (1963)	Observ.	8 months	33	–	65	50% patients had 50% reduction, 9% had no red., 5% had higher secretion	–	–	3
McIntyre (1966)	Controlled study	3 months	Control 19 Gastric freezing 89	–	–	no difference between groups at end of 3 mos.	–	–	–
Lubos (1966)	Controlled study	12 months	Control 17 Gastric freezing 171	–	6 6	no difference between groups	–	–	–
Perry (1964)	Randomized double blind	6 months	Control 20 Gastric freezing 20	–	57 30	difference between groups not significant at end of 3 & 6 mos.	–	–	–

Rose (1964)	Randomized double blind	5 months	Control	17	–	29		difference between groups significant*	–	–	–
			Gastric freezing	19		75					
Wangensteen (1965)	Randomized double blind	6 months	Control	30	44	21		difference between groups significant* at end of 2 months but not at 6 mos.	–	–	–
			Gastric freezing	30	47	47					
Harrell (1967)	Randomized double blind	18 months	Control	24	–	46	4	significant depression at end of 6 mos. in gastric freezing group.	–	–	–
			Gastric freezing	28		76 end 1 yr	25 end 2 yr				
Zikria (1967)	Randomized double blind	24 months	Control	8	–	25	12.5	not significantly different at end of 6 months	–	–	–
			Gastric freezing	8		0 end 1 yr.	0 end 2 yr.				
Ruffin (1969)	Randomized double blind	24 months	32 in true freezing		39	34	without reaching an end point	no statistically significant difference between groups	–	–	–
			78 in sham freezing		41	38					

1. Type of study: Observ. = observational study.
   Patients were treated with freezing without random assignment or use of a control group.
   Controlled study.
   Patients treated with gastric feezing are compared with a group of patients on medical or surgical treatment of duodenal ulcer. Patients in either group are not chosen at random.
   Randomized double-blind study.
   Randomly the patients are assigned to the control and the experimental groups. Sham freezing is the treatment received by those in the control group. Neither the patients nor the attending physicians are aware of the type of treatments received.
2. Complete relief is defined as no recurrence in symptoms of duodenal ulcer at the time of the follow-up examinations (except otherwise indicated).
3. Almost all subjects had reduction in acid immediately following the freeze.
4. All deaths were said to be due to causes other than freezing.

*Difference between groups significant at $p \leqslant 0.05$.

patients in the sham and 80 in the experimental freezing group, the other five randomized double-blind studies had 8 to 30 patients in the two groups. The lengths of follow-up varied between 6 to 24 months. Of these five randomized studies (Perry et al., 1964; Rose et al., 1964; Wangensteen et al., 1965; Harrell et al., 1967; Zikria et al., 1967) two (Rose et al., 1964; Wangensteen et al., 1965) demonstrated that patients treated by gastric freezing fared better than those without the treatment, while the other three indicated little difference between the sham and the treatment groups.

DISCUSSION OF STUDIES

It was difficult to judge these findings. The confusion was caused by the lack of a basis of comparison. There was no uniformity in terms of types of studies, sample sizes, freezing temperatures, lengths of follow-up, and patient selection. The type of patients studied ranged from male veterans (Perry et al., 1964) with severe duodenal ulcer to subjects examined at an outpatient clinic (Lubos et al., 1966). In addition, "the treatment of ulcer is highly affected by other 'personal factors,' such as seasonal variation, environmental stress, the use of (or abstinence from) stimulants" (Hitchcock et al., 1964). Therefore, the evaluation of efficacy of the procedure from observational and controlled studies was especially difficult. Another difficulty with both the observational and the controlled studies stems from the possibility that the patients receiving gastric freezing were likely to have sought the treatment when the disease was at its worst. The natural regression effect of the disease may therefore bias the real treatment effect due to freezing. (The regression effect is a tendency of variable measures to bounce back from extremes toward their means. This is a mathematical phenomenon and does not depend on the subject matter of the investigation.)

The randomized double-blind studies did not agree even though random assignment of patients should control for the placebo and the regression effects. The varying results of the five randomized double-blind studies mentioned before could be attributed to two shortcomings in the design of the studies involved.

POWER OF THE TESTS

Incongruence of small significance levels with small sample size. In the five double-blind studies, the investigators used a significance level of 0.05 to determine whether the gastric freezing patients fared better than those in sham freezing. However, in experiments with small sample sizes (all five studies had no more than 30 patients in each treatment group), using a significance level as small as 0.05 will likely guarantee an insignificant result. Larger significance levels (α-levels) are called for in such cases. However, increasing the α-level also increases the likelihood that the true null hypothesis might be erroneously rejected. The investigator might strike a balance after careful study of the power of the test and consideration of the losses and gains incurred from the various outcomes (An excellent discussion of this is found in Mosteller and Bush (1954).)

The power of the test is the probability that the test will lead to the rejection of the null hypothesis which, in our studies, states that the two treatments are equally effective. Thus, the higher the power, the more likely is the effect sought to be confirmed. The power of a statistical test depends upon three parameters: the significance level, the sample size, and the effect size (i.e., the difference δ in the proportions cured) between patients with improvement in the two treatment groups. When we assess the proportion of successes in a sample of size *n*, we say that the proportion of successes is a binomial random variable. The word binomial refers to the two categories for patients, success or failure. And the distribution of the proportion of success in a sample of a given size is called a binomial distribution. Consider the results from the two treatment groups as two different binomials with equal sample sizes and unequal *P*'s (P_G, P_S: the true proportions of patients with improvements in the gastric and sham freezing groups respectively; $\delta = P_G - P_S$). Tables 12-2a to 12-2d show the sample sizes and powers for different combinations of α, δ, and *P*'s, as computed by Cohen (1969). The sample sizes and their corresponding powers appear in adjacent columns of the table.

Table 12-2a. $\alpha = 0.025$ (one-tailed)

		δ**					
		0.1		*0.2*		*0.3*	
		Sample Size	*Power (%)*	*Sample Size*	*Power (%)*	*Sample Size*	*Power (%)*
		10	10	10	20	10	47
		20	16	20	35	20	72
	0.1	30	21	30	49	30	86
		50	32	50	71	50	97
		100	56	100	94	100	>99.5
		10	7	10	15	10	27
		20	10	20	24	20	48
	0.3	30	12	30	34	30	64
		50	17	50	52	50	85
		100	29	100	81	100	99
P_S^*		10	7	10	15	10	31
		20	10	20	24	20	54
	0.5	30	12	30	34	30	70
		50	17	50	52	50	89
		100	29	100	81	100	99.5
		10	7	10	20	10	69
		20	10	20	35	20	94
	0.7	30	12	30	49	30	99
		50	17	50	71	50	99.5
		100	29	100	94	100	99.5

*P_S = proportions with complete relief in sham freezing group.
P_G = proportions with complete relief in gastric freezing group.
**$\delta = P_G - P_S$ = difference in proportions of patients with complete relief in the two groups.
Tables 2a–2c are abridged from Tables 6.21, 6.3.2, 6.3.3, 6.3.5 in Cohen, *Statistical Power Analysis for the Behavior Sciences*, Academic Press, 1969, by permission of the author and publisher.

Table 12-2b. $\alpha = 0.05$ (one-tailed)

		δ					
		0.1		*0.2*		*0.3*	
		Sample Size	*Power (%)*	*Sample Size*	*Power (%)*	*Sample Size*	*Power (%)*
		10	17	10	30	10	47
		20	24	20	47	20	72
	0.1	30	31	30	61	30	86
		50	44	50	80	50	97
		100	68	100	97	100	> 99.5
		10	12	10	23	10	38
		20	16	20	35	20	60
	0.3	30	19	30	46	30	75
		50	26	50	64	50	91
		100	41	100	88	100	> 99.5
P_S		10	12	10	23	10	42
		20	16	20	35	20	66
	0.5	30	19	30	46	30	80
		50	26	50	64	50	94
		100	41	100	88	100	> 99.5
		10	12	10	30	10	79
		20	16	20	47	20	97
	0.7	30	19	30	61	30	> 99.5
		50	26	50	80	50	> 99.5
		100	41	100	97	100	> 99.5

The practice of using very small α, such as 0.05, results in power values being relatively small, all other things being equal. For example, for $\alpha = 0.05$, $\delta = 0.1$, $P_S = 0.1$, $n = 30$, power is 31%; whereas for $\alpha = 0.2$, $\delta = 0.1$, $P_S = 0.1$, $n = 30$, power is 60%. A small power implies a large probability of making a type II error. This error is the probability of accepting the null hypothesis when it is false. Similarly, the use of small sample sizes also leads to small powers of the test. Hence, by using *both* a small sample size and a small α, one can be sure that the probability of detecting a statistically significant result is very small indeed.

VARIATIONS IN STUDIES

Possible lack of uniform procedures for handling the patients after the freezing. Under the double-blind study design, one could expect similar experiences in both the freezing and the sham groups. However, Rose et al. (1964) and Harrell et al. (1967) reported that only 53 and 50%, respectively, of their control groups would be willing to undergo similar treatment again as compared with the 94 and 80% of their experimental groups. This significant discrepancy between the groups suggests a lack of uniform procedure for handling the patients after the freezing. In fact, of the five studies considered, only Wangensteen et al. (1965) and Zikria et al. (1967) kept their patients at the hospital for at least 2 and 7

Table 12-2c. $\alpha = 0.1$ (one-tailed)

		δ					
		0.1		*0.2*		*0.3*	
		Sample Size	*Power (%)*	*Sample Size*	*Power (%)*	*Sample Size*	*Power (%)*
		10	27	10	44	10	61
		20	37	20	62	20	82
	0.1	30	45	30	74	30	92
		50	59	50	89	50	99
		100	80	100	99	100	> 99.5
		10	20	10	35	10	52
		20	26	20	49	20	73
	0.3	30	31	30	61	30	85
		50	39	50	76	50	96
		100	55	100	94	100	> 99.5
P_S		10	20	10	35	10	56
		20	26	20	49	20	77
	0.5	30	31	30	61	30	88
		50	39	50	76	50	97
		100	55	100	94	100	> 99.5
		10	20	10	44	10	88
		20	26	20	62	20	99
	0.7	30	31	30	74	30	> 99.5
		50	39	50	89	50	> 99.5
		100	55	100	99	100	> 99.5

days, respectively. Perry et al. (1964) appointed physicians for evaluating the results of the patients at home. Rose et al. (1964) and Harrell et al. (1967), however, sent their patients home, and the follow-up evaluations were done by the patients' own regular physicians. Consequently, the Rose and Harrell studies lack control of the post-treatment effects precisely at the period–shortly after the freezing–when the psychological effects were likely to be strongest. Information on the desire of patients to repeat the procedure is not reported by the other investigators who had retained the patients at the hospital after receiving the treatment. The Ruffin et al. (1969) study, in which the patients were kept at the hospital for at least 3 days after the treatments, did not report information on this desire either. So, the initial discrepancy remains largely unexplainable.

If we now regard the five studies together as a group (i.e., with a sample size of 99 in the sham and 105 in the control), the overall conclusion did not favor the freezing at the usual significance levels. (Weighted standard normal deviate for the 5 studies taken as a group is 1.07.) A test for agreement among the five investigations gives a highly significant chi-square of 59.4 on 4 degrees of freedom, which indicates that the studies disagree with one another–that is, cannot be regarded as 5 repetitions of the same study on samples from the same population. Because of the conflicting reports, some physicians continued to employ the procedure. Others abandoned the use of gastric freezing.

Table 12-2d. $\alpha = 0.2$ (one-tailed)

		δ					
		0.1		*0.2*		*0.3*	
		Sample Size	*Power (%)*	*Sample Size*	*Power (%)*	*Sample Size*	*Power (%)*
		10	42	10	62	10	79
		20	52	20	78	20	93
	0.1	30	60	30	87	30	97
		50	72	50	95	50	> 99.5
		100	88	100	> 99.5	100	> 99.5
		10	36	10	53	10	71
		20	43	20	68	20	88
	0.3	30	49	30	78	30	94
		50	58	50	89	50	99
		100	74	100	98	100	> 99.5
P_S		10	36	10	53	10	74
		20	43	20	68	20	89
	0.5	30	49	30	78	30	95
		50	58	50	89	50	99
		100	74	100	98	100	99.5
		10	36	10	62	10	89
		20	43	20	78	20	99
	0.7	30	49	30	87	30	> 99.5
		50	58	50	95	50	> 99.5
		100	74	100	> 99.5	100	> 99.5

THE COOPERATIVE RANDOMIZED CLINICAL TRIAL

The report of the cooperative study initiated in 1963 appeared in July 1969 (Ruffin et al., 1969) and the debate over the actual benefits of gastric freezing ended, at least for the moment. The study had been conducted by the joint effort of five institutions: University of Chicago School of Medicine, Duke University Medical Center, Louisiana State University School of Medicine, Scott and White Clinic, and Vanderbilt University School of Medicine. The wide acceptance of the study was largely attributed to the investigators' great care in controlling extraneous factors which might have biased the results. All five institutions used identical patient selection criteria, freezing procedure, collection of data, and evaluation of results. Both study groups–freeze and sham (control)–in each institution were similar in characteristics of average age, average duration of ulcer, past clinical history of ulcer.

The freezing procedures employed in the control and the experimental group were identical except for the temperature of the coolant circulating in the balloon. The sham freezing even used the same apparatus as the true freezing. Patients in both groups experienced the cold tube in the mouth and the upper esophagus. However, in the sham procedure, the coolant was *not* allowed into the balloon placed in the stomach; instead, two small auxiliary tubes filled the balloon with tap water at 37°C. In this manner, the only difference in the treatments received can be fairly attributed to the cooling alone.

From 24 months' observation of the total of 160 patients in the study (82 in freeze group and 78 in sham group), the investigators concluded that "at no time was there a significant difference in the two groups at any period of follow-up" in all clinical and laboratory observations.

But by 1969, a large number of patients had already been through the gastric freezing treatment. In 1964 White et al. (1964) estimated that 1,000 machines had been used on 10,000 to 15,000 patients. By the time of the publication of Ruffin's evaluation of the treatment, the number of machines in use had risen to 2,500 (Fineberg, personal communication). In the absence of any working machinery of public policy decision-making or FDA regulations concerning innovation and adoption of a new procedure, the evaluations and sanctions of procedures fell upon the shoulders of the medical profession. Through the collaborative effort on a carefully randomized investigation, the physicians reached a consensus whereupon the use of gastric freezing for the treatment of duodenal ulcer was discontinued. This process is an example of the medical profession's successfully evaluating and regulating the use of its own innovative treatments.

SUMMARY

The acceptance and rejection of gastric freezing for the treatment of bleeding duodenal ulcers are reviewed as an example of a therapeutic innovation widely adopted before proof of its value was available. This acceptance was ultimately reversed when the convincing results of randomized, controlled trials became available. These trials were conducted independently by concerned physicians seeking to establish the therapeutic value of gastric freezing.

Acknowledgments

I owe to Dr. John Gilbert and Professor Frederick Mosteller my introduction to this issue. They have given me much encouragement by their continued interest. I especially want to thank Professor Mosteller who along with Dr. Benjamin Barnes, offered many valuable suggestions during the progress of the work.

References

Artz CP, McFarland JB, Barnett WO: Clinical evaluation of gastric freezing for peptic ulcer. Ann Surg 159:758, 1964

Barner HB, Collins CH, Jones TI, et al: Clinical gastric "freezing." Am J Dig Dis 11:625, 1966

Berg M, Geisel A, Necheles H: The treatment of duodenal ulcer by gastric freezing: clinical and physiological observations. Am J Gastroenterol 42:593, 1964

Bernstein EF, McFee AS, Goodale RL Jr, et al: Treatment of post gastrectomy stomal ulcer by gastric freezing. Arch Surg 87:13, 1963

Bernstein EF, Goodale RL Jr, McFee AS, et al: Interim report on results of gastric freezing for peptic ulcer: present indications, limitations, and clinical achievement. JAMA 187:436, 1964

Brown CR, Taylor L: Failures of gastric hypothermia in treatment of peptic ulcer diathesis. J Abdom Surg 5:57, 1963

Cohen J: Statistical Power Analysis of the Behavior Sciences. Academic Press, New York, 1969

Editorial: Current status of gastric freezing. N Engl J Med 269:755, 1963

Fineberg H: Personal communication

Harrell WR, Rose H, Fordtran JS, et al: Gastric hypothermia for duodenal ulcer: a long term controlled study. JAMA 200:290, 1967

Heineken TS, Rich RE, Greifinger W, et al: Gastric freezing: preliminary report on ten cases. Am J Gastroenterol 39:648, 1963

Hightower NC, Bernstein EF: Panel symposium: Gastric freezing. Presented at Sixty-fourth Annual Meeting of American Gastroenterological Association, San Francisco, Calif., May 1963

Hitchcock CR, Bitter JE, Sutherland RD: Clinical evaluation of gastric freezing for duodenal ulcer. JAMA 188:409, 1964

Holland RH, Morkovin D: Clinical notes: complications of gastric freezing. JAMA 186:863, 1963

Karacadag S, Klotz AP: Secretory comparison of gastric freezing and radiation therapy. Am J Gastroenterol 42:604, 1964

Kirsner JP: Facts and fallacies of current medical therapy for uncomplicated duodenal ulcer. JAMA 187:423, 1964

Kukral JC: Gastric ulcer: an appraisal. Surgery 63:1024, 1968

Lubos MC, Viril LC, Klotz AP: A controlled study of outpatient gastric freezing. Am J Dig Dis 11:266, 1966

Manlove CH: Complications after gastric hypothermia. Am J Surg 109:185, 1965

McIntyre JA, Jalil S, Deitel M: Gastric secretory changes resulting from gastric hypothermia. Br J Surg 53:439, 1966

McIntyre JA, Brindis R. Clinical course after gastric freezing: long term follow-up of 74 patients and a review of the literature. Can J Surg 12:210, 1969

Mosteller F, Bush RR: Selected quantitative techniques, Handbook of Social Psychology. Gardner Lindzey ed. Addison-Wesley, Reading, Mass., 1954

Nichols EO: Gastric freezing in small clinic. Priv Clin and Hosp of Texas 4:5, 1963

Perry GT, Dunphy JV, Fruin RC, et al: Gastric freezing for duodenal ulcer: a double-blind study. Gastroenterology 47:6, 1964

Peter ET, Bernstein EF, Sosin H, et al: Technique of gastric freezing in the treatment of duodenal ulcer. JAMA 181:760, 1962

Rose H, Fordtran JS, Harrell R, et al: A controlled study of gastric freezing for the treatment of duodenal ulcer. Gastroenterology 47:10, 1964

Ruffin JM, Grizzle JE, Hightower NC, et al: A co-operative double-blind evaluation of gastric "freezing" in the treatment of duodenal ulcer. N Engl J Med 281:16, 1969

Scott HW, O'Neill JA, Snyder HE, et al: An evaluation of the long term results of gastric freezing for duodenal ulcer. Surg Gynecol Obstet 121:723, 1965

Walker CO: Chronic duodenal ulcer, Gastrointestinal Disease: Pathophysiology, Diagnosis, Management. MH Sleisenger and JS Fordtran eds., W.B. Saunders Co., Philadelphia, Pa., 1973

Wangensteen OH, Root HD, Jensen CB, et al: Depression of gastric secretion and digestion by gastric hypothermia: clinical use in massive hematemesis Surgery 44:265, 1958

Wangensteen OH, Peter ET, Nicoloff DM, et al: Achieving "physiological gastrectomy" by gastric freezing: a preliminary report of an experimental and clinical study. JAMA 180:439, 1962

Wangensteen SL, Barker HG, Smith RB, et al: Gastric "freezing." A double-blind study. Am J Dig Dis 10:420, 1965

White RR, Hightower NC, Adalid R: Problems and complications of gastric freezing. Ann Surg 159:765, 1964

Zikria BA, De Jesus RS, Cunnick WR, et al: Gastric "freezing"—a clinical double-blind study. Am J Gastroenterol 47:208, 1967

13

The rise and fall of internal mammary artery ligation in the treatment of angina pectoris and the lessons learned

Ernest M. Barsamian

In 1880 Langer suggested that "the heart can also be nourished with blood through collateral circulation when one or both branches of the coronary arteries are made impervious as a result of an atheromatous process." Extracardiac anastamoses of the coronary arteries to the internal mammary arterial circulation had been demonstrated in dogs (Hudson et al., 1932). In 1939 Fieshi of Genoa injected india ink into the internal mammary artery of cadavers and demonstrated communications to the periaortic and peripulmonary vasculature. Although no direct communications to the heart were seen, Fieshi suspected that vascular connections did exist between the internal mammary and coronary arteries. He further conjectured that bilateral ligation of the internal mammary arteries in the second intercostal space would cause hypertension proximal to the ligature and would shunt blood through the pericardiophrenic artery via collaterals into the coronary circulation. Two surgeons, Zoja and Cesa Bianchi, ligated both internal mammary arteries of a patient with a long history of angina following myocardial infarction. The patient's angina improved, and he was reported to be well two years later.

Fieshi's work went unnoticed during World War II. In 1953 Battezzati, also of Genoa, while reviewing references on coronary perfusion, discovered Fieshi's forgotten publication and, together with Tagliaferro, reported and confirmed the earlier work of Fieshi (Battezzati et al., 1955). Soon Battezzati was performing this operation routinely, and other surgeons in Europe (Jelinek and Quintzo, 1958; Rieben, 1958; Rieben and Stiefel, 1958) and the United States (Glover et al., 1957) followed suit.

CHARACTERISTICS OF THE OPERATION

The operation of internal mammary artery* ligation is unique in the following ways:

1. In the annals of surgical treatment few operations have gained as wide attention over such a short span of time as the operation of ligating the mammary arteries for the relief of angina pectoris.
2. This operation continued to gain wide acceptance even amidst much controversy.
3. Rarely has any operation had its usefulness questioned at the zenith of its popularity in as decisive a test as that to which the mammary artery operation was subjected. Indeed, as a result of the test based on a sham operation, mammary artery ligation was discarded even more rapidly than it was adopted.
4. Finally, the mammary artery ligation has a classic status as the operation that forced recognition of the placebo effect of treatment–whether medical or surgical–as no other form of treatment had demonstrated quite so decisively. Because of this very simple and clear-cut demonstration of the placebo effect, the logical demand for controlled studies of surgery gained recognition and acceptance.

FACTORS IN POPULARITY OF THE OPERATION

What made this operation popular? Before we answer this question, we should know how a surgeon decides whether to operate. In general, every time a surgeon is faced with this question, consciously or subconsciously he has to weigh answers to the following four questions:

1. What is the natural history of the disease from which the patient suffers?–that is, what is the expected outcome in the absence of treatment?
2. What is the risk of surgery in terms of morbidity and mortality? In other words, how safe is the surgery?
3. Is surgery curative or palliative? One would accept a higher risk for an operation that is curative than for one that is only palliative.
4. Are the chances favorable that a better operation or other method of treatment will be ready for use if surgery is postponed for a reasonable period of time, and can surgery safely be postponed?

The answers to these questions will determine whether an operation will gain wide acceptance. Thus if it is safe, if it is curative, and if the prognosis without surgery is ominous, surgery will be recommended by even the most cautious physician. Although safety was, perhaps, the most important single factor, additional considerations help explain the immediate popularity of mammary artery ligation. By order of importance, these are:

1. *Safety:* An operation that carries a high risk of mortality or morbidity is avoided by surgeons, not only because a basic tenet of the Hippocratic Oath is to do no harm, but the realistic appraisals of internists in practice consistently

*Hereafter referred to as mammary artery.

develop referrals to a surgeon that are in number inversely related to the incidence of deaths and complications in his practice. The internal mammary artery ligation was safe and could be done under local anesthesia. It did not entail entering any of the body cavities and was relatively free of intraoperative complications or postoperative physiological derangements. It could be done quickly with no blood loss. With small incisions and minimal retraction, there was little postoperative pain.

By contrast, direct surgical removal of the obstructing lesion in the coronary artery, whether by endarterectomy or by resection and grafting of the occluded segment, did not at that time gain acceptance because it was too risky, even though it clearly offered a more direct approach than any of the other operations which had been devised for the restoration of the blood supply to the ischemic myocardium.

2. *Simplicity:* An operation that is simple to learn and simple to perform, such as the mammary artery ligation, will be adopted quickly by a large number of surgeons. Surgeons by and large are busy people, and few who are well established in successful practice may be in a position to invest the time and effort necessary to learn a complex and difficult procedure. Such innovative activities would initially be less rewarding than the alternate continued use of familiar procedures. For example, only a handful of surgeons has attempted the total correction of transposition of the great vessels, Whipple's procedure for carcinoma of the pancreas, or the splenorenal venous shunt for portal hypertension, although many years have passed since these difficult and complex operations were first described.

Some operations, though relatively safe, are not simple. A good example is the Vineberg Procedure, which implants the mammary artery in the ischemic myocardium. Vineberg wrote and talked about his operation for over ten years before it received some acceptance (Vineberg, 1946; Vineberg and Jewett, 1947; Vineberg and Niloff, 1950; Vineberg and Miller, 1951; Vineberg et al., 1955; Vineberg and Walker, 1957).

3. *Applicability:* A surgical procedure, even though safe and simple, cannot gain immediate wide acceptance if it is not applicable to a large segment of the population. Coronary artery disease is one of the commonest lethal diseases, and few symptoms are as demanding of attention and relief as angina pectoris. Mammary artery ligation appeared to provide a solution.

4. *Effectiveness:* A major determinant of the ultimate acceptance of an operation for cure or palliation is the end result. Yet effectiveness is a distant fourth as the basis for the early popularity of an operation. Although responsible surgeons obviously care if their patients are improved postoperatively, all too often the assessment following an operation is difficult and subjective. If an "authority" states that an operation is effective (see Chapter 8), then this judgment is apt to be accepted, especially if the operation is also simple and safe.

Since determining the effectiveness of the mammary artery ligation was difficult and initially inconclusive, the wide applicability of the simple and safe operation that brought initial relief of angina proved irresistible, and it caught on like wildfire. The many previous procedures to induce collaterals to the heart from extracardiac sources, including poudrage, which introduces foreign material such as asbestos into the pericardial sac, ligation of the coronary sinus, and retrograde perfusion via the coronary sinus and omental grafts to the heart, etc. (Beck, 1935; Thompson and Raisbeck, 1942; Beck, 1948), reflected the quandry of the surgeons and their desperation. They were ready to adopt any safe surgical modality that would relieve angina. Finally, an enthusiastic report published in the *Reader's Digest* (Ratcliff, 1957) made many patients aware of this procedure and sent them to surgeons asking for the operation. (It is, perhaps, surprising that between 1955 and 1960 there were still patients with angina whose mammary arteries were not ligated!)

ASSESSMENT OF OPERATIONS FOR ISCHEMIC HEART DISEASE

The effectiveness of many operations is difficult to assess at the time of their introduction. This is, in part, because physicians have no incentive to document the effectiveness of medical therapy in various subclasses of a disease until an alternative therapy, such as an operation, becomes available. Once the operative therapy has been introduced into practice, the surgeon may find himself already convinced of its effectiveness, while the physician may remain skeptical. Each, under these circumstances, is apt to consider a random trial unethical.

Such assessment is particularly difficult in surgery for coronary artery insufficiency where, except for the electrocardiogram, which may be helpful but is apt to be inconclusive, the only available index of improvement is the highly variable symptom of angina. Proof of effectiveness should ideally include demonstration that the operation is followed by an increase in collateral circulation to the heart. In addition, the increase must be shown to be greater than that resulting from the disease itself, since the myocardial ischemia of coronary artery disease is a powerful growth stimulant of collateral coronary arteries. Coronary angiography was not available at the time when mammary ligation was introduced, but even today the task would be an exceedingly difficult one.

In general, besides relief of angina, the other desirable clinical indices for improvement (prolongation of life, prevention of arrhythmias, prevention of myocardial infarction, improvement of ventricular function, and ability to exercise) following surgical treatment of coronary artery disease could not be analyzed twenty years ago; the natural history of coronary artery disease was unknown, because surgeons had failed initially to conduct proper prospective double-blind studies, or because adequate instrumentation for proper assessment of cardiac function was unavailable.

THE SHAM OPERATION

By 1958 several experimental studies had cast doubt on the earlier enthusiasm of Battezzati in Italy and Glover in this country. Sabiston and Blalock (1958) showed that internal mammary artery ligation had no protective effect in experimental coronary artery occlusion in animals. Similarly, Hurley and Eckstein (1959) could show no effect of ligation of the mammary arteries on the retrograde flow of the occluded circumflex artery in dogs, nor was there any electrocardiographic change when the central mammary artery was clamped. Skeptical clinical reports began to appear.

Fish et al. (1958) told 24 patients with angina before surgery that the operation was experimental, that it had no physiologic basis, and that surgeons did not know if angina would be relieved following surgery. This was, of course, a deliberate departure from the customary positive suggestion with which therapy is offered. The importance of suggestion is apparent from the results. After an initial improvement the angina returned to its preoperative level in all but 4 patients, who showed moderate improvement. Adams (1958) reported 2 patients who improved following placement of untied ligatures around the internal mammary arteries. Subsequently, he occluded the arteries by tying the ligatures, but the patients had no further subjective improvement. This unique observation, including the use of the patient as his own control–though limited to 2 patients–suggested to Adams that the operation was no more than a form of placebo.

To settle the controversy, Cobb et al. (1959) and Dimond et al. (1958) almost simultaneously carried out controlled studies on patients with angina. In these two studies a total of 35 patients (17 in Cobb's study and 18 in Dimond's) were assigned to one of two treatment groups by a random process. One group of patients in each study received the operation of mammary artery ligation while the other group received a sham operation, an operation which outwardly looked like mammary artery ligation, but in which the arteries were not ligated. For mammary artery ligation, which was usually carried out under local anesthesia, an incision two inches long was made in the skin over the second intercostal space just lateral to the sternum. The incision was carefully developed into the deeper tissues until the mammary artery was identified in the parasternal space superficial to the pleura. Two ligatures of 00 silk were passed around the artery and tied. The incision was then closed in layers.

In the sham operation, the patient was prepared in exactly the same way, the local anesthesia and the skin incision were identical, and the mammary artery was similarly exposed in the parasternal area. However, the artery was not ligated. The incision was then closed in layers. Since all the steps were identical between the real operation and the sham operation except for the omission of ligation of the mammary artery in the latter, any difference in the results between the two groups of patients could be attributed to the occlusion or patency of the mammary artery. Thus, if the group with the mammary artery ligated fared better, the assumption would be that there is a physiologic basis for the relief of angina, namely, increased coronary artery flow through enhanced collaterals developed proximal to the ligature of the mammary artery. On the other hand, if there were no significant differences in the amount of improvement between the two groups, then the ligation of the mammary artery could not be considered to have any direct beneficial effect on angina. If neither group improved, then one would conclude that the operation was of no value.

As it turned out, the result of these controlled studies showed that there was some improvement in angina in both groups of patients–those having the real operation as well as those having the sham operation. Furthermore, the improvement was not significantly different between the two groups. In Cobb's study, 8 patients who had their mammary arteries ligated had a 34% subjective improvement in the first six months following operation compared to a 42% subjective improvement in the 9 patients who had the sham operation. In Dimond's study, 10 of 13 patients who had their mammary arteries ligated reported significant improvement while all 5 who had the sham operation reported significant improvement.

PLACEBO EFFECT OF SURGERY

What is the explanation for the similar improvement in both groups? In the studies on mammary artery ligation almost all the patients had typical angina with positive exercise tolerance tests. This symptom was relieved to an equal degree by the real and sham operations. However, the sensation of chest pain or angina is not a reliable index of the severity of coronary artery disease for two reasons. The first is that the threshhold for pain varies among all persons. And second, even if the pain threshhold were to be held constant, the same severity of coronary artery disease is not likely to produce the same degree of angina. Indeed, angina occurs in only about 20% of patients with coronary artery disease, and, furthermore, a small percentage of patients actually *lose* their angina following myocardial infarction, i.e., when their coronary artery disease becomes more severe.

Angina is related not only to exercise but also to emotional stress. Often patients have anginal attacks sitting in their favorite chair watching television. Some degree of emotional overlay is present in most patients with angina, and the knowledge that the anginal pain is related to heart disease will in itself produce significant concern and emotional disturbance for many patients. All these variables make angina, and its relief, a fickle index in the assessment of any treatment—medical or surgical—devised to improve myocardial ischemia. Finally, to add to the complexity of analyzing angina is the variability in how the physician defines angina and in how the physician interprets the patient's described symptoms.

The electrocardiogram after exercise in the vast majority did not improve following mammary artery ligation or sham operation, even though angina improved. However, in some, the electrocardiogram did improve, but it is well known that changes diagnostic of ischemic myocardium may appear from time to time in electrocardiograms in patients with angina and that such ischemic changes may also clear with or without treatment. Furthermore, the improvement noted in some of these patients could be the result of enforced rest in the hospital.

Improvement could also be the result of the powerful psychodynamics inherent in the surgeon's approach and in the expectation on the part of the patients that surgery will improve them. This expectation was strengthened by the fact that these patients had usually been treated ineffectually for prolonged periods by medical means. They naturally were hopeful and eager for relief and more than willing to undergo any therapy which might provide it. Thus, they were specially conditioned to respond to the placebo effect of surgery.

The fact that patients who had the sham operation clearly reported improvement in their angina demonstrated conclusively the placebo effect of surgical treatment. Numerous operations in the past had appeared to have nonspecific beneficial effects, but the recognition of these as a placebo effect was accelerated by the experience with mammary artery ligation and by the subsequent publication by Beecher of "Surgery as Placebo," in which this term was first used (Beecher, 1961).

DISCUSSION

It is ironic that the considerations of safety and simplicity that facilitated the introduction of mammary artery ligation were also responsible for its rapid downfall. An easy and relatively safe operation to perform, it was equally easy and safe to carry out in sham. The opportunity was, indeed, a unique one, as reflected by the fact that no other randomized comparison of an operation with a sham operation has been recorded in the English surgical literature.*

The improvement enjoyed by patients who had the sham operation enhanced healthy skepticism concerning improvements claimed after more complicated operations for angina. It was disquieting to realize that improvement after any operation might be attributable to a psychological and emotional reaction to surgery and to the many other dramatic events during hospitalization, rather than to physiological mechanisms.

In this light, one might contemplate the possible need for a comparison of coronary artery bypass graft with a sham operation. How much of the relief of angina which follows this operation might also be a placebo effect? A sham operation for coronary artery saphenous vein bypass graft might consist of completion of the bypass graft and then tying it off. This would surely be considered unethical, despite the strong scientific interest in the results of a controlled study of the saphenous vein bypass. Indeed, by present-day standards, even the sham studies of internal mammary ligation as they were performed would not be considered ethical. In Cobb's study (1959) the patients were informed that the operation was being evaluated, but were not informed of the double-blind nature of the study nor of the possibility that some would be subjected to a sham operation. This was acceptable practice then; but with more precise delineation of the rights of patients and of the ethical and legal issues demanding informed consent, it is not acceptable practice now. (For an interesting discussion of the ethical dilemmas encountered in the use of any placebo in experiments or in patient care, see Bok, 1974.)

CONCLUSION

The significance of the classic investigation of mammary artery ligation is twofold: first, it demonstrated unequivocally the existence of the placebo effect of surgical treatment. Second, by questioning the reliability of the usual clinical evaluation of any operation designed to relieve angina, the demand for properly controlled studies gained impetus and spread to other surgical and medical pro-

*See Chapter 12 for an equally successful experimental use of a nonoperative sham.

cedures, such as portasystemic shunts, radical mastectomies, and all forms of chemotherapy of cancer.

Today's ethical standards require informed consent be given freely by each patient. By these standards, the sham operation could not have been done, since a sham procedure, by definition, withholds from the patient the nature of his treatment. Yet, I believe that even more serious ethical questions can and should be raised concerning the introduction of new surgical procedures of alleged benefit without proper controlled trials, as discussed by Gilbert, McPeek, and Mosteller in Chapter 9.

The life cycle of the internal mammary artery operation in the United States from rise to fall was less than three years. This short life cycle is a vivid demonstration of the efficiency of a properly designed study in answering difficult questions about the value of a surgical procedure.

SUMMARY

The surgical innovation of internal mammary artery ligation for angina pectoris provides a unique example of why ineffectual operations may be accepted and of the testing of an operation by comparison with a properly selected control group of patients. These control patients had a sham operation, and the similar clinical improvement following the sham operation or the ligation of the artery established the possibility of a surgical placebo effect.

Acknowledgment

I wish to thank Dr. Benjamin A. Barnes and Dr. John P. Bunker for the helpful suggestions they have made in editing this chapter.

References

Adams R: Internal-mammary-artery ligation for coronary insufficiency. An evaluation. N Engl J Med 258:113, 1958

Battezzati M, Tagliaferro A, De Marchi G: La legature delle due arterie mammarie interne nei disturbi di vascolarizzazione del miocardio. Minerva Med 46:1178, 1955

Beck CS: The development of a new blood supply to the heart by operation. Ann Surg 102:801, 1935

Beck CS: Revascularization of the heart. Ann Surg 128:854, 1948

Beecher HK: Surgery as placebo. A quantitative study of bias. JAMA 176:1102, 1961

Bok S: The ethics of giving placebos. Scientific American 231:17, 1974

Cobb LA, Thomas GI, Dillard DH, et al: An evaluation of internal-mammary-artery ligation by a double-blind technic. N Engl J Med 260:1115, 1959

De Marchi G. Battezzati M, Tagliaferro A: Influenze della legatura delle arterie mammarie interne sulla insufficienza miocardica. Minerva Med 47:1184, 1956

Dimond EG, Kittle CF, Crockett JE: Evaluation of internal mammary artery ligation and sham procedure in angina pectoris. Circulation 18:712, 1958

Dimond EG, Kittle CF, Crockett JE: Evaluation of internal mammary artery ligation and sham operation for angina pectoris. Am J Cardiol 5:483, 1960

Fish RG, Crymes TP, Lovell MG: Internal-mammary-artery ligation for angina pectoris. Its failure to produce relief. N Engl J Med 259:418, 1958

Glover RP: A new surgical approach to the problem of myocardial revascularization in coronary artery disease. J Arkansas Med Soc 54:223, 1957

Glover RP, Davila JC, Kyle RH, et al: Ligation of the internal mammary arteries as a means of increasing blood supply to the myocardium. J Thorac Cardiovasc Surg 34:661, 1957

Hudson CL, Moritz AR, Wearn JT: The extracardiac anastomoses of the coronary arteries. J Exp Med 56:919, 1932

Hurley RE, Eckstein RW: Effect of bilateral internal mammary artery ligation on coronary circulation in dogs. Circ Res 7:571, 1959

Jelinek R, Quintzo G: Belkrag zur chirurgishen. Klin Wschr 70:3, 1958

Langer L: Die foramina thebesii im herzen des menschen. Sitzungsberichte. Akad Wissensch Math Naturwissensch Cl Vienna 82:25, 1880

Meade RH: Surgery for coronary artery disease, A History of Thoracic Surgery. Charles C. Thomas, 1961, p 480

Ratcliff JD: New surgery for ailing hearts. Reader's Digest 71:70, 1957

Rieben von W: Surgery of angina pectoris. Helv Chir Acta 25:298, 1958

Rieben von W, Stiefel GE: Bilateral ligation of internal mammary artery. Schweiz Med Wochenschr 88:388, 1958

Sabiston DC Jr, Blalock A: Experimental ligation of the internal mammary artery and its effect on coronary occlusion. Surgery 43:906, 1958

Thompson SA, Raisbeck MJ; Cardio-pericardiopexy; the surgical treatment of coronary arterial disease by the establishment of adhesive pericarditis. Ann Intern Med 16:495, 1942

Vineberg AM: Development of an anastomosis between the coronary vessels and a transplanted internal mammary artery. Can Med Assoc J 55:117, 1946

Vineberg AM, Jewett BL: Development of an anastomosis between the coronary vessels and a transplanted internal mammary artery. Can Med Assoc J 56:609, 1947

Vineberg AM, Niloff PH: The value of surgical treatment of coronary artery occlusion by implantation of the internal mammary artery into the ventricular myocardium. An experimental study. Surg Gynecol Obstet 91:551, 1950

Vineberg AM, Miller GG: Internal mammary coronary anastomosis in the surgical treatment of coronary artery insufficiency. Can Med Assoc J 64:204, 1951

Vineberg AM, Munro DD, Cohen H, et al: Four years' clinical experience with internal mammary artery implantation in the treatment of human coronary artery insufficiency including additional experimental studies. J Thorac Cardiovasc Surg 29:1, 1955

Vineberg AM, Walker J: Six months' to six years' experience with coronary artery insufficiency treated by internal mammary artery implantation. Am Heart J 54:851, 1957

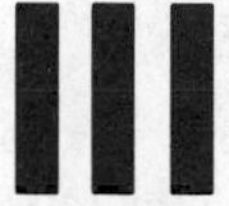

ASSESSMENT OF COSTS, RISKS, AND BENEFITS OF ESTABLISHED PROCEDURES

In Part II we compared the assessment of surgical innovation by trial and error with that which can be achieved by careful clinical trials. If trial and error seems a hazardous and inordinately slow way of determining whether an operation is valuable or useless, it must be remembered that most of the useful operations performed today were introduced and assessed by trial and error. In the chapters that comprise Part III we attempt to assess the risks and benefits of several commonly performed and well-established operations.

We find that the analysis often confirms strongly held surgical opinion, and when it does, we gain experience and confidence in the analytic method. On the other hand, when medical or surgical doubt exists, we find that the analysis may help to provide new insights or to identify where new clinical data are needed. Inguinal herniorrhaphy is an example of an operation for which the indications are widely agreed upon. Yet Neuhauser's analysis in Chapter 14 casts doubt on elective inguinal herniorrhaphy in the elderly as a life-prolonging procedure, and we conclude that the unchallenged status of this operation is based on its effectiveness in improving the quality, rather than the quantity, of life of the patient.

Our confidence in the herniorrhaphy analysis rests heavily on the reliability of the clinical data used. In Chapter 15 Gilbert discusses this issue and presents a method of analysis to test the sensitivity of results to particular values which may not be accurately known, such as the rate of strangulation in unrepaired hernias. Sensitivity analysis also allows us to estimate the effects of critical variables such as age and preoperative physical status. Thus, in Chapter 16, by Fitzpatrick, Neutra, and Gilbert, and 17, by Bunker, McPherson, and

Henneman, we see that the predicted effects on life expectancy of cholecystectomy for "silent" gallstones and of hysterectomy for uterine dysfunction depend heavily on age and preoperative physical status.

In contrast to elective inguinal herniorrhaphy, the indications for cholecystectomy for "silent" or minimally symptomatic gallstones and for elective hysterectomy for symptomatic relief are subject to considerable medical disagreement. Our analyses indicate that in the good risk young or middle-aged patient these two operations increase life expectancy, whereas in older and poorer risk patients, life expectancy is shortened. In both circumstances the change in life expectancy is small. We conclude that the decision to operate in the poorer risk group should be based primarily on considerations of the expected effect on quality of life. In general, few systematic data correlating the effects of surgery with the subsequent quality of life have been collected, and it is for this reason that uncertainty and disagreement persist concerning the indications for many operations.

Another kind of problem is presented by Neutra in Chapter 18. Outcome, in his analysis of appendectomy, can be measured in terms of case fatality, days of convalescence, and costs, all of which can be readily and reliably measured. At issue here is the degree of preoperative diagnostic discrimination and its effect on postoperative mortality and morbidity. Neutra's analysis demonstrates the resulting conflict between a diagnostic strategy that minimizes mortality and one that minimizes morbidity and costs.

Part III closes with Chapter 19 in which McPherson and Fox consider the effectiveness of breast cancer therapy as an example of a well-studied disease whose treatment has remained highly controversial. Setting aside recent developments in chemotherapy, they consider the controversy that has centered on the question of radical versus simple mastectomy. This example is useful because it illustrates what can happen when controlled trials, for whatever reason, are not carried out. In addressing the relative costs, risks, and benefits of the alternative procedures, we are impressed by differences in costs and risks which are large and important, while the accompanying benefits, if they exist at all, are too small to measure. For this disease and choice of treatment, we conclude that the issue is not just that clinical data are inadequate, but rather that the fundamental biological questions underlying rational therapy remain unanswered.

14

Elective inguinal herniorrhaphy versus truss in the elderly

Duncan Neuhauser

The appropriateness of elective inguinal herniorrhaphy in the elderly is not at issue in the current surgical literature. The last known article insisting on the use of a truss as a preferred alternative to surgery in old age appeared in 1947 (Thomas, 1947; see also Coyte, 1942). A typical recent evaluation of the truss is:

"There are very few cases in which (nonoperative mechanical devices) are necessary or desirable. They are for timid people who do not wish to face up to the realities of any situation. Early operation is so simple that it is by all means the method of choice. [Koontz, 1963]"

This elective operation is advised in the elderly because it may save life by avoiding the high mortality associated with obstruction and strangulation and improve the quality of life by relief of pain or avoiding an uncomfortable truss (Williams and Hale, 1966; Guillen and Aldrete, 1970; Ponka and Brush, 1974).

This chapter reviews the available data in order to see what effect the choice of truss versus elective herniorrhaphy has on the life expectancy of a 65-year-old person. After this, quality of life will be considered. To answer the question of life expectancy, one needs to know the mortality rates associated with (a) elective and (b) emergency surgery, (c) the probability of recurrence of the hernia after operation, (d) the yearly probability of strangulation, and (e) the life expectancy of the patient. Given this information, we can calculate the average effects of using a truss and thus running the risk of obstruction followed by an

Supported in part by a Grant from the Robert Wood Johnson Foundation and the Commonwealth Fund and a USPHS Grant (GM-1-8674).

Table 14-1. 1971 Medicare discharges and operative deaths by age with and without obstruction.

		Total	*Age 65-74*	*Age 75+*
Inguinal Hernia without Obstruction (ICDA 550)	% with Surgery	93.6%	95%	91.4%
	Probability of Mortality at Operation	.00519	.00336	.00881
Inguinal Hernia with Obstruction (ICDA 552)	% with Surgery	88.3%	88.9%	87.9%
	Probability of Mortality	.0469	.0365	.0544
Total Discharges		84,995	54,300	30,695

Source: Social Security Administration, Department of Health, Education and Welfare. (See Table 14-4, Appendix)

emergency operation and its high mortality, or of having an immediate elective operation with its low mortality and the risk that the hernia will recur and need additional elective operations.

As usual with such questions, the data fall short of the ideal. The most that can be said of the data used here is that they are the best available in the literature.

MORTALITY FOR ELECTIVE INGUINAL HERNIORRHAPHY IN THE 65-YEAR-OLD

Table 14-1 gives the total number of inguinal hernia patients in the Medicare program (65+) for 1971 and shows operative mortality rates for unobstructed (elective) hernia of .00336 for ages 65-74 and .00881 for ages 75+. Other reported mortality rates are:

Source	*Operative Mortality Rate*	*n*	*Age*
Ziffren (1972)	.002	–	60–69
Ponka and Brush (1974)	.005	200	70+
Vaughn (1964)	.023	300	60–95
Andersen and Ostberg (1972)	.006	668	70+
Guillen and Aldrete (1970) (Review of 5 Studies)	.021	428	Various Elderly

MORTALITY FOR EMERGENCY HERNIORRHAPHY

Apparently, different definitions of emergency herniorrhaphy prevail in the literature. Maingot's (1961) classification is shown in Figure 14-1. An emergency would include obstruction and perhaps incarceration.

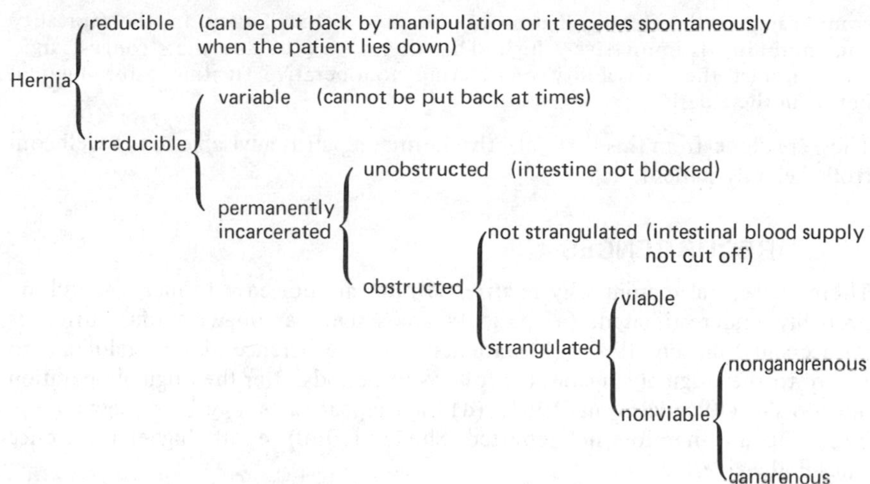

Figure 14-1. Typology for severity of inguinal hernia.

Source: Rodney Maingot: *Abdominal Operations.* 4th Edition, 1961, New York: Appleton-Century-Crofts, p. 899.

Table 14-1 shows the Medicare mortality for obstructed hernias as .0365 for ages 65-74 and .0544 for ages 75 and over. Other studies report:

Source	*Operative Mortality Rate*	*n*	*Age*
Beller and Colp (1926)	.109	46	61+
Frankau (1931)	.197	233	60+
Guillen and Aldrete (1970)	.132	68	Elderly
Andersen and Ostberg (1972)	.138	225	Elderly

We have no good explanation as to why the Social Security data shown in Table 14-1 present lower operative mortality rates than those found in the surgical literature cited above. The Social Security data are based on discharge status and not 30-day postoperative status. They are recent and may reflect improvement in surgical skill. They may reflect definitions of elective and emergency operations. The Medicare data reflect the universe of elderly patients, while the literature reports nonrepresentative samples. Strangulated hernias may have a higher mortality than incarcerated hernias, and the literature may include differing proportions of these events.

The rationalization for elective herniorrhaphy has apparently been based on the nine- and tenfold ratio in mortality rates compared with emergency surgery, without consideration of the risk of incarceration and strangulation. To cite Williams and Hale (1966):

"Since this study has not examined what percentage of inguinal hernias become complicated in the elderly, it can only be shown that if they do, the mortality and morbidity is impressively high. This finding is probably the strongest argument against the advisability of electing nonoperative treatment for inguinal hernia in the elderly."

They conclude from this that "elective hernial repair is advisable in the well controlled elderly patient."

RECURRENCES

There are several reasons why recurrence rates are not easy to measure and are probably underestimated: (a) patients are sometimes unaware of recurrences (Grace and Johnson, 1937); (b) patients with a recurrence may be reluctant to return to the original surgeon, (c) follow-up periods after the original operation are too short (Postlethwait, 1964); (d) high repeat rates may be somewhat embarrassing and therefore not reported. Shelley (1940) reports higher recurrence rates in the elderly.

Source	*Recurrence Rate After First Operation*	*Age*	*n*
Shelly (1940)	20.0	61–80	–
Grace and Johnson (1937)	25.8	50+	1032 (65% follow-up)

Apparently, recurrence rates have been falling. The following studies do not break down rates by age.

Postlethwait (1971)	1–10%	(Review of Literature)
Rostad (1968)	0.5–30%	(Review of Literature)
Gaster (1970)	20%	
Iles (1965)	0.6–8.6%	
Quillinan (1969)	10%	
Koontz (1962)	15–25%	
Zimmerman and Anson (1967)	20–30%	
Ponka and Brush (1974)	2%	(Incomplete Follow-Up)

The current consensus of writers seems to suggest a 10% recurrence rate. Second recurrences apparently occur with higher probability.

Source	*Second Recurrence Rate*
Grace and Johnson (1937)	34%
Thieme (1971)	33%
Clear (1951)	39%
Postlethwait (1971)	8%

Table 14-2. Time of recurrence after previous herniorrhaphy (all ages).

Years following operation	*Postlethwait (1971)*	*Mehnert, et al. (1963)*	*Postlethwait (1964)*	*Fallis (1937)*	*Thieme (1971)*
0–1		33%			29%
0–5	57.1%		68.8%	67.5%	60%
0–10	78.4%		82.2%	81.5%	
All Years	100%	100%	100%	100%	100%
n	300	122	250	200	226

Third and more recurrences have been reported (Shelley, 1940). Fortunately, the analysis that follows is not particularly sensitive to these variations in recurrence rates so we can live with some error here. A 30% second recurrence rate seems reasonable.

When does the recurrence take place? Five studies are summarized in Table 14-2. These studies suggest that 30% of recurrences will appear within one year. 35% within years one to five, and the remaining 35% thereafter.

LIFE EXPECTANCY OF THE 65-YEAR-OLD HERNIA PATIENT

In the United States in 1969 a 65-year-old man could expect to live an additional 13 years and a 65-year-old woman 16.5 years (Statistical Abstract of the United States, 1972). Assuming 90% of the patients are men (Ponka and Brush, 1974; Grace and Johnson, 1937), then the average life expectancy of the 65-year-old hernia patient is 13.3 years.

YEARLY PROBABILITY OF INCARCERATION AND STRANGULATION

The usually cited rate of strangulation of 4% with a range 1.7–6% is not very helpful because it is not based on a time period (Koontz, 1963; Maingot, 1961; Zimmerman, 1963). No writer on hernias was encountered who inquired into this critical variable in judging the usefulness of this operation.

To obtain such a yearly probability, we must seek a population where elective herniorrhaphies are nonexistent. It is likely that nonoperated patients today are an adverse selection of the population (Andersen and Ostberg, 1972) and may yield very biased estimates of the probability of strangulation in the average patient.

Paul Berger's 1880–84 sequence of patients in Paris fits our needs better (Berger, 1896). Dr. Berger ran a truss clinic in an era when elective herniorrhaphies were not done. In fact, emergency herniorrhaphies were done on only a fraction of strangulated patients. His method was to ask each of 10,000 patients who came to be fitted for a truss *avec le plus grand soin* ("with the greatest care") when the hernia had first appeared, and whether or not the patient had undergone an accident (strangulation or incarceration). The accident had to be severe enough for the patient to remember it.

Of all men and women with inguinal hernias, 1.43% remembered having an accident. Of course, those patients who died from the accident would not have reached Dr. Berger. His data show an 8.5% mortality rate for accidents. To correct for this, it would be appropriate to increase the rate by 10%,* so that 1.5% of patients (all ages) have had accidents.

This is not a rate per year of risk, however. On Berger's sequence, 8,633 patients over age 10 had a mean age of onset of 43.1 years and a mean age of presentation at his clinic of 51.3 years. For these patients, there were 242 accidents (plus 10% correction factor), yielding a probability of accident per hernia year of 0.0037. Of Berger's patients, over 90% were for inguinal hernias. Since the other hernia patients had a higher accident rate per patient, the above figure slightly overestimates the risk of accident.

Fortunately, Neutra of the Harvard School of Public Health and Velez of the Medical School at Cali have been able to collect specific strangulation rates for modern-day Cali, Colombia, where almost no elective hernia operations are performed (Neutra, personal communication). A population survey gave data of the hernia years at risk per 1,000 population by age. Hospital records gave the number of incarcerations and strangulations that were operated upon. From these two figures, yearly probabilities of strangulation and incarceration were obtained. For all ages, the yearly probability was .00290, and for those over 65 it was .00291.

There are two reasons why the Berger and Neutra probabilities may be overestimates. First, both hernia populations very likely include people with and without trusses. Presumably, a truss reduces the probability of strangulation, although no data to support this contention were found. If the entire population were wearing trusses, these probabilities might be lower.

The second reason that these may be overestimates is that for some patients their first awareness of their hernia is when it incarcerates or strangulates. Frankau (1931) reports this to be the case in 10.2% of his series of 654 strangulated hernias of all ages. These patients should be excluded from the numerator of the yearly probability estimates. Our analysis has not adjusted for this in order to be conservative in favor of the elective operation.

According to Beller and Colp (1926), "the length of time that a patient has a hernia bears no relationship to the incidence of strangulation." According to Williams and Hale (1966), "there are no reliable guides for predicting which will become complicated." If emergencies were predictable, the analysis that follows would be different. We will consider the effect of assuming that strangulation will occur within the first year following the occurrence of the hernia.

THE ANALYSIS: TRUSS VERSUS ELECTIVE OPERATION

In order to simplify our analysis, the following assumptions have been made. The effect of relaxing these assumptions will be discussed later.

Two sets of numbers have been used. The first uses those values which system-

*10% was chosen instead of 8.5% in order to be conservative.

atically place the benefit of the doubt in a direction favorable to the elective operation. (This is the conservative test of the hypothesis that the truss prolongs life.) The second set of numbers is based on what seems the most reasonable and reliable data.

The patient is assumed to be 65 years old and in the absence of hernia associated mortality will live 13.3 years. This, of course, is an average, and some patients could at age 65 be predicted to live more or less than this average. On the average, patients older than 65 have a shorter life expectancy so if we fail to demonstrate the life saving nature of the elective operation for the average 65-year-old, we have also done the same for older patients.

Strangulation is assumed to be an independent event that occurs if operated upon only once. The probability of strangulation is so low that the error here is exceedingly small. The decision analysis that follows is not at all sensitive to multiple strangulations.

All strangulated and incarcerated hernias go to surgery. All recurring hernias in the elective branch go to surgery.

Only truss versus elective operation is considered. There are insufficient data to consider a "do nothing" third alternative.

For the elective branch, the decision will be to operate without delay. For this reason, the chance of strangulation in the elective branch is negligible.

Given the patient has a truss, if a strangulation occurs, it will occur midway between day 1 and death 13.3 years later.

Given a .0037 yearly probability of strangulation, then for 13.3 years the cumulative probability of strangulation is:

$$1 - (1 - .0037)^{13.3} = .0481$$

Given a .00291 yearly probability of strangulation, then the cumulative probability of strangulation is:

$$1 - (1 - .00291)^{13.3} = .0380$$

THE VALUE OF A YEAR OF LIFE

The simplest democratic assumption is to give the value of 1.0 to each and every year of life. A more sophisticated approach would be to value each year of life beyond age 65 at less and less under the assumption that the year 65-66 is on the average to be preferred to the year 75-76. Years of life saved in the future have not been discounted. By not making either of these adjustments, we give the benefit to the elective operation which risks losing proportionally more younger years of life.

THE DECISION TREES

The decision trees are shown in Figures 14-2 and 14-3 for the conservative test and the most reasonable estimates respectively (Raiffa, 1970; McCreary, 1967). The decision tree starts on the left with the "choice node" square which is the

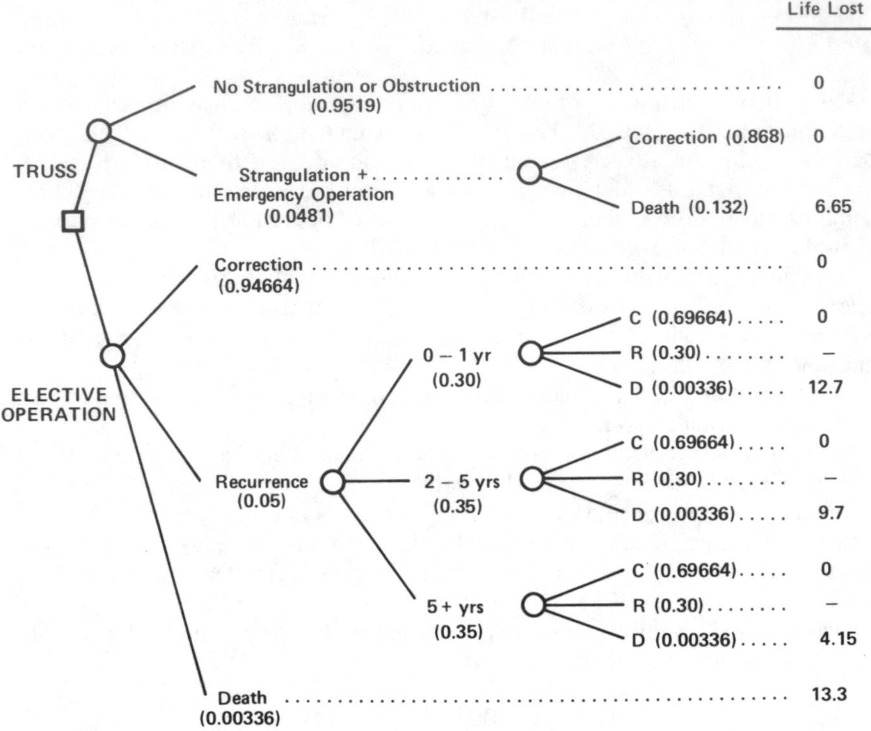

Figure 14-2. Decision tree: truss versus elective operation in the 65-year-old—the conservative test (benefit of the doubt given in favor of the elective operation).

Calculation of Expected Values (Probabilities × Years of Life Lost)

Truss	(.0481)(.132)(6.65) = .0422		
Elective Operation:	First Operation	(.00336)(13.3)	= .04469
	Recurrences:	(.05)(.30)(.00336)(12.7)	= .00064
		(.05)(.35)(.00336)(9.7)	= .00057
		(.05)(.35)(.00336)(4.15)	= .00024
	Total for Elective Operation		= .04614

departure point for the two "branches" of truss and elective herniorrhaphy. The circles indicate "chance nodes" and indicate the unpredictable events that can befall the patient. Probabilities for these events are assigned and must sum to 1.00. To the right are the "payoffs" which are the average years of life lost. These trees have not been fully "grown" in that third recurrences have been excluded for the reason that they have a negligible effect on the results. Thus, the payoffs for these three branches are left out. Multiplying the probabilities by the payoffs gives the "expected value" for each branch. Here, the expected value is the average years of life lost for the average patient undergoing the events that the branch defines. The expected values are then summed for the

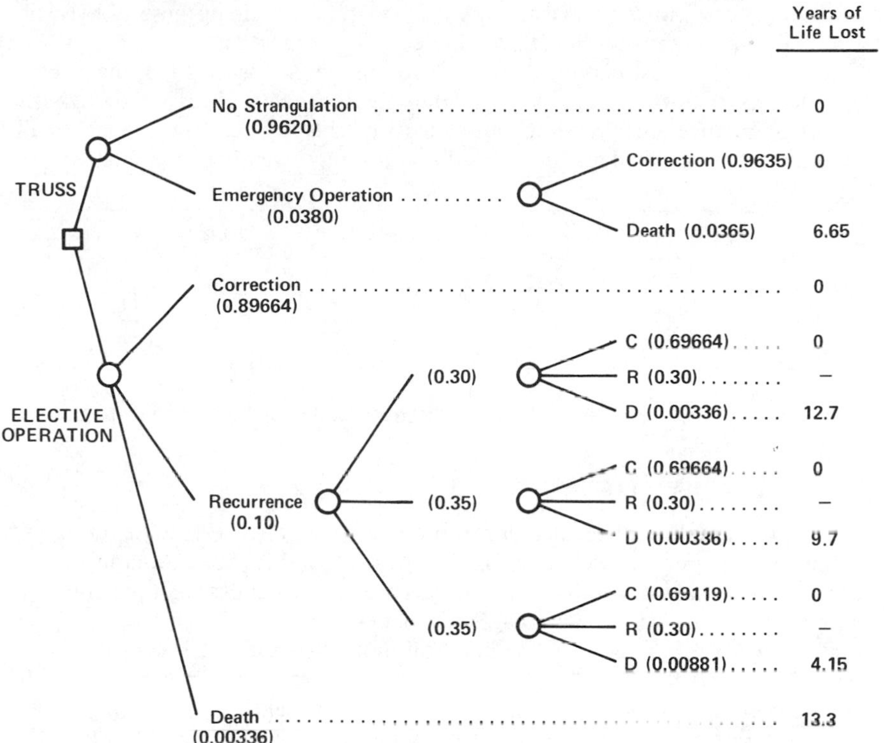

Figure 14-3. Decision tree: truss versus elective operation in the 65-year-old—most reasonable comparison.

Calculation of Expected Values

Truss	(.0380)(.0365)(6.65) = .00922		
Elective Operation:	First Operation	(.00336)(13.3)	= .04469
	Recurrences:	(.10)(.30)(.00336)(12.7)	= .00128
		(.10)(.35)(.00336)(9.7)	= .00114
		(.10)(.35)(.00881)(4.15)	= .00128
	Total for Elective Operation		= .04839

two choices, truss and elective operation, to obtain the overall expected value. The higher this value the greater the average loss of life.

RESULTS

The Conservative Test shows that the elective operation has a higher loss of life than the truss for the 65-year-old. Since life expectancy declines with age we have therefore shown that the same is true for the average person who is older than 65. The conservative test has been used to make the strongest case for the elective operation because this is the standard of surgical practice uniformly proposed by the current surgical literature. In spite of this purposeful bias, the elective operation fails to show that it increases life expectancy.

Turning to the most reasonable comparison shown in Figure 14-3, the elective operation has a mortality that is 5 1/2 times greater than the truss. Although this is a large relative difference in outcome, the absolute differences are small. Translating the expected loss of years of life into days we obtain:

			Expected Days of Life Lost
Truss	.00922 × 365	=	3.37
Elective Operation	.04839 × 365	=	17.66
Difference in favor of truss		=	14.29

The absolute difference is 14.29 days which, spread over 13.3 years, is negligible.

QUALITY OF LIFE

Because the absolute difference in mortality is so small, the issue of quality of life becomes important. Some hernias are painful, and for some, wearing a truss is inconvenient and uncomfortable. Other hernias are painless and patients may not even know they have a hernia. Some patients do not wish to have an operation, while for other patients, an operation that will avoid 13.3 years of wearing a truss is well worth it.

One noted Boston surgeon who once used a truss said they are "dirty, tight, uncomfortable, hot and smelly," and he would not wish the elderly, who suffer as it is, to be compelled to use them. Another surgeon, 69 years old and retired, had a painless hernia and preferred to avoid an operation. For him, the truss was the preferred choice. But whatever the patient's choice, it is apt to be strongly felt. Inguinal hernia in men is likely to have strong sexual implications, and the wearing of a truss may represent a humiliating affront to self-image, to be concealed along with false teeth, and to be corrected even at considerable risk.

This raises the interesting philosophical question. Would you prefer a shorter high-quality life or a longer low-quality life? It is not clear that there is one right answer to this. It would seem that the correct approach would be to present these two alternatives to the patient and let him decide. It might be helpful to have the patient try a truss for a month or two to see what it is like.

COMPLIANCE

Will the patient wear the truss? Should he? For all we know, it may not be necessary for some elderly people to wear a truss. This might be the most fruitful area for research. What is the yearly probability of strangulation or obstruction with and without a truss? For the sedentary elderly, a truss may not be necessary. This may have an important effect on the quality of life, which apparently is the real issue here.

COSTS

The elective route is clearly more costly to the government but not perhaps for the insured patient. Using the Medicare data, the costs can be estimated as follows:

	Length of Stay × *Per Diem Cost*	+ *Surgeon's Fee*	= *Total*
Elective Operation	8.9 × $100	+ $300	= $1,190
Emergency Operation	11.1 × $100	+ $300	= $1,410
Cost of Truss (estimate)			= $50

Since the emergency operation occurs on the average 6.65 years in the future, discounting by 10%, the present value of the emergency operation is $770.* The discounted value of the average first recurrence is $539. Therefore, the average costs of the two branches are:

		Costs 10% Discount Rate	*Costs No Discounting*
Truss 50 + (.0380) (770)	=	79.26	103.58
Elective Operation 1190 + .10 (539) (one recurrence)	=	1,243.90	1,309.00
Difference:		$1,164.64	$1,205.42

For the 76,505 elective operations paid for by Medicaid, this would reduce their total costs from $95,164,569 to $6,063,786, a savings of $89 million per year. However, this may allow the elderly to die in other more expensive ways.

For this $95.1 million, the net total effect on life expectancy is to eliminate a maximum of 3073 years of life in the elderly per year.**

The interesting public policy question is whether this is worth it, since we are not paying to prolong life but, if anything, to improve quality of life. There are many nonhealth care substitutes that the government could provide to the elderly that might improve quality even more. For example, the government could prove $89 million worth of free movies or reduced subway fares. The choice is not obvious. Another approach would be to offer the patient a choice: the elective operation or $1,164.64 in cash and a free truss.

THE PERFECT SURGEON

What is the upper limit in improved mortality that could be obtained from the elective operation? How much return could we possibly get from making an all out effort to improve this choice? To assess this, the perfect surgeon is worthy of our consideration. He or she would have zero elective mortality and zero

*Other discount rates could be used, but as the analysis shows, costs are not particularly sensitive to the discount rate.

**Maximum because this assumes all the elderly have a 13.3 year life expectancy without the risk associated with their hernia.

recurrence rate.* The difference in costs would then be $1,190 less $79.26 or $1,110.74, and the savings in mortality would be .00922 years per patient. This is a cost-per-year of life saved of $120,471. We will never be able to reduce the costs below this rather high amount.

SENSITIVITY ANALYSIS

For small changes in some of the variables, the mortality results may be different. The only variable that seems likely to change the results is the yearly probability of strangulation. It is not the patient's calendar age that matters, rather, it is his life expectancy. Some patients might be expected to live more than 13.3 years. What length of expected life would make the elective operation preferable?

Given the .00291 yearly probability of strangulation, surprisingly, age does not make much difference in the choice. At a life expectancy of 64 more years, the truss still has a lower mortality. At a life expectancy of 80 years, the elective operation only saves 2 days in life in this 80-year time span. This sounds as if elective operation is never life-saving. We hesitate to go so far. One reason is that with such a long life expectancy, the choice now becomes sensitive to the time of strangulation. If the strangulation is most likely in the two decades following the onset of the hernia, then the truss will shorten life. Another reason for hesitancy is that we have no knowledge of the relative operative mortality rates for earlier ages. We would like to defer judgment about the benefits of elective operation in the young until further data are available.

MODELING THE DECISION PROCESS

The reader is urged to "plug in" his own values to this analysis and find out what happens to the results.

Consider, for example, the idea that if a hernia is to strangulate, it will do so soon after it appears. The logic behind this idea is that at first the opening is small and more likely to obstruct and strangulate. No evidence sufficient to support or deny this hypothesis was found. However, we can restructure our analysis accordingly. To approximate this, we can change the payoff associated with truss → strangulation → death from 6.65 to 12.8 years of life lost. This assumes that strangulation, if it is to occur, will in the year after occurrence of the hernia. The expected value of the truss for the most reasonable comparison (Figure 14-3) then becomes:

$$(.0380)\,(.0365)\,(12.8) = .01775$$

which is still much below the expected value for the elective operation (.04839).

Thus, this has a negligible effect on the result.

*Some recurrences may not be due to surgical failure but rather to the patient's condition. The assumption here is that elimination of all recurrences is the limit. Neither zero mortality nor zero recurrence is possible.

The analysis, as shown, assumes that each year of life has equal value. The year 65-66 is given the same value as the year 75-76. Other alternatives are possible but do not effect the results greatly. For example, valuing the year 65-66 at 1.0, valuing the year 66-67 at .95, the year 67-68 at .90, and so on, yields a result not much different from that shown in Figure 14-2. The more the early years are weighted heavily, the more the truss is preferred. But weighting the later years heavily does not make the elective route preferable. However, these variations combined with considerations of quality of life associated with the use of a truss might shift the choice for some individuals.

DECISION ANALYSIS, RANDOMIZED CLINICAL TRIALS, AND CLINICAL JUDGMENTS

Would it be worth investing in the definitive randomized clinical trial to compare truss with elective operation in order to avoid reliance on doubtful data gathered from here and there? Given the sample size required to show a statistically significant difference in life expectancy and the decade or two required for follow-up, such a trial may well be an excessive expenditure. It might be more useful to study the yearly probability of strangulation, if the analysis is so sensitive to this variable. Perhaps the one remaining question of major interest is the differential yearly probability of strangulation with and without a truss.*

Although this decision can be analyzed in much more detail, it will never be a complete substitute for the physician's clinical judgment. For example: How well does this patient understand the alternatives? What is the estimate of this patient's risk, life expectancy, recurrence rates, and such? Will a truss interfere with this patient's sex life? Does the patient fear surgery or look forward to it?

Is this patient a sedentary city dweller or a physically active worker who lives two days away from the nearest surgery? Is this a patient who desperately wishes to live for 2 more years but is indifferent to living or dying thereafter?

Although all these considerations could be included in a decision analysis that would be specific to each patient, the best approach may be to have the physician aware of the basic alternatives presented here. Knowing this, the thoughtful physician has enough good sense to use this analysis as a departure point for the consideration of each patient, one by one.

Because the formal analysis here does not take quality of life into account, does that mean it is unimportant? Not at all. In fact, the analysis, by demonstrating the trivial differences in mortality, shows the possibly overwhelming importance of quality of life to this decision. There are two reasons why this analysis has only explicitly considered mortality. First, mortality can be generalized to all patients, while an analysis based on quality of life trade-offs would be meaningful for only one patient at a time. Second, the impact of this analysis was felt to be greater because of the concreteness of its payoffs measured in loss of life.

*The value of decision analysis may be that it pinpoints those areas where clinical research should be pursued; where a limited research budget might be committed. It is doubtful that this question of differential yearly strangulation, with and without a truss, would come to anyone's mind as the major unanswered question without proceeding through this analysis.

SUMMARY

The best available data on elective inguinal herniorrhaphy indicate that this does not prolong life in the elderly. It may or may not improve the quality of life. The only really important variable that will change this is the yearly probability of strangulation.

What has changed this picture from an era of 30 or more years ago is the surgeon's ability to reduce the mortality of the emergency operation. Surgeons are now so skillful that they have eliminated the need for the elective operation to save lives in the elderly.

APPENDIX

Table 14-3. Summary of data used for analysis of truss versus hernia.

	*Conservative Test**	*Most Reasonable Comparison*
Yearly Probability of Strangulation and Obstruction	.0037	.00291**
Mortality associated with Elective Operation	.00336	.00336
Mortality associated with Late Recurrence	.00336	.00881
Mortality associated with Obstruction	.132	.0365
First Recurrence Rate	.05	.10
Second Recurrence Rate	.20	.30
Time of Recurrence:		
0–1 Years	.30	.30
2–5 Years	.35	.35
5+ Years	.35	.35

*Bias in favor of elective operation.

**This, too, is conservative because it does not adjust for strangulations that are simultaneous with the first appearance of the hernia.

Table 14–4. Number of Medicare discharges and average length of stay by age for discharges from short-stay hospitals with inguinal hernia with and without obstruction (ICDA 550 and 552), January–December 1971.

	Total		*65–74*		*75 +*	
Diagnosis and discharge characteristics	*Number of discharges*	*Average length of stay*	*Number of discharges*	*Average length of stay*	*Number of discharges*	*Average length of stay*
Inguinal hernia without obstruction (ICDA 550)						
Total	76,505	8.9	50,755	8.3	25,750	10.1
One diagnosis	48,415	7.8	32,925	7.5	15,490	8.6
Two or more diagnoses	28,090	10.8	17,830	9.9	10,260	12.4
With surgery	71,615	8.9	48,080	8.3	23,535	10.0
Without surgery	4,890	10.0	2,675	9.1	2,215	11.1
Discharged alive	76,110	8.9	50,585	8.3	25,525	10.0
Discharged dead	395	14.8	170	8.9	225	19.3
Operative Mortality	.00519		.00336		.00881	
Inguinal hernia with obstruction (ICDA 552)						
Total	8,490	11.1	3,545	10.5	4,945	11.5
One diagnosis	4,615	9.2	1,950	8.6	2,665	9.6
Two or more diagnoses	3,875	13.4	1,595	12.9	2,280	13.6
With surgery	7,495	11.4	3,150	10.8	4,345	11.9
Without surgery	995	8.6	395	8.6	600	8.6
Discharged alive	8,110	11.0	3,420	10.3	4,690	11.5
Discharged dead	380	13.5	125	17.8	255	11.3
Operative Mortality	.0469		.0365		.0544	

Source: Social Security Administration, Department of Health, Education and Welfare.

References

Andersen B, Ostberg J: Long term prognosis in geriatric surgery: 2–17 year follow-up of 7922 patients. J Am Geriatr Soc 20:255, 1972

Beller A, Colp R: Strangulated hernia from the standpoint of the viability of the intestinal contents. Arch Surg 12:901, 1926

Berger P: Résultats de l'Examen de Dix Mille Observations de Hernies. Paris, Extrait du neuvième congres français de chirurgie 1895, 1896

Clear J: Ten year statistical study of inguinal hernias. Arch Surg 62:70, 1951

Coyte R: The non-operative treatment of hernias: trusses and belts. Practitioner 149:312, 1942

Fallis LS: Recurrent inguinal hernia: an analysis of 200 operations. Ann Surg 106:363, 1937

Frankau C: Strangulated hernia: a review of 1487 cases. Br J Surg 19:176, 1931

Gaster J: Hernia: One Day Repair. New York, Hafner Publishing Company, 1970

Glassow F: Recurrent inguinal and femoral hernia: 3000 cases. Can J Surg 7:284, 1964

Grace RR, Johnson VS: Results of herniotomy in patients of more than 50 years of age. Ann Surg 106:347, 1937

Guillen J, Aldrete JA: Anesthetic factors influencing morbidity and mortality of elderly patients undergoing inguinal herniorrhaphy. Am J Surg 120:760, 1970

Iles JDH: Specialisation in elective herniorrhaphy. Lancet 1:751, 1965

Koontz AR: Resection of the cord in inguinal hernia repair. Current Medical Digest 29:65, 1962

Koontz AR: Hernia. New York, Appleton-Century-Crofts, 1963

Maingot R: Abdominal Operations. 4th edition, New York, Appleton-Century-Crofts, 1961, p 899

McCreary E: How to grow a decision tree. Think 33:13, 1967

Mehnert JH, Brown MJ, Kroutil W, et al: Indirect recurrences of inguinal hernias. Am J Surg 106:958, 1963

Ponka JL, Brush BE: Experiences with the repair of groin hernia in 200 patients aged 70 or older. J Am Geriatr Soc 22:18, 1974

Postlethwait RW: Recurrent inguinal hernia. Am J Surg 107:739, 1964

Postlethwait RW: Causes of recurrence after inguinal herniorrhaphy. Surgery 69:772, 1971

Quillinan RH: Repair of recurrent inguinal hernia. Am J Surg 118:593, 1969

Raiffa H: Decision Analysis. Reading, Massachusetts, Addison-Wesley, 1970

Ravitch M: Repair of Hernias. Chicago, Yearbook Medical Publishers, 1969

Rostad H: Inguinal hernia in adults. Acta Chir Scand 134:49, 1968

Shelley HJ: Incomplete indirect inguinal hernias: a study of 2462 hernias and 2337 hernia repairs. Arch Surg 41:747, 1940

Social Security Administration, Office of Research and Statistics: Personal communication. Based on one in twenty sample of discharges.

Statistical Abstract of the United States. Washington DC, Government Printing Office, 1972, Table 72, p 56

Thieme ET: Recurrent inguinal hernia. Arch Surg 103:238, 1971

Thomas TM: The use and abuse of trusses. Practitioner 159:388, 1947

Vaughn AK: quoted in Nyhus LM and Harkins HN: Hernia. Philadelphia, JB Lippincott Company, 1964

Williams JS, Hale HW: The advisability of inguinal herniorrhaphy in the elderly. Surg Gynecol Obstet 122:100, 1966

Ziffren SE: Surgery after sixty? Emergency Medicine 4(7):74, 1972

Zimmerman LM: External and internal abdominal hernias. Am J Gastroenterol 40:405, 1963

Zimmerman LM, Anson B: Anatomy and Surgery of Hernia. Second edition. Baltimore, Williams and Wilkins, 1967

15

Sensitivity analysis of elective herniorrhaphy

John P. Gilbert

One method of investigating the implications of policy decisions simulates the process under consideration by using a computer program, and then uses this program to determine the effects of different policies. This procedure is, of course, only as good as the algorithm used in the program, and so, to be convincing, this underlying model should be accurately and explicitly defined. Factors not included in the model cannot influence the results obtained. If an explicit model of the process can be faithfully translated into a computer program, the computer can be used to explore the effects of an almost endless variety of input parameters upon the model. Such programs can be used in several ways. One of these, the one considered here, is to investigate the sensitivity of the outcome to the particular values used in the analysis. A second use tests how well the theoretical understanding of a process, as exemplified by the computer program, can predict the outcomes observed in practice.

METHODS

To illustrate these ideas a computer program is described that simulates the model set up by Neuhauser in Chapter 14 for analyzing the relative risk of elective herniorrhaphy versus wearing a truss for patients with inguinal hernias.

Preparation of this paper has been facilitated by Grant #GM 15904 of the National Institute of General Medical Sciences.

The input parameters used are:

(1) Pr {D|Elec. S.} The probability of death from elective herniorrhaphy.
(2) Pr {D|Emer. S.} The probability of death from emergency herniorrhaphy.
(3) Pr {Str.|truss} The probability that a patient with a truss will require emergency surgery within a year.
(4) Pr {Rec.|1st year} The probability that a hernia that has been repaired will recur within the first year following surgery. This is assumed to be higher than the rate for later years.
(5) Pr {Rec.|1+ years} The probability that a hernia will recur within one year, given that it did not recur during the first year.

The program differs from his model in that it performs detailed calculations by yearly intervals rather than making the approximation that everyone survives to the expected life of the group. It also makes slightly different assumptions about the probability of recurrence after corrective surgery because Neuhauser does not give annual rates. In this illustration the program has been run using only the annual death rates for males. They constitute the majority of hernia patients. An advantage of the program is that it calculates the survival curves of the groups under consideration rather than just their expected life spans.

As implemented the program has two possible oversimplifications. One is that time intervals used are years, and so the program does not provide for the possibility that a person might have more than one recurrence within a given year. The other is that the probability of recurrence is taken to be high for the first year after each operation and low thereafter. A better model might have a more gradual change. However, as Neuhauser points out, relatively few data exist on how this risk changes as a function of time after operation, or on the risk of recurrence as a function of the patient's age at time of operation.

The general program can simulate many different diseases. It works by following an imaginary cohort of patients from the age when they are assumed to have developed their disease until they have all died from one cause or another. The course of the cohort is computed at yearly intervals and their life expectancy is calculated from the numbers surviving for each year of the time period. Depending upon the disease process being modeled, each patient is considered to be in one of the definite number of states at the start of each year. These states describe the patient's condition in terms of the disease studied, such as alive and free of disease, alive with metastases, dead, and so forth. For each pair of states we assume that we know the probability that a patient who was in the first state at the beginning of the year will be in the second state at the end of the year, and vice versa. Some of these transition probabilities will, of course, be zero. The program proceeds recursively computing from the number of patients in each state at the beginning of the first time period the number who will be in each state at the beginning of the second time period. These results are then used to compute the number in each state for the following time period and this is repeated, until all patients have died.

By running the program repeatedly, using different values for the transition probabilities that determine the chances that a patient will move from one state to another, the sensitivity of the model to these parameters can be determined. To apply this program to the specific model employed by Neuhauser for the study of inguinal herniorrhaphy we assume that at any particular time a patient must be in one of four states or categories. These are:

(1) Alive with hernia, presumably using a truss, and at risk of strangulation and emergency surgery.

(2) Alive with a hernia that has been repaired within the last year, and therefore at a higher risk of recurrence.

(3) Alive with hernia that was repaired more than one year previously and therefore at a lower risk of recurrence.

(4) Dead from other causes or from the surgical mortality of herniorrhaphy.

When the program starts, everyone is in state 1 and is presumed to be at age 65. The program first applies the appropriate mortality rate for this age group and deducts the appropriate number of deaths and enters them in category 4. The next step depends upon whether a policy of elective surgery or a policy of using a truss is being simulated. The elective surgery policy will be outlined first and then the truss policy.

ELECTIVE SURGERY

The total surviving population in state 1 is given elective surgery, and the proportion of them not surviving (determined by Pr{Death|Elective Surgery}) is added to those already in state 4. The survivors are entered into state 2. During each succeeding iteration, the number of deaths from all other causes is computed using the death rate appropriate to that age group (65 for the first iteration, 66 for the second, etc.). All survivors in state 2 are subject to the possibility of a recurrence at the "high" rate and so this proportion of them is also subject to reoperation and its attendant mortality. The survivors of reoperation stay in category 2. The proportion of patients in category 2 who do not suffer from recurrence move to category 3. Those patients already in category 3 are subject to recurrence at the "low" rate. The proportion who have recurrences is then further subject to operative mortality with the proportion surviving reoperation being added to category 2. The deaths go to category 4. Thus, for each year from age 65 to 100, when everyone is considered to have died, the program takes the number of people expected in each state and computes how many would be expected to be in each state the following year.

TRUSS THERAPY

The population given a truss rather than elective surgery is handled in a similar manner. All patients start in category 1 and are subject to the same death rate from other causes. The survivors in category 1 are further subject to strangulation requiring emergency surgery with a probability Pr{Strangulation|Truss}; of these, a proportion dies determined by Pr{Death|Emergency Surgery}. These are added to category 4. The survivors of emergency surgery are tallied in category 2. On successive iterations, patients move from category 2 with a high risk to category 3 with a low risk of recurrence, unless they have a recurrence or die. The patients in categories 2 and 3 are treated exactly as they were in the elective surgery model. The principal difference is that, in the truss model, patients remain in category 1 until they require emergency surgery due to strangulation or they die of other causes.

RESULTS

Using the data presented by Neuhauser in his Table 14-3, all combinations of parameter values were tried. The results for these 16 different simulations are presented in Table 15-1. Each row presents a comparison of the life expectancy of patients treated by elective surgery with that of those treated with a truss only. The first five columns give the values of the input parameters used in the model while the last column is the difference in the expectation of life computed in days. The first row uses the parameters of Neuhauser's "conservative" test, the last row corresponds to his "most reasonable" test, while the other rows show the effects of various combinations of these two sets of values. In general the computer simulation seems to be about one day more favorable to the elective surgery than Neuhauser's calculations. This may be due to the effect of recurrences in the truss patients who have had their hernias repaired following strangulation. This possibility is not allowed for in his model. In any case these results do not change the general thrust of his findings, and they provide some indication of the effects of the individual parameters.

Table 15-1. Difference in the expectation of life for patients age 65 treated with elective surgery or using a truss.

Parameter Values					
Pr(Death Emer. S.)	*Pr(Str. Truss)*	*Pr(Rec. 1st Yr)*	*Pr(Rec. 1+ Yrs)*	*Pr(Death Elec. S.)*	*Difference Days**
0.13200	0.00370	0.01500	0.00500	0.00336	1
0.13200	0.00370	0.01500	0.01000	0.00336	1
0.13200	0.00370	0.03000	0.00500	0.00336	1
0.13200	0.00370	0.03000	0.01000	0.00336	0
0.13200	0.00291	0.01500	0.00500	0.00336	3
0.13200	0.00291	0.01500	0.01000	0.00336	3
0.13200	0.00291	0.03000	0.00500	0.00336	3
0.13200	0.00291	0.03000	0.01000	0.00336	3
0.03530	0.00370	0.01500	0.00500	0.00336	12
0.03530	0.00370	0.01500	0.01000	0.00336	12
0.03530	0.06370	0.03000	0.00500	0.00336	12
0.03530	0.00370	0.03000	0.01000	0.00336	12
0.03530	0.00291	0.01500	0.00500	0.00336	13
0.03530	0.00291	0.01500	0.01000	0.00336	13
0.03530	0.00291	0.03000	0.00500	0.00336	13
0.03530	0.00291	0.03000	0.01000	0.00336	13

*The value given is the expectation of life for truss patients less that of surgical patients, hence positive values favor the truss group.

Table 15-2. Deaths by age intervals for cohorts of 10,000 patients starting at age 65 and using parameters of the "most reasonable" model.

	Number of Deaths in			
Age Interval	*Surgery Group (A)*	*Truss Group (B)*	*A - B*	*Cumulative Difference*
65*	34		34	34
65-69	1487	1494	-7	27
70-74	2144	2153	-9	18
75-79	2329	2337	-8	10
80-84	2049	2055	-6	4
85-89	1378	1381	-3	1
90-94	537	538	-1	0
95-99	41	41	0	0

*This line shows deaths associated with the initial elective surgery separated from other sources of mortality.

Table 15-2 gives the deaths predicted by the model for starting cohorts of 10,000 patients in 5-year time intervals using the parameters of the "most reasonable" model. The column showing the cumulative difference indicates that although the truss group has higher mortality in every time period this is not enough to offset the initial mortality of the elective surgery.

To give a feeling for the effect of patient age the program was rerun for a population of patients who had their hernias at age 45. To allow for the better surgical experience of younger patients the death rates of both elective and emergency surgery have been made increasing linear functions of age. The value at age 45 is taken as two-thirds that of age 65, and for each year of age over 45 it increases by one-fortieth of the rate of 45. Thus at age 65 these death rates are the same as those used in Table 15-1, while at older ages they are slightly higher. These results are presented in Table 15-3. This table emphasizes the importance of the death rate of emergency repair of strangulated hernias on the expectation of life of the truss group. This suggests that the access to emergency care should be considered before recommending the use of a truss.

The effect of the physical status of a patient at the time of diagnosis, which would affect the mortality rate of elective surgery, has not been investigated here since it can be calculated directly using the Neuhauser model.

DISCUSSION AND SUMMARY

A computer program that simulates the course of a disease process by determining how patients would progress from one disease state to another over the course of time, and that concurrently applies the relevant age-specific mortality rates to the group being followed, has been described. The model is determined by the transition probabilities that control the movement from each disease state

Table 15-3. Difference in the expectation of life for patients age 45 treated with elective surgery or using a truss.

Parameter Values					*Differ-ence Days***
*Pr(Death Emer. S.)**	*Pr(Str. Truss)*	*Pr(Rec. 1st Yr)*	*Pr(Rec. 1+ Yrs)*	*Pr(Death Elec. S.)**	
0.08800	0.00370	0.01500	0.00500	0.00240	-36.
0.08800	0.00370	0.01500	0.01000	0.00240	-33.
0.08800	0.00370	0.03000	0.00500	0.00240	-35.
0.08800	0.00370	0.03000	0.01000	0.00240	-33.
0.08800	0.00291	0.01500	0.00500	0.00240	-23.
0.08800	0.00291	0.01500	0.01000	0.00240	-21.
0.08800	0.00291	0.03000	0.00500	0.00240	-22.
0.08800	0.00291	0.03000	0.01000	0.00240	-20.
0.02357	0.00370	0.01500	0.00500	0.00240	10.
0.02357	0.00370	0.01500	0.01000	0.00240	12.
0.02357	0.00370	0.03000	0.00500	0.00240	10.
0.02357	0.00370	0.03000	0.01000	0.00240	12.
0.02357	0.00291	0.01500	0.00500	0.00240	13.
0.02357	0.00291	0.01500	0.01000	0.00240	16.
0.02357	0.00291	0.03000	0.00500	0.00240	14.
0.02357	0.00291	0.03000	0.01000	0.00240	16.

*The death rates used in these calculations increase with the age of the patient. The values shown are the initial values for age 45.
**The value given is the expectation of life for truss patients less that of surgical patients, hence positive values favor the truss group.

to every other. By varying these parameters it is possible to investigate their effects on the outcome of the process easily and inexpensively. The program also makes it possible to monitor the proportions of patients in each state over time.

This program has been applied to the model describing patients with inguinal hernia at age 65 given in Chapter 14. The results of the program followed those presented there and the effects of varying each combination of the parameters were investigated. The effects of these policies on a younger group of patients, age 45, were also presented.

When such models can be derived that properly represent the medical situation under study, they provide a quick way to investigate the sensitivity of policy decisions to factors that are not accurately known, such as the strangulation rate of unrepaired hernias.

Acknowledgment

The author is indebted to the editors for their comments and to Mrs. Rowena Foss for her typing.

16

Cost-effectiveness of cholecystectomy for silent gallstones

Garry Fitzpatrick
Raymond Neutra
John P. Gilbert

Ingelfinger (1968) has estimated that in America today, there may be as many as 15 million persons carrying gallstones or approximately 7.4% of the entire population and 12% of the adult population.* Judging from the Framingham study of a predominantly Caucasian population (Friedman et al., 1966), approximately 3.9% of adult Caucasians in America between the ages of thirty and sixty-two harbor medically diagnosed gallstones. Bainton, et al. (1976) in Wales have recently published the results of a radiological survey of a random sample of the population; 9.2% of persons 45–69 years of age had radiological evidence of gallstones. Among Ingelfinger's estimated 15 million stone carriers about 4,000 deaths related to benign and 4,000 deaths related to malignant gallbladder disease occur each year (Vital Statistics of the U.S., 1970). The majority of these deaths occur in persons above the age of 50.

Removing gallbladders in America is a costly business. Assuming $2,000 as a minimum reasonable estimate for overall hospital and medical expenses for an uncomplicated cholecystectomy and an additional $1,000 loss of income by the patient during convalescence, the national cost for the approximately 400,000 operations on diseased gallbladders exceeds $1.2 billion annually.

When gallstones become clinically symptomatic, causing acute cholecystitis, ascending cholangitis, or obstructive jaundice, there is no reason to question the benefits of surgical intervention. Often the relief of the severe pain associated

*According to the 1970 Census, the total population of the United States was 203,210,000. Approximately 126,000,000 were age 20 or over.

with symptomatic gallstones is, in itself, sufficient benefit. When gallstones are asymptomatic or producing minimal symptoms–incidentally discovered, perhaps, during routine x-ray examinations or during abdominal surgery for some other condition–the decision whether to remove the gall bladder prophylactically is a difficult one concerning which there is considerable medical disagreement. It is to this decision that the following analysis is directed.

THE PROBLEM

In order to compare the efficacy of surgical with symptomatic medical management of silent gallstones we need to know the positive and negative outcomes of the two treatments and their probabilities. For lack of usable data on morbidity and convalescence, we have restricted ourselves to the outcomes of death under the two options. Therefore, this analysis cannot be definitive.

RISKS OF OPERATIVE MANAGEMENT OF SILENT GALLSTONES

The mortality for surgery of the gallbladder a half-century ago was estimated at 6.6% by Heuer (1934). Surgery at that time was limited largely to patients whose disease was in an advanced stage, and most of the deaths were attributed to biliary cirrhosis and liver failure as a result of longstanding calculous disease. Heuer based his estimate of operative mortality on reports which appeared in the American and European literature between the years 1923 and 1932. Between 1932 and 1950 Glenn and Hays (1952) reported an operative mortality of surgery for benign biliary tract disease of only 1.8%. Their report was based on the experience of a single institution (the New York Hospital) which specializes in diseases of the gallbladder, and which may be different from the average surgical experience. This point exemplifies a difficulty frequently encountered in this review. The majority of reports on the subject of gallbladder surgery come from the country's largest institutions, whose surgeons are more highly specialized than the national average. On the other hand, such institutions receive more difficult cases referred from other hospitals, and these patients cannot be regarded as random samples from the general population.

During the following decade (1950-62), there were 39 deaths following 2,358 operations for biliary tract disease at the New York Hospital (Glenn and McSherry, 1963), an overall mortality not much different from that of the previous 20 years. However, when deaths were analyzed according to duration of disease and magnitude of procedure, there was found to be a striking difference in mortality rates observed between acute and "chronic" cases (Table 16-1). The mortality for removal of the gallbladder was 2.3% if carried out in the presence of acute cholecystitis. When cholecystectomy was carried out for chronic biliary tract disease–usually in relatively healthy patients with minimally symptomatic gallstones–the mortality was only 0.3%.

The report of such a low operative mortality for elective cholecystectomy for chronic disease convinced physicians and surgeons of the advantage of early surgery for quiescent or minimally symptomatic gallstone disease. More recent

Table 16–1. Case fatality rates for biliary tract operations.

Operation Performed	*Number*	*Deaths*	*% Mortality*
Cholecystectomy			
acute	266	6	2.3
chronic	1,444	4	0.3
Common bile duct exploration			
alone	139	3	2.2
with cholecystectomy	388	11	2.8

The risk of death varies greatly according to the duration of disease and magnitude of the procedure. (Adapted from Glenn and McSherry, 1963, with permission of the authors and publisher.)

mortality studies from Finland (Seiro and Asp, 1966), America (Seltzer et al., 1970), and Sweden (Boquist et al., 1972) have shown reductions in overall mortality to 0.9%, 1.6%, and 0.9%, respectively. Another recent report from a community hospital in Canada (Mylne and Karnauchow, 1974) gave an overall mortality of 1.1%. The American and Canadian reports are interesting for their age-adjusted figures which demonstrate that the risk is markedly reduced when the operation is performed on those under 50 years of age (Table 16–2).

The publication of the National Halothane Study in 1969 provided for the first time a large series of gallbladder operations which relate operative risk to three patient variables: age, sex, and preoperative physical status. As part of the Halothane Study, data from 13,420 cholecystectomies and 5,870 common bile duct explorations were analyzed according to these variables, subdivided in the following manner: (1) age 0 to 49, from 50 to 69, and over 69; (2) sex, male or female; and (3) preoperative physical status, A (good) or B (poor). Physical status category A combined the standard risk classifications 1, 2, and 5 as defined by the American Society of Anesthesiologists. (ASA 1 is good risk elective; ASA 2 is good risk elective but with moderate systemic disease, for example, moderate diabetes or moderate hypertension; and ASA 5 is good risk emergency.) Category B combined ASA risks 3, 4, and 6 (ASA 3 signifies severe systemic disease, ASA 4 advanced or premorbid systemic disease, and ASA 6 advanced severe disease undergoing emergency surgery). For convenience in the present analysis, we have used only data from patients subjected to halothane anesthesia.

The mortality data used in our analysis are reproduced in Table 16–3. Note

Table 16–2. Case fatality rates for cholecystectomy in three different age groups.

Age	*American*	*Canadian*
Over 60	3.4%	3.1%
50–60	1.0%	1.1%
Under 50	0.24%	0.17%

The risk of death rises steeply with age. (Seltzer et al., 1970, by permission of *Surgery, Gynecology and Obstetrics* and of the author. Mylne and Karnauchow, 1974, with permission of the publisher.)

Table 16-3. Case fatality rates for cholecystectomy and for cholecystectomy with common bile duct exploration by age, sex, and preoperative physical status.

Physical Status	*Cholecystectomy Alone*				*Cholecystectomy plus Common Bile Duct Exploration*			
	A		*B*		*A*		*B*	
Age	*Female*	*Male*	*Female*	*Male*	*Female*	*Male*	*Female*	*Male*
Under 50	0.054%	0.104%	1.256%	2.398%	0.213%	0.411%	4.826%	8.92%
50 to 69	0.280%	0.539%	1.714%	3.258%	1.010%	1.932%	6.017%	11.00%
70+	1.307%	2.494%	5.161%	9.511%	1.833%	3.481%	7.194%	13.02%

The case fatality is strongly dependent on the anesthetic risk category regardless of age. The good risk "A" categories have case fatalities 10 to 20 times lower than the case fatalities of the high risk "B" categories. (Bishop and Mosteller, 1969, with permission of the authors.)

that mortality is almost twice as high for men as for women in all categories. Note also that mortality is very low in good risk patients under 50 years of age, increasing markedly in the older age groups. Thus, for patients in Physical Status Category A (good risk), the risk of death following cholecystectomy is five times greater over 50 years of age than below 50. Over 70 years of age, the risk of death following cholecystectomy is increased an additional fivefold. A third important point is that preoperative physical status also markedly affects postoperative mortality. Under 50 years of age, for example, the mortality risk of cholecystectomy is approximately 23 times greater for patients in poor preoperative physical condition (Physical Status Category B) than for patients in good preoperative condition (Category A). Fortunately, the majority of patients fall into the two good risk categories: the numbers of patients with ASA risks 1, 2, and 3 are in the ratio of 10 to 5 to 1. Finally, it should be noted that the mortality for combining a common bile duct exploration with cholecystectomy is, on the average, about four times greater in all groups, reflecting the greater technical difficulty and more frequent and serious complications associated with this operation.

Thus, the risk of elective cholecystectomy alone, carried out in healthy young patients, is low; and the risk of cholecystectomy, at an older age in a patient who is perhaps now in poorer physical condition and who may now require common duct exploration for an obstructing stone and jaundice, is very much higher. But before recommending cholecystectomy for silent stones to avoid the increased risk of surgery when the patient is older and perhaps sicker, we need to know the probability that surgery will, in fact, be required for subsequent disease. That is, we need to know the natural history of silent gallstones managed expectantly.

RISKS OF SYMPTOMATIC MANAGEMENT OF SILENT GALLSTONES

An early attempt at assessing the complication rate for silent gallstones was carried out by Comfort et al. (1948) using a series from the Mayo Clinic of 998 cases of gallstone disease found incidentally at laparotomy for other conditions. Follow-up letters were sent to 184 patients and 112 were finally considered suitable for study. Over a 20-year period 46% of the 112 patients developed symptoms. Half of these symptomatic patients eventually underwent cholecystectomy with a mortality of 13%. In another frequently quoted study, Lund (1960) at the Copenhagen County Hospital tried to determine the incidence and fate of silent gallstones by long-term follow-up of patients in whom stones were discovered by cholecystography.* Approximately 50% of the women and 30% of the men developed severe symptoms or complications at a later date. Surgery was required in 23% of the patients developing symptoms.

A well-controlled study attempting to determine the fate of nonoperated gallstones was reported more recently by Wenckert and Robertson (1966). All

*This is not really a study of silent stones, as most of these patients had some symptoms to warrant a cholecystogram; rather it is a series of mildly symptomatic, unoperated gallstones.

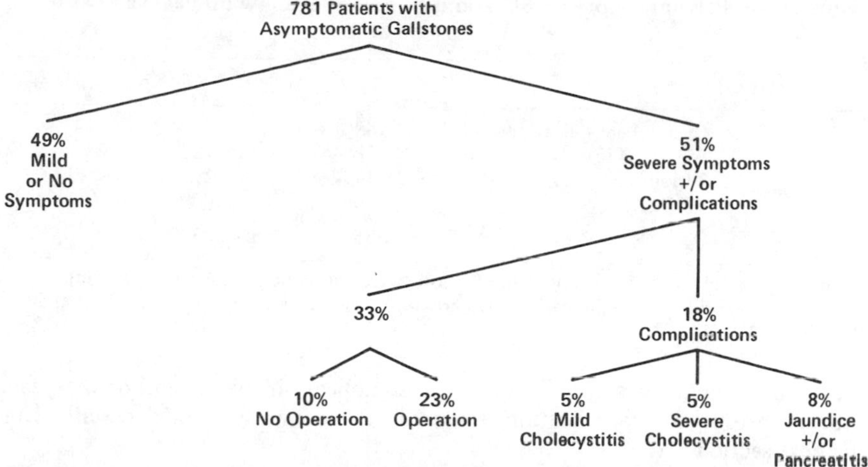

Figure 16–1. The fate of patients with minimally symptomatic gallstones in Malmo, Sweden.

By the end of 11 years 49% of patients had not yet had a complication or an episode of severe pain. (From Wenckert and Robertson, 1966, with the permission of the author.)

patients with positive cholecystograms done in Malmo over a 12-month period in 1951–52* were followed for eleven years. Six hundred and sixty-two cases were excluded because their symptoms were severe enough at the time of x-ray to warrant operation within a year. The remaining 781 patients were followed for 11 years; 49% had mild or no symptoms, 33% had severe symptoms, and 18% had complications (Figure 16–1). The 144 patients who developed complications were further subdivided. There were 39 patients with severe cholecystitis, 59 with jaundice and/or pancreatitis, and 42 with mild acute cholecystitis. The three other patients had cancer of the gallbladder and one had obstruction. Among these 144 patients with complications, there were 10 deaths (6.9%). There were 173 patients with biliary colic severe enough to warrant surgery. Two of these patients died, a case fatality of 1.16%. The overall case fatality for patients requiring surgery over the 11-year interval was, thus, 12/317, or 3.79%.

In these several studies of silent gallstones, we have differing estimates of the likelihood of escaping complications. Comfort et al. (1948) report 54% of patients symptom free at 20 years. Lund (1960) does not specify the period of follow-up. In the Malmo study, the overall probability of escaping complications in an 11-year period was 49%. If the yearly probability of escaping complications has been constant over that interval, we can solve for that probability by taking the eleventh root of .49, which is 93.7%. Its complement, 6.3%, is the

*During this period, it was the policy of the Malmo General Hospital, Department of Surgery, to offer conservative treatment for patients with only occasional uncomplicated attacks.

Table 16-4. Percentage of complications in patients below 60 years and at or above 60 years of age.

Age	*< 60*	*≥ 60*
Escaped complication	48%	53%
Biliary colic only	38%	18%
Serious complications	14%	29%
TOTAL	100%	100%
	n = 558	n = 223

Although the chance of escaping complications were the same for the two age groups, the proportion of severe complications was greater in the older age group. (Wenckert and Robertson, 1966)

probability that a person will develop a complication by the end of the year. This probability of complication is used in the computer model described in the next section.

The Malmo study also provides data on the risk of complication and its severity as a function of age. The data, which are reproduced in Table 16-4, divide the population into only two age groups, those below 60 and those at or above 60 years of age. The probability of escaping complication does not change much with age, but the proportion of serious complications increases with age. The way this phenomenon has been dealt with in the computer model is explained in the section on methodology.

The question of the relationship of stones to cancer has been hotly debated for years. Gallstones are present in 85-90% of operated cases of carcinoma of the gallbladder (Vadheim et al., 1944; Thorbjarnarson and Glenn, 1959; Gerst, 1961). Both gallstone disease and carcinoma of the gallbladder are three times more common in females. There is, in most cases of gallbladder cancer, a long-standing history of biliary colic, chronic cholecystitis, and biliary stasis, and the geographical frequency of the two diseases is similar. But do these associations alone implicate gallstones in the etiology of cancer, or might not the malignancy be the cause, rather than the effect of gallstones?

Two or three points are clear about gallbladder cancer. It is a disease of the age group over 50 years; over 90% of cases occur after the sixth decade (Adson, 1973). Advanced incurable lesions are found in 68-77% of cases (Adson, 1973; Vaittinen, 1970), and potentially curative cholecystectomy is possible in only one of four patients with malignant disease of the gallbladder. Diagnosis is difficult, symptoms are nonspecific and the average length of survival of patients who die of cancer of the gallbladder averages only 4 to 5 months. This very poor prognosis has led many surgeons to advocate prophylactic cholecystectomy for silent stones as an "anticancer" operation.

The surgical literature presents rather high estimates of the cancer risk among gallstone patients. The extensive collected data of Vaittinen (1970) suggest the risk may be as great as 1.4% per year. This figure, however, was obtained by taking the ratio of gallbladder cancers found to the number of operations performed for gallstones each year. This denominator is far too small, since the vast number of patients with unknown gallstones is also presumably at risk of

Table 16–5. The probability of gallstones in gallbladder cancer patients and population controls.

	Cancer	*No Cancer*
Gallstones	.85	.08
No Gallstones	.15	.92

The proportion of gallbladder cancer patients who have gallstones is much higher than the proportion in the population at large. Using these figures, the annual incidence rate of gallbladder cancer, and Bayes Theorem, we estimate the rate of gallbladder cancer in persons with stones to be only 22/100,000 per year.

developing cancer. Thus, Vaittinen's figure tends to overestimate the incidence of gallbladder cancer in people with cholelithiasis.

A more appropriate estimate can be made by contrasting the probability of gallstones in cancer patients with the probability in the general population. Various authors (Vadheim et al., 1944; Thorbjarnarson and Glenn, 1959; Gerst, 1961) have reported the incidence of gallstones in cancer patients to be 85%; the prevalence of gallstones in the general adult population is 8% (Friedman et al., 1966). Using these reasonably firm data (Table 16–5), we can estimate the gallbladder cancer death rate in persons with cholelithiasis.

There were 2,555 deaths in 1970 from gallbladder cancer among an adult population of 126 million in the United States. Therefore, the overall probability of death from cancer of the gallbladder is 2.03/100,000. To determine the probability in adult stone carriers of developing cancer, we applied Bayes Theorem (McNeil et al., 1975) and calculated an annual incidence in patients with gallstones of 21.56/100,000. Using life table methods, we calculate that the risk to people with gallstones of developing gallbladder cancer over a 20-year period is only 4.3/1,000. The 11-year risk is 2.36/1,000. This would predict 2 cases in the Malmo cohort of 781 patients with silent stones; the observed number was 3. This is a very small risk and does not appear to justify the removal of gallbladders solely as a cancer prevention. The cancer risk was, however, included in the rate of complication reported in the Malmo study (Wenckert and Robertson, 1966). In our model, cancer patients are included together with all other complications and the total group subjected to the overall case fatality rate.

THE ANALYSIS

Decision Analysis: The Individual Patient

The surgeon has two options when considering a patient with minimally symptomatic gallstones. He can operate now and run a small risk of depriving some people of their remaining life, or he can wait and hope that no gallstone complications will have occurred by the time the patient dies. If complications do occur, the patient has a higher chance of dying because he will be older, because he may have developed some chronic cardiorespiratory condition in the interim and, finally, because the case fatality from emergency gallbladder surgery is higher than the case fatality for elective surgery. On the other hand, he has lived to an older age than the person who died from elective surgery.

In this analysis we will be comparing the two options as to the years of life saved rather than as to the expected number of deaths. We do this because we realize that ten deaths which occur at age 50 deprive the patients of more years of life than ten deaths which occur at age 90.

We had initially tried to approach this problem using a decision tree of the sort used by Neuhauser for strangulated inguinal hernia in Chapter 14. The rate of gallstone complications (6.3% per year) is much higher than the risk of strangulation (0.2% per year), and this high rate of complication significantly changes the size of the population still at risk within a few years of follow-up. We preferred to simulate this situation as closely as possible and elected to use a modification of the computer simulation program devised by one of us (JPG) and reported in Chapter 15.

In the simulation we assess the effects of elective surgery or medical management on patients of different age, sex, and anesthetic risk for each category. Two cohorts of 10,000 persons are submitted respectively to the "operate now" and "wait and see" options. The operated group loses immediately a number of patients as a result of the elective operation. After that, the appropriate age-sex specific death rate for all causes depletes the cohort until at age 110 there are no survivors. Standard death rates were used because unpublished life insurance data (Single Medical Impairment Study, New York Life, 1972, unpublished) show no excess risk after cholecystectomy. In the unoperated group the general death rate is also at work, depleting the cohort year after year. In addition to this there is the 6.3% risk of complications each year which results in an operation whose case fatality depends on the age of the patient. Patients who have had a complication and have survived the subsequent operation are no longer at risk of further complications, but they are, of course, still subject to the overall risk of death. Patients in the poor risk simulations were considered not only to have higher operative death rates, but also to have a greater risk of dying from other causes than those given in the standard mortality tables.

The model is thus determined by four classes of parameters: (1) The first is the death rate associated with elective surgery at the age, sex, and risk status under consideration. The second parameter (2) is the age-specific death rate associated with surgery *for complications* which a patient with this sex, initial age, and risk status would experience. Thus, the probability of dying from a complication depends on the age at which it occurs. These two classes of parameter were based on data from the National Halothane Study. The third class of parameter (3) is the age-sex-anesthetic risk-specific mortality rates for all causes. For good risk patients national life tables (National Center for Health Statistics, 1975) were used. For poor risk patients these were modified as explained in the methodological note (*vide infra*). The final parameter (4) is the probability of a complication in a year. This was 6.3% derived from the Malmo study as discussed in the previous section.

The results of the modeling, in terms of expected days of life saved by surgery or by medical management are shown in Table 16-6 for each age, sex, and anesthetic risk category considered. The most striking finding is that the losses and gains are small, the largest being of the order of a month of life saved. We interpret this to mean that the decision to operate for minimally symptomatic gallstones can be governed by considerations of morbidity and the patient's

Table 16-6. Days of life expectancy gained by surgery or by a "wait and see" policy for minimally symptomatic gallstones.

	Age	*Good Risk*	*Poor Risk*
MEN	49	S 16*	W 33**
	60	S 7	W 37
WOMEN	49	S 15	W 4
	60	S 11	W 14

*S = Surgery is preferred.
**W = Waiting is preferred.
Poor risk patients gain up to a month of life by waiting. Good risk patients gain one or two weeks by surgery. The losses and gains are not great.

Table 16-7. Theoretical "5-year plan" of prophylactic cholecystectomy (poor risk patients).

Age	*(1)* Medically Managed Survivors	*(2)* % of Medically Managed Survivors Who Have Had a Complication	*(3)* Surgically Managed Survivors	*(3) - (1)* Surgical Survivors Minus Medical Survivors
60-64	10,000	0	9,829	-171
65-69	7,289	27.6%	7,247	-42
70-74	4,525	47.7%	4,544	19
75-79	2,139	62.3%	2,167	28
80-84	616	72.9%	628	12
85-89	79	81.0%	81	2
90-94	3	100.0%	3	0
95-99	0	–	0	0

When the survival of one cohort of patients managed medically is compared with that of another cohort managed surgically, one sees that the medically treated group has more survivors at the end of the first decade of follow-up. A higher mortality in the medically treated group causes a deficit in survival in subsequent periods, but does not cancel the benefits gained by deferring operation in this high risk group.

peace of mind rather than by fear of mortal events. Having said this, we emphasize that good risk men and women stand to *lose* two weeks of life if a "wait and see" policy is adopted. Poor risk men and women *gain* as much as a month by adopting this policy.

An example of the expected gains and losses is presented in Table 16-7 which shows the survivors for 5-year intervals in the surgically and medically managed cohorts of poor risk 60-year-old females. In the first two 5-year periods, the surgically managed patients have fewer survivors; after this, their survival is superior but not sufficiently so to counterbalance the earlier loss of life expectancy. In the same table, we show the proportion of survivors in the medically managed group who have experienced a gallbladder complication. This proportion who have had the complication rises sharply and eventually reaches 100%.

How sensitive are these results to the estimated rate of complication adopted from the Malmo study? By substituting different rates of complication, we found that 49-year-old good risk females would *gain* from the "wait and see" policy only when the rate of complication fell from 6.3% per year to 0.8% per year. This is equivalent to an 11-year attack rate of 8% rather than the 51% observed at Malmo. None of the studies have cited a complication rate this low.

At the other extreme we found that a complication rate of 9% per year would be necessary in order to make elective surgery as attractive as medical management for the 60-year-old poor risk patient. This is equivalent to a 65% probability of complications in 11 years, a figure higher than the 51% reported in the Malmo study. We see that fairly large fluctuations in the rate of gallstone complications does not change our conclusion about the rather minimal gains or losses in days of life which result from selecting a surgical or medical approach to the management of silent gallstones.

SOME SOCIETAL CONSIDERATIONS

We have seen that there is some small benefit to be expected from removing silent gallstones from young low-risk patients. How costly would pursuing this benefit be if we consider it on a national level? For this analysis we need to know the prevalence of silent stones in the population and its distribution by age and risk. This prevalence is difficult to estimate for a number of reasons. First, many of the studies have been based on the incidence of gallstones found in autopsy material (Torvik and Høivik, 1960), which largely overestimates the prevalence of gallstones due to the preponderance of older people in autopsy series. Second, apart from the well-known associations of gallstones in females with increasing parity, obesity, and advanced age (Friedman et al., 1966), there are striking differences in the incidence of gallstones among different races in the United States (Comess et al., 1967; Cunningham and Hardenbergh, 1956; Yamase and McNamara, 1972; Erickson, 1972).

There appear also to be geographic and regional differences in the prevalence of cholelithiasis, quite apart from ethnic population differences (Plant et al., 1973; Milner and Hewitt, 1972; Comess et al., 1967; Sampliner et al., 1970). This raises the question of how the data are collected. Many authors have used gallbladder surgery rates as an index of the prevalence of gallbladder disease in an area. It has been amply demonstrated (Lewis, 1969; Bunker, 1970; Mylne and Karnauchow, 1974; Plant et al., 1973; Milner and Hewitt, 1972; Wennberg and Gittelsohn, 1973; Vayda, 1973) that there are up to tenfold differences in cholecystectomy rates between not only different countries, but also among regions within the same province or state (Table 16–8). Estimation of prevalence rates from rates of cholecystectomy in these situations would be very misleading.

Third, even when one uses radiologic data rather than operative rates, the study is subject to bias from the beginning because the majority of people referred for cholecystography have epigastric or abdominal symptoms at least suggestive of cholelithiasis. They are not truly asymptomatic, or otherwise would not have been referred to the radiologist.

Bainton et al. (1976) have estimated that 9.2% of the adult population have gallstones. This gives about 11.6 million persons in the country with biliary calculi. The cholecystectomy rate for the United States in 1971 was 185/100,000

Table 16-8. Regional differences in cholecystectomy rate.

Location or Country	*Year*	*Rate**	*Size of Sample*	*Reference*
England and Wales	1967	4.9	48,391,000	(Vayda, 1973)
England and Wales	1966	6.1	48,075,000	(Bunker, 1970)
Luton, England	1971	7.0	250,000	(Plant et al., 1973)
Rennes, France	1965	8.0	208,465	(Plant et al., 1973)
Vermont, U.S.A. (Lowest incidence area)	1969–1971	11.6	9,583	(Wennberg and Gittelsohn, 1973)
Kansas, U.S.A. (Lowest incidence area)	1965	12.1	95,000	(Lewis, 1969)
United States	1971	18.5	205,000,000	(Bunker, 1970)
Canada	1968	31.1	20,744,000	(Vayda, 1973)
Vermont, U.S.A. (Highest incidence area)	1969–1971	37.2	10,900	(Wennberg and Gittelsohn, 1973)
Kansas, U.S.A. (Highest incidence area)	1965	42.3	44,000	(Lewis, 1969)
Kapuskasing, Canada	1971	43.7	12,835	(Plant et al., 1973)
Windsor, Canada	1971	45.8	236,904	(Plant et al., 1973)

*Expressed as cholecystectomies per 10,000 population.

The marked variations in cholecystectomy rates even within one state suggest that the operative rate reflects patterns of health care utilization more than it does the prevalence of gallstones in the population.

(Blanken, 1974), and this would represent about 400,000 cholecystectomies a year. Thus, only 3.4% of the patients with stones are currently operated on each year.

If we were to screen all 50-year-olds and all 60-year-olds every year, we would detect the prevalent stones at age 50 and the stones which had appeared over the subsequent decade of high incidence. From current Census figures (Bureau of the Census, 1974) we estimate that some 4 million persons would then receive a cholecystogram each year for this screening program. At a cost of $50 per cholecystogram this would amount to $200 million a year. Based on the prevalence of gallstones in these age groups in Bainton's study (1976), some 368,000 cases of gallstones would be found. If all were operated, and if we assume direct medical expenses of $2,000 and income losses of $1,000, there would be an additional cost of $1.1 billion. Consideration of an investment of this magnitude in order to prolong life by one or two weeks should, of course, take into account the many other demands on medical resources, as discussed in Chapter 2.

CONCLUSIONS

On the basis of the foregoing analysis, the decision to operate for a silent gallstone ought not to be based solely on life expectancy, but should be heavily influenced by other considerations such as the risk of morbidity, and the patient's peace of mind. Our analysis has not dealt with these issues. Even the mortality analysis deserves further exploration. We have used the National Halothane Study case fatality for "cholecystectomy with exploration of the common bile duct" to estimate the probability of death given a serious complication. This figure may be too low, and if this is the case, a higher figure would make surgery more attractive. We have not separated out the contribution of gallbladder cancer to the survivorship curves in the treatment groups, an analysis which would be of interest. The presentation here must, therefore, be viewed as a selective review of the literature with a preliminary modeling and sensitivity analysis.

The model used in the analysis promises to be of continued use for it will allow us to examine the sensitivity of our results to changes in the parameters. In particular, we will explore the importance of changes in the operative case fatality as a function of the age of the patient and the extent of the procedure. The model will allow us as well to examine the occurence of complications over time and the cost and convalescence associated with them. This further analytic work is in progress.

Acknowledgments

The authors gratefully acknowledge the constructive criticisms of Drs. William V. McDermott, Jr. and Francis D. Moore of the Department of Surgery, Harvard Medical School. Many thanks are due to Mrs. Pamela Brown, Worcester City Hospital, for typing of the original manuscript, and to Natalie Katz Fisher of The Stanford University School of Medicine, for editing and typing of the final manuscript.

METHODOLOGICAL NOTE

Four classes of parameters were used in the computer model on which our conclusions are based. We now discuss the way the parameter values used in the model were derived.

Mortality from All Causes

For the good risk groups, the age-specific mortality rates were obtained from national life tables (DHEW Pub. No. (HRA) 75-1150). The poor risk groups were subjected to higher mortality rates that were computed from the standard rate for each age using the formula:

$$m_{PI} = 1 - \exp\,[\ln(1 - m_{GI}) \times 5]$$

where

m_{PI} is the mortality for poor risk patients at age I and

m_{GI} is the mortality for good risk patients at age I.

This function changes a mortality rate of 0.01 to 0.049, 0.20 to 0.672, and has the effect of changing the life expectancy of a 40-year-old male from 25 years to 17. The factor "5" in the formula was derived from unpublished insurance data on persons with chronic bronchitis whose rate of mortality is five times that of the general population of the same age and sex (Single Medical Impairment Study, New York Life, 1972).

The Death Rate for Elective Surgery

The elective surgery death rate was obtained from the Halothane data (Bishop and Mosteller, 1969). (See Table 16-3.) The rate for age 60 was taken to be that given for the interval 50 to 70. The data given for the interval 0 to 49 were taken as an estimate of the rate for age 45 (since relatively few cases occur before 30), and interpolated value was taken for the age 49 using the formula:

$$\text{Elec mort 49} = \exp[(2 \times \ln(\text{mort 44}) + \ln(\text{mort 60}))/3].$$

The Death Rate for Surgery After a Complication

The probability of death given a complication was estimated for age 45 and age 75. The estimation procedure for age 45 was as follows. The Malmo study (Wenckert and Robertson, 1966) reports the proportion of complications which were serious and nonserious in persons below age 60. To the "serious" group we applied the Halothane Study's probability of death for the serious procedure "cholecystectomy with common duct exploration;" to the second group, "nonserious," we applied the probability of death for the less serious procedure "cholecystectomy without common duct exploration." The resultant overall probability of death given a complication at age 45 was thus a weighted average of the two probabilities of death, the weights being the proportion of complications which were respectively "serious" and "nonserious." A similar procedure was followed for persons aged 75, using death rates for patients 70 and over. The proportion of complications which were "serious" and "nonserious" in the two age groups is shown in Table 16-4.

An exponential function was fitted to the probability of death at these two ages and this function was then used to estimate the probability of death following complication for each intervening age. The form of the function was:

$$\text{Prob of death} = \exp[A + B(\text{age} - 45)]$$

where

A = ln(probability of death at age 45)

and

B = [ln(probability of death at age 75) - ln(probability of death at age 45)] /30, where the number "30" is the number of years (75-45) in the interval.

The Yearly Probability of Complications

The 11-year probability of escaping a complication in Malmo (Wenckert and Robertson, 1966) was 0.49. If the yearly probability of escaping complications was constant over that 11-year period, it can be estimated by solving for it in the formula:

$$\text{Probability of escaping complications in 11 years} = (\text{Probability of escaping for one year})^{11}.$$

Taking logarithms of both sides of the equation, we have:

$$\ln \Pr(\text{escaping for 11 years}) = 11 \times \ln \Pr(\text{escaping for 1 year})$$

or

$$\ln \Pr(\text{escaping for 1 year}) = \ln \Pr(\text{escaping for 11 years})/11$$

$$= \ln(.49)/11 = -.06485.$$

Taking the antilog, we get a 93.7% chance of escaping complications in a year, or a 6.3% chance of getting a complication in a year.

References

Adson MA: Carcinoma of the gallbladder: A symposium on surgery of the biliary tree. Surg Clin North Am 53:1203, 1973

Arnold DJ: 28,621 cholecystectomies in Ohio: Results of a survey in Ohio hospitals by the Gallbladder Survey Committee, Ohio Chapter, American College of Surgeons. Am J Surg 119:714, 1970

Bainton D, Davies G, Evans K, Gravelle I: Gallbladder desease prevalence in a South Wales industrial town. N Engl J Med 294:1147, 1976

Bishop YMM, Mosteller F: Smoothed contingency table analysis. The National Halothane Study. Edited by JP Bunker, WH Forrest Jr., F Mosteller, et al. National Institutes of Health, National Institute of General Medical Sciences, Bethesda, Md., 1969, pp 259–266

Blanken GE: Surgical operations in short-stay hospitals, United States–1971. Vital and Health Statistics, Series 13–No. 18, DHEW Publication No. (HRA) 75–1769, Rockville, Md., National Center for Health Statistics, November 1974

Boquist L, Bergdahl L, Andersson A: Mortality following gallbladder surgery: A study of 3,257 cholecystectomies. Surgery 71:616, 1972

Bunker JP: Surgical manpower: A comparison of operations and surgeons in the United States and in England and Wales. N Engl J Med 282:135, 1970

Bureau of the Census: Estimates of the population of the United States. Series P-25, No. 529, September 1974, Table 1, p 4

Comess LJ, Bennett PH, Burch TA: Clinical gallbladder disease in Pima Indians: Its high prevalence in contrast to Framingham, Massachusetts. N Engl J Med 277:894, 1967

Comfort MW, Gray HK, Wilson JM: The silent gallstone: A ten to twenty year follow-up study of 112 cases. Ann Surg 128:931, 1948

Cunningham JA, Hardenbergh FE: Comparative incidence of cholelithiasis in the Negro and White races. Arch Intern Med 97:68, 1956

Erickson WG: Cholecystectomy and the American Indian: A 10 year comparative study. Rocky Mt Med J 69:33, July, 1972

Friedman GD, Kannel WB, Dawber TR: The epidemiology of gallbladder disease: Observations in the Framingham study. J Chronic Dis 19:273, 1966

Gerst PH: Primary carcinoma of the gallbladder: A 30 year summary. Ann Surg 153:369, 1961

Glenn F, Hays DM: The causes of death following biliary tract surgery for non-malignant diseases. Surg Gynecol Obstet 94:283, 1952

Glenn F, McSherry CK: Etological factors in fatal complications following operations upon the biliary tract. Ann Surg 157:695, 1963

Heuer GH: The factors leading to death in operations upon the gall-bladder and bile-ducts. Ann Surg 99:881, 1934

Ingelfinger FJ: Digestive disease as a national problem. V. Gallstones. Gastroenterology 55:102, 1968

Lewis CE: Variations in the incidence of surgery. N Engl J Med 281:880, 1969

Lund J: Surgical indications in cholelithiasis; prophylactic cholecystectomy elucidated on the basis of long-term follow-up in 526 nonoperated cases. Ann Surg 151:153, 1960

McNeil BJ, Keeler E, Adelstein SJ: Primer on certain elements of medical decision making. N Engl J Med 293:211, 1975

Milner J, Hewitt D: The occurrence and treatment of gallbladder disease in Ontario. J Chronic Dis 25:73, 1972

Mylne GE, Karnauchow PN: Cholecystectomy and related procedures in two community hospitals. Can J Surg 17:20, 1974

National Center for Health Statistics: United States Life Tables, 1969, 1971. DHEW Publication No. (HRA) 75-1150, 1975

Plant JCD, Percy I, Bates T, et al: Incidence of gallbladder disease in Canada, England and France. Lancet 2:249, 1973

Sampliner RE, Bennett PH, Comess LJ, et al: Gallbladder disease in Pima Indians. N Engl J Med 283:1358, 1970

Seiro J, Asp K: Surgical treatment of the biliary tract: Morbidity and mortality. Int Surg 45:258, 1966

Seltzer MH, Steiger E, Rosato FE: Mortality following cholecystectomy. Surg Gynecol Obstet 130:64, 1970

Thorbjarnarson B, Glenn F: Carcinoma of the gallbladder. Cancer 12:1009, 1959

Torvik A, Høivik B: Gallstones in an autopsy series: Incidence, complications and correlations with carcinoma of the gallbladder. Acta Chir Scand 120: 168, 1960

Vadheim JL, Gray HK, Dockerty MB: Carcinoma of the gallbladder: A clinical and pathologic study. Am J Surg 63:173, 1944

Vaittinen E: Carcinoma of the gallbladder: A study of 390 cases diagnosed in Finland 1953-1967. Ann Chir Gynaecol Fenn 59 Suppl 168:7, 1970

Vayda E: A comparison of surgical rates in Canada and in England and Wales. N Engl J Med 289:1224, 1973

Wenckert A, Robertson B: The natural course of gallstone disease: Eleven-year review of 781 nonoperated cases. Gastroenterology 50:376, 1966

Wennberg J, Gittelsohn A: Small area variations in health care delivery. Science 182:1102, 1973

Yamase H, McNamara JJ: Geographic differences in the incidence of gallbladder disease: Influence of environment and ethnic background. Am J Surg 123: 667, 1972

17

Elective hysterectomy

John P. Bunker
Klim McPherson
Philip L. Henneman

The National Center for Health Statistics estimates that 690,000 hysterectomies were performed in 1973 in the United States. This represents a rate of 647.7 per 100,000 females,* a rate higher than that for any other major operation, and a rate which, if continued in the future, would result in loss of the uterus by more than half the female population by age 65. How many of these hysterectomies were carried out for standard, conventional indication is not known, but it has been frequently alleged that hysterectomy is carried out unnecessarily in many patients.

A major basis for this concern is the large variation in rates for hysterectomy in different populations. Hysterectomy rates in the United States and in Canada are more than double those in Great Britain (Bunker, 1970; Vayda, 1973). Similar large differences are observed within the United States itself, with two- and three-fold variations in hysterectomy rates reported among hospital service areas in both Vermont and Maine (Wennberg and Gittelsohn, 1973, 1975). It seems unlikely that the prevalence of gynecological disease varies to any such large degree, and therefore we assume either that hysterectomies are being performed for markedly varying indications, or that access to gynecological care varies widely, or both.

Wennberg and Gittelsohn (1973) have demonstrated a strong correlation be-

*Calculated on the basis of the entire female population of all ages. When corrected for women who have already undergone hysterectomy, a rate of 706.3 per 100,000 females at risk is obtained. (See Appendix 17-I.)

Supported in part by a grant from the Robert Wood Johnson Foundation.

tween numbers of surgical specialists and the numbers of operations performed in Vermont. We assume that this effect holds for the country as a whole. One might entertain the possibility that the issue is entirely one of unmet need for hysterectomy in the areas of low rates were it not for the very high overall or average rates. But whatever the contribution of access, it is clear that the indications leading to hysterectomy must vary considerably, and that a patient with a gynecological complaint might be advised to undergo hysterectomy if she lived in one geographic area, but might receive nonsurgical treatment, or no treatment, if she lived in a different one. What are the characteristics of such a patient?

Professional opinion appears to vary widely, some gynecologists advocating hysterectomy for low back pain or for birth control, others urging that indications be limited to a small set of distinct pathologic conditions (Table 17-1). Between these two extremes is a broad spectrum of symptoms and indications for hysterectomy. The borderline or "marginal" case, the patient who is apt to undergo hysterectomy in one medical community but not in another, might be described as follows: she is 40 to 50 years of age, premenopausal, and in good general health. Her menses are somewhat irregular in frequency, and the severity of associated symptoms may debilitate her for several days. She has had two or three episodes of profuse menstrual bleeding for the control and diagnosis of which emergency curettage was performed. She complains of some fatigue, but is only slightly anemic and has not required transfusion. Papanicolaou examinations, performed yearly, have been negative. She expresses a fear of pregnancy, desires sterilization, but prefers to avoid major surgery.

For such a patient, hysterectomy (complete hysterectomy, with or without removal of ovaries and Fallopian tubes) offers a number of potential benefits. These benefits must be weighed against attendant costs and risks, and it is the uncertainty inherent in the measurement and prediction of both risks and benefits which presumably underlies the marked variations in professional

Table 17-1. Indications for hysterectomy.

1. Malignancies of the vagina, cervix, uterus, ovaries, or fallopian tubes.
2. Nonmalignant diseases of the uterus causing symptoms, e.g., fibroids causing pressure on bladder with consequent frequency; uterine pain or bleeding not responsive to hormonal therapy or uterine pain or bleeding in women in whom hormonal therapy is contraindicated.
3. Nonmalignant diseases of the tubes and ovaries where the uterus is not primarily involved in disease, but where the uterus is removed because of its anatomic proximity to these diseased adnexi or appendages, e.g., chronic advanced tubal infection, extensive endometriosis.
4. Late complications of childbirth including conditions secondary to diseases of supporting structures, e.g., cystocele, rectocele, procidentia.
5. Removal of the uterus in nongynecologic pelvic surgery where necessary to encompass disease originating elsewhere, e.g., uterine involvement in colon cancer or in an abscess secondary to diverticulitis.
6. Obstetrical catastrophies, e.g., uncontrollable postpartum bleeding, uterine rupture, uncontrolled uterine sepsis developing from septic abortion, etc.

opinion and practice. How well these risks and benefits can be identified it is now our purpose to examine.

The objective of hysterectomy, under the circumstances we have postulated, is the relief of a condition which does not threaten life. The operation itself, however, does affect life expectancy, and we will consider this effect first.

The risk of death in a healthy 40-year-old woman during elective hysterectomy or in the immediate postoperative period is small. We estimate this to be 1:2000 or less, which is equivalent to a loss of 6.9 days of the 38-year life expectancy of a 40-year-old woman ($0.0005 \times 38 = 0.019$ year = approximately 6.9 days; see Figure 17-1 and Appendix 17-II). To this we add the risk to life of late complications, the greatest being intestinal obstruction secondary to intra-abdominal adhesions. Assuming a 1% incidence of intestinal obstruction severe enough to require operative relief in the ten years following hysterectomy (or any abdominal operation), and a 1% mortality for its surgical relief (emergency laparotomy), there is an additional loss of 1.3, or a total of 8.2 days' loss of life expectancy for the 40-year-old woman undergoing elective hysterectomy.

Against any losses in life expectancy, we can weigh those gains which accrue secondary to the removal by hysterectomy of a variety of threats to life which our patient would otherwise face. The most prominent among these are the risks of death from cancer of the cervix, the corpus, and (if the ovaries are removed together with the uterus) the ovary. Added to these are small additional risks of death as a result of curettage, should excessive uterine bleeding occur in the future requiring this operation, and of pregnancy, whether or not allowed to proceed to term and delivery. Hormonal therapy which might be given for the management of excessive menstrual bleeding or for contraception is an additional risk of concern (Shapiro, 1975; Smith et al., 1975; Ziel and Finkle, 1975). We do not include it, however, since hormonal therapy following hysterectomy presumably entails the same risk.

The sum of threats to life prevented by hysterectomy, as listed above, is approximately 22 days for the average 40-year-old woman (see Figure 17-1). Elective hysterectomy and oophorectomy thus might be expected to increase the life expectancy of our 40-year-old woman in good physical health by 22 less 8 days, a net increase in life expectancy of 14 days. If hysterectomy alone is performed, leaving the ovaries intact (and thus a potential site of future cancer), the estimated increase in life expectancy is reduced to 4½ days. These calculations are, of course, based on approximations and average values, and our assumptions are subject to errors. If the risks of surgical death should be double those we have assumed, the estimated small gain in life expectancy is reduced from 14 to 7 days. On the other hand, it is likely that we have underestimated the life-extending effect of hysterectomy, since there is a reported twofold or greater increase in risk of future uterine malignancy in women who have a history of abnormal bleeding (Hammond et al., 1968). Taking this into account, the increase in life expectancy resulting from hysterectomy might be as much as a month.

We conclude that the effect of hysterectomy on the life expectancy of a 40-year-old woman in good general health is small and uncertain, but appears to be slightly favorable. However, it is important to bear in mind that in real life these

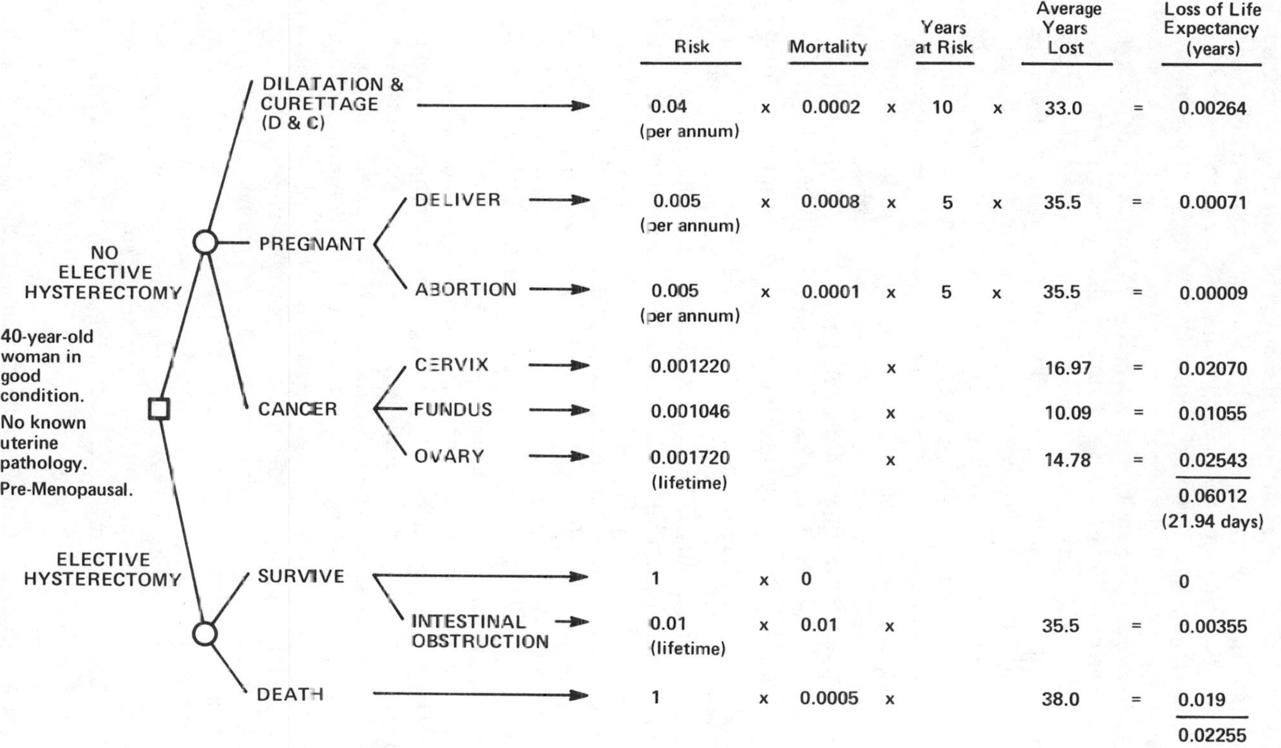

Figure 17-1. Decision tree: elective hysterectomy versus nonsurgical management. Estimated loss of life expectancy with and without hysterectomy and oöphorectomy in 40-year-old woman in good general health; has had two or three episodes of profuse menstrual bleeding, requiring D & C; no known uterine pathology. (See Appendix 17–II for source of values.)

few days of life expectancy are not being given to or taken away from all patients. A very small number of women lose their entire life expectancy because of surgical mortality, and a somewhat larger—but still quite small—number lose several years of life at an older age from cancer in the absence of hysterectomy. Patient preferences are presumably strongly influenced by these considerations. Thus, death as a consequence of elective hysterectomy comes at an age when a woman is apt to have many responsibilities as a mother, homemaker, or worker, and when her enjoyment of life may be large. Even if she chooses not to undergo hysterectomy, she may never develop cancer, or it may occur only many years in the future, at a time when responsibilities and enjoyment of life are apt to be less, and when our ability to detect and treat cancer might be improved. On the other hand, death from cancer is widely feared, and many might gladly undergo a small risk of death today to lessen the risk of cancer in the future.

What are the other benefits and risks—advantages and disadvantages—of hysterectomy? It is at least certain that hysterectomy will relieve menstrual discomfort and inconvenience. Fatigue from chronic blood loss and anemia, and some of the unpleasant symptoms of the premenopausal syndrome should be improved (the onset of the menopause will, of course, be immediate). The patient will also be relieved of any fears she may have of pregnancy or of uterine and ovarian malignancy.

Relief of symptoms should lead to an improved sense of well-being; how much of an improvement in the quality of life an individual patient will enjoy following hysterectomy is not certain, however, for there are a good many potential unpleasant side effects associated with this operation. The recovery from the operation itself is apt to be somewhat more prolonged than that following many other elective abdominal procedures, and it may be several months before the patient feels that she can return to her preoperative level of activity. Complications are common and troublesome, most notably urinary tract infections, which are reported in a high percentage of women following hysterectomies.

The most serious common sequelae, however, are probably in mood and psyche (Polivy, 1974). Depression requiring psychiatric attention is a recognized sequel of hysterectomy. Its frequency and significance are uncertain, since it appears that many of the patients receiving psychiatric care postoperatively have been under psychiatric care preoperatively, and that similar depression often follows natural menopause. In attempting to weigh the benefits and risks of a procedure intended to improve the quality of life, however, the possibility of major or minor psychiatric sequelae is of genuine concern. An indeterminate number of women are troubled, in addition, by feelings of loss of womanhood and of attractiveness, further reducing the net quality of life benefits of hysterectomy. Unfortunately, there are no data on how many women consider that they have, on the whole, benefited from hysterectomy, and how many have not. In the absence of such data, we tentatively conclude that elective hysterectomy for relief of symptoms in a healthy 40-year-old woman is justifiable on the basis of known risks and benefits.

Let us now consider how our analysis and conclusions might be altered under different circumstances. An older patient, or one in less favorable preoperative physical status, for example, would face a larger anesthetic and operative risk.

The magnitude of this increased risk has been documented in the National Halothane Study. Thus, the risk of operative or postoperative death for the seven operations classified as "low death rate operations," including hysterectomy, was ten times greater for patients of physical status Risk 2, who are defined as having "moderate complicating systemic disturbance, nonemergency," than for patients in Risk 1, defined as having "no complicating systemic disturbance, nonemergency" (Moses, 1969).

We have specified our 40-year-old patient in the foregoing analysis to be in Risk 1. A similar patient, if moderately severe hypertension were present, would qualify as Risk 2, and the loss of life expectancy following elective hysterectomy would presumably be ten times greater than in our calculation. Similarly, there was an approximately twofold increase in operative mortality for each additional decade after the age of 40 for the seven "low death rate" operations. For a 50-year-old woman suffering from moderately severe hypertension, therefore, elective hysterectomy would present very different implications for life expectancy.

The average life expectancy for a 50-year-old woman is 29 years; in the presence of moderately severe hypertension this is reduced to 26.4 years (Weinstein and Stason, 1976). We estimate that elective hysterectomy for this patient entails a very much larger loss in life expectancy, 81 days, whereas the sum of the several risks of not operating electively are 22 days, almost exactly the same as at age 40 (see Figure 17-2 and Appendix 17-II). Thus, life expectancy is now shortened, rather than lengthened. But, of course, it was not to prolong life that elective hysterectomy was proposed for our first hypothetical patient; it was for the relief of symptoms. A loss of life expectancy must be considered part of the price paid in exchange for the anticipated improvement in the quality of life.

From the foregoing, it is apparent that we can provide at least rough approximations of some of the risks and benefits of elective hysterectomy, and, indeed, it can be assumed that somewhat similar considerations are taken into account as part of each individual surgical decision. The decision is customarily made by the surgeon, often with relatively little participation from the patient. Indeed, some patients appear to prefer not to participate; yet under the clinical circumstances we have postulated above, it is the patient herself who should be in the best position to judge the severity of discomfort and disability, and to decide whether the prospect of future relief is sufficient to justify the immediate costs and risks of hysterectomy.

The costs in morbidity and mortality the patient must pay. The costs in dollars, however, are rarely paid directly by the patient, and, therefore, are not apt to enter into the physician's recommendation or the patient's decision. It is Society as a whole that pays an increasing proportion of the medical costs, and, under national health insurance, will presumably pay all of them.

The costs are substantial. Deane and Ulene (1976), in comparing cost effectiveness of hysterectomy and of tubal ligation for sterilization, estimate the net costs of hysterectomy, at a discount rate of 5%, to be $5,432 for a 40-year-old woman (based on estimated medical costs, number of days of disability, value of days of work lost as a result of operation, reduction in future days lost, medications, Pap smear tests, and sanitary supplies).

The costs of hysterectomy were calculated by Deane and Ulene to be greater

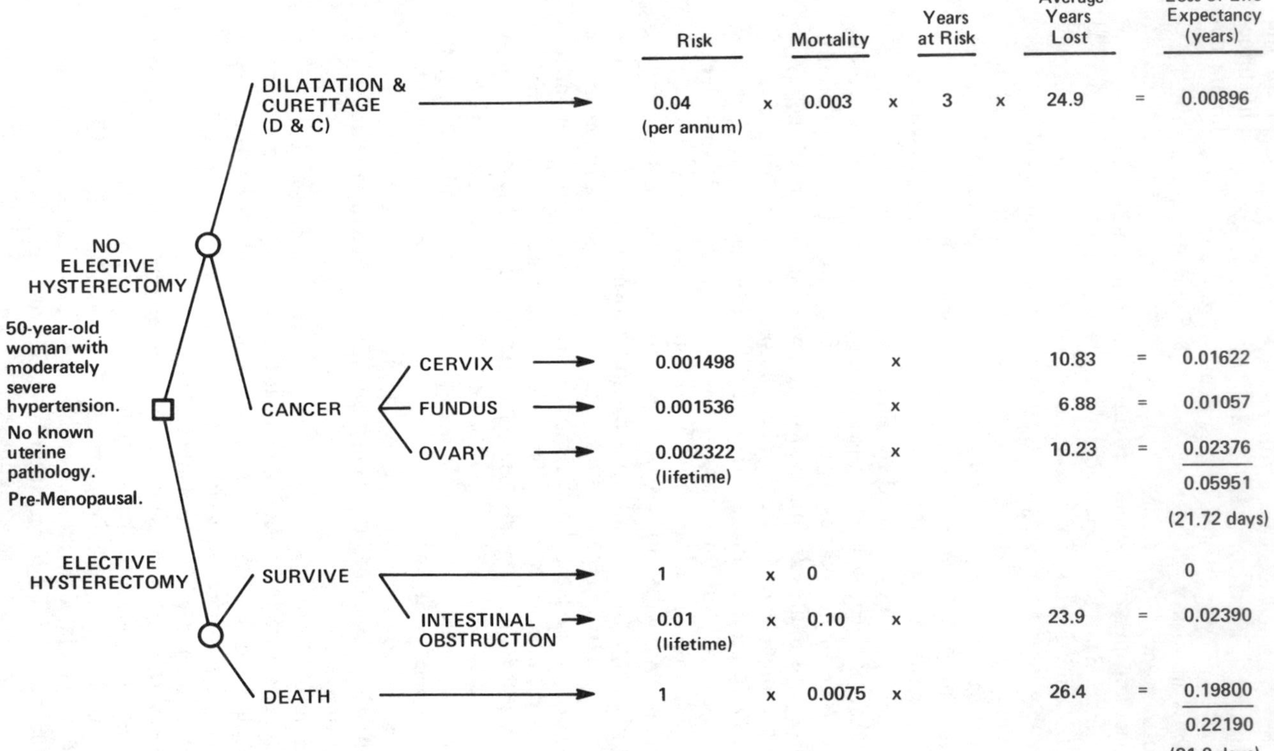

Figure 17-2. Decision tree: elective hysterectomy versus nonsurgical management. Estimated loss of life expectancy with and without hysterectomy and oöphorectomy in 50-year-old woman with moderately severe hypertension; has had two or three episodes of profuse menstrual bleeding, requiring D & C; no known uterine pathology. (See Appendix 17–II for source of values.)

than those of tubal ligation for all ages, at discount rates of 5% or greater. Their conclusion was that "when a reasonable discount rate is applied, the rational choice is tubal ligation at any age from Society's point of view. This conclusion applies to all women who would accept sterilization by either hysterectomy or tubal ligation, except for those for whom there is an overwhelming risk to one or both of the procedures."

Sterilization is only one of the several considerations in the present analysis of the cost-benefit appropriateness of elective hysterectomy in the symptomatic premenopausal woman, and accordingly it is to other benefits that we must look for justification of costs. One other such benefit, as we have seen, is an estimated small increase in life expectancy, achieved primarily by precluding future cancer of the uterus. We have estimated this increase in life expectancy to be two weeks to a month at the most. Converting this into dollars per year of life saved results in a cost well in excess of that which Neuhauser suggests, in Chapter 2, that Society might be willing to pay. Indeed, as Cole has concluded from his analysis of costs and risks of prophylactic hysterectomy, "hysterectomy for cancer prophylaxis does not appear justifiable. The gains are uncertain and small and the potential health losses are great" (Cole and Berlin, 1976).

We return, then, to the question of quality-of-life benefits, for which elective hysterectomy was undertaken. The answer to this question cannot at present be provided, since these benefits have not been documented. The first order of business, therefore, is to collect comprehensive data on the outcomes of elective hysterectomy. Even with these data in hand, however, it cannot be assumed that easy answers can be provided. The individual patient may consider that the quality-of-life benefits of hysterectomy are sufficient to offset attendant risks; indeed, based on the extremely high hysterectomy rates reported for physicians' wives, who should be reasonably well informed "consumers," it seems likely that many women will make this choice (Bunker and Brown, 1974).

Society may take a somewhat different view. If and when it is agreed to make "necessary" medical care available to every citizen as a right, Society must decide what is necessary and what is unnecessary. There can, of course, be little question as to the necessity of hysterectomy in the treatment of cancer of the endometrium, large, painful, or bleeding fibroids, or uterine prolapse. At issue will be the allocation of public funds for a procedure when it appears to be more of a convenience or luxury than a necessity, and in competition with growing demands for funds to pay for other medical procedures, many of which may present stronger claims.

SUMMARY

Hysterectomy rates vary two- and threefold between developed countries and within the United States. From this we conclude that a patient with gynecological complaints who undergoes hysterectomy in one geographic area might receive nonsurgical treatment, or no treatment, if she lived in another geographic area. This patient is apt to be 40 to 50 years of age, premenopausal, and in good general health. Her menses are irregular and she has had two or three episodes of profuse menstrual bleeding for which D & C was required. There is no demonstrable uterine pathology. Since indications for hysterectomy are borderline, we call her the marginal surgical patient.

Elective hysterectomy and oöphorectomy in such a patient, we estimate, will increase her life expectancy approximately two weeks, and perhaps as much as a month, primarily by precluding future cancer of the uterus and ovaries. For the patient who is less healthy or older—for example, a 50-year-old woman with moderate hypertension—life expectancy is shortened by elective hysterectomy as a result of a greatly increased risk of surgery.

The principal benefits of elective hysterectomy, it is assumed, are improvements in the quality of life. Menstrual discomfort and inconvenience will be relieved, but these benefits may be offset by a variety of unpleasant sequelae associated with hysterectomy and castration. There are no data on what proportion of women, on the balance, are benefited by elective hysterectomy. While the benefits are unmeasured and uncertain, the costs are large. These costs are rarely paid by the patient. Society, if it is to pay the costs, must decide whether to allocate public funds for a procedure if it appears to be more of a convenience or luxury than a necessity.

Acknowledgments

The authors wish to express their thanks to Ann B. Barnes, M.D.; Byron Wm. Brown, Ph.D.; Philip Cole, M.D.; Valentina C. Donahue, M.D.; Malkah T. Notman, M.D.; and George M. Ryan, M.D. for their review of this chapter and for their valuable suggestions; and to Mr. A.L. Ranofsky for providing data from the National Center for Health Statistics.

APPENDIX 17-I. OPERATION RATE ADJUSTMENT FOR POPULATION-AT-RISK

All surgical rates reported by the National Center for Health Statistics are for total male and/or female populations. Yearly rates for specific procedures are based on data abstracted by the National Discharge Survey from a national probability sample of the hospital records of discharged patients; rates are estimated using the Census population and expressed per 100,000 population. For operations that involve the removal of an organ, no corrections are made for those people in the population (i.e., the denominator of the rate of surgery) who have undergone the operation previous to the year of the survey and, hence, are no longer at risk. For procedures which are performed frequently, the difference in sample size and number at risk can be large. Therefore, figures reported by the National Center for Health Statistics should be adjusted if they are to be used as measures of the "risk" of coming to surgery. We illustrate a method of adjusting rates of hysterectomy as an example of the quantitative importance of correcting for population at risk.

The National Center has reported an operation rate of 647.7 hysterectomies per 100,000 female population for 1973; this is an increase of 33% over the 1968 reported rate (National Center for Health Statistics, 1973 and 1975). An estimate

Table 17-2. Proportion of women with operative menopause by 1960-62. Data from a probability sample of U.S.A. women.

Age at time of response	*Total*	*Operative meno-pause*	*Proportion of women having had operative menopause (P_i)*
18-24	534	1	.0019
25-34	746	25	.0335
35-44	784	91	.1161
45-54	705	173	.2454
55-64	443	120	.2709

Source: National Center for Health Statistics: Vital and Health Statistics, Data from The National Health Survey, Age at Menopause, United States 1960-1962 by Brian MacMahon and Jane Worcester, Public Health Service Pub. No. 1000–Series 11–No. 19.

of the total U.S. population at risk of coming to surgery is calculated by subtracting from the Census population that proportion of the population having undergone hysterectomy prior to the year being considered. Estimates of these proportions are obtained from the National Health Survey of age at menopause taken in 1960-62 (MacMahon and Worcester, 1966) and are presented in Table 17-2. These must be considered to be underestimates since they do not take into account the subsequent increase in hysterectomy rates noted above.

Subject to this limitation, we calculate, by Equation 1 below, rates of 527.1 and 706.3 hysterectomies per 100,000 female population-at-risk for the years 1968 and 1973, respectively.

$$R = \frac{O_T}{N'_T} \times 100{,}000 \qquad (1)$$

where:

R = crude risk of operation per 100,000 female population,

O_T = total number of hysterectomies performed on U.S. women in given year,

N'_T = total U.S. female population at risk for given year,

and:

$$O_T = \sum_{i=1}^{k} O_i,$$

$$N'_T = \sum_{i=1}^{k} N'_i = \sum_{i=1}^{k} N_i(1 - P_i),$$

with:

k = number of age intervals,

O_i = annual number of hysterectomies performed on U.S. women* in *i*th age interval ($i = 1,2, \ldots k$),

N'_i = annual U.S. female population at risk in *i*th age interval,

N_i = Census female population in *i*th age interval, for given year,

and

P_i = proportion of women with operative menopause by 1960-62 (Table 17-2).

The crude rate calculated from Equation 1 is not as informative as a cumulative probability curve presenting the risk of organ removal as a function of age. Such curves were used by Fairbairn and Acheson (1969), and also by Bunker and Brown (1974), though neither pair of authors adjusted their national rates as advocated here. Using our method of adjusting for the population at risk, age-specific risks of organ removal by the end of any age interval can be approximated from the following formula:

$$H_x = 1 - \prod_{i=1}^{x} (1 - L_i R_i) \qquad (2)$$

where:

H_x = risk of organ removal by the end of *x*th age interval,

L_i = number of years in *i*th interval, and

R_i = annual risk of organ removal in *i*th age interval, as calculated by:

$$R_i = \frac{O_i}{N'_i}.$$

The curves in Figure 17-3 depict the cumulative probability that a woman will undergo a hysterectomy in this country computed from Equation II, were she to be subjected throughout her life to the estimated age-specific rates for the years 1968 or 1973, and adjusted by the method described. Therefore, were the country to maintain the rate of hysterectomy as reported for 1973, at least half of the women in this country would have a hysterectomy by the age of 65.

We suggest that the National Center for Health Statistics utilize available past and current data on persons at risk in its probability samples to determine rates of surgery for populations at risk, and publish cumulative probabilities of organ removal as a function of age, with calculated standard errors, for those procedures that are performed frequently. At present, the estimation of population at risk

*Age-specific hysterectomy rates provided by Mr. A.L. Ranofsky, National Center for Health Statistics.

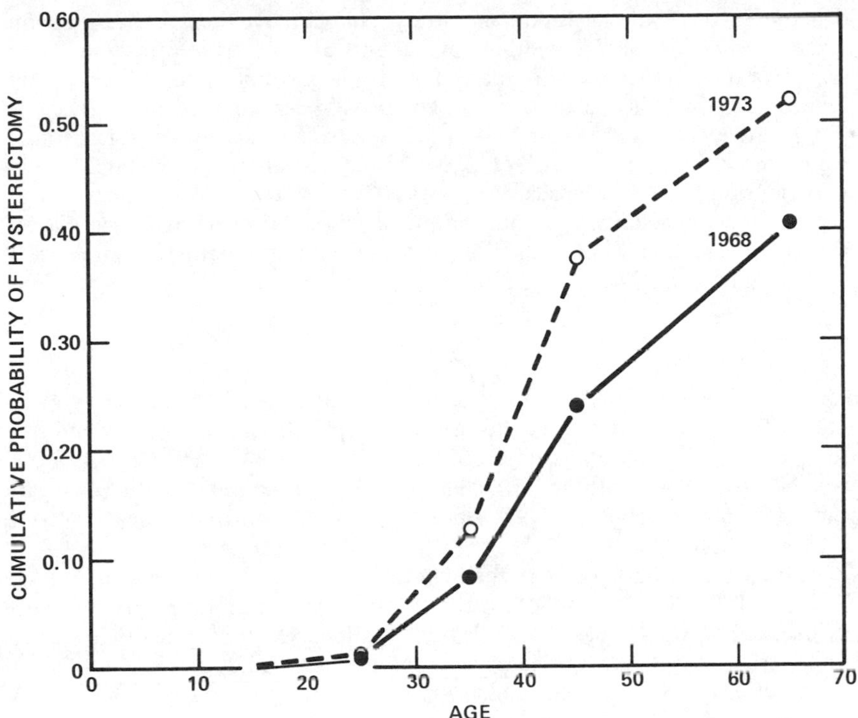

Figure 17-3. Cumulative probability of hysterectomy as a function of age.
Cumulative probability that a woman would undergo hysterectomy in the United States were she to be subjected throughout life to the estimated age-specific hysterectomy rates for the years 1968 and 1973 reported by the National Center for Health Statistics and corrected by the method described.

can only be approximated. With the passage of time and the accumulation of a more historical data base, the calculation of cumulative probabilities of organ removal can be made with increasing confidence.

APPENDIX 17-II. VALUES USED IN DECISION TREES

The values used in the decision tree of Figures 17-1 and 17-2 were chosen in the following manner:

D & C

Risk: In 1973 the D & C rate was 17.9 per 1,000 for women aged 34 to 45 and 13.3 per 1,000 for women 46-64 (National Center for Health Statistics, unpublished statistics). We assume the likelihood of D & C for both patients is at least double that for the population as a whole and we assign a value of 0.04.

Mortality: In the National Halothane Study the operative mortality rate for the seven "low-death rate" operations in patients aged 10 to 49, in "good" preoperative physical status (ASA risk 5), performed as emergencies, was approximately .0002.* We assign this risk to the 40-year-old women in excellent preoperative condition (Figure 17-1). On the basis of age and physical status, we estimate the mortality risk of a 50-year-old woman with moderately severe hypertension to be 15 times greater, or 0.003.

Years at risk: For women aged 40, the median age of natural menopause is 50. For premenopausal women aged 50, the median age of natural menopause is 53 (MacMahon and Worcester, 1966).

Pregnancy

Risk: In 1973 there were 31,862 live births in women aged 40 to 44 and a population of 5,898,000 women in this age bracket, a "risk" of pregnancy and full-term delivery of approximately .005. There were 1,942 births in 6,173,000 women aged 45-49, with no births reported beyond the age of 50; we disregard these few births beyond age 45, since they do not contribute measurably to the calculation.

Mortality: During the same year, the maternal mortality of women 40 to 44 was 78.5 per 100,000 live births (based on 25 deaths) and 154.5 per 100,000 live births at ages over 45 (based on 3 deaths) (National Center for Health Statistics, unpublished data). We assign a value of 80 per 100,000 (0.0008) risk of maternal death for a 40-year-old woman in excellent general health.

Abortion

Risk and Mortality: There are no reliable data for predicting a value for the likelihood of operative abortion, and we arbitrarily assign a value of .005. The mortality of legal abortion in New York City from mid-1970 to mid-1972 was 5.0 per 100,000 for women of all ages (Tietze et al., 1973). We assume that the mortality would be at least twice this value in women over 40 and assign a value of 0.0001. We have less confidence in the assigned risk and mortality values for abortion than for other values used; the contribution to the analysis and conclusions is, however, too small to be of concern, as can be seen in Figure 17-1.

Cancer of Cervix, Fundus, and Ovary

Mortality Risk: Age-specific death rates from these three causes were taken from: Vital Statistics of the United States, 1968, Volume II, Mortality, U.S. Department of Health, Education and Welfare, Rockville, Maryland, 1971, and from the U.S. Census figures for 1968. These denominators were adjusted for the proportion of women having undergone elective hysterectomy by each 5-year age group. These figures were taken from Appendix I. Figure 17-3,

*This is a "fitted" rate based on a smoothed contingency table analysis (Bishop and Mosteller, 1969).

leaving those women at risk of cancer of these sites. Therefore, the mortality risk was taken as the number of women dying after age 40 divided by the estimated number of women with intact wombs aged 40 or more.

Average Years Lost: Given the age-specific death rates for each site the average age of death for fatal cancers was calculated by life table analysis and the average number of years lost obtained by subtraction from the average age of death of the 40-year-old female population.

Hysterectomy

Mortality Risk: The overall operative mortality for hysterectomy in the National Halothane Study was .0027. The effect of variations of age and preoperative physical status was examined for groups of operations. Hysterectomy was included among the seven "low death-rate" operations. The operative mortality for elective low death-rate operations in females of ages 10 to 49 and in "good" preoperative physical condition (ASA risk 1 and 2) varied between .00035 and .00074 for the five anesthetic groups studied, and therefore we assign a value of .0005 for a 40-year-old woman in excellent physical condition. For a 50-year-old woman with moderately severe hypertension, we estimate that there is a twofold increase in risk on the basis of age, and a tenfold increase on the basis of physical status. These risks are not additive, however, and we therefore estimate a 15-fold increase, or 0.0075.

Intestinal Obstruction

There appear to be few data on the risk of intestinal obstruction following hysterectomy. In one series of 300 abdominal hysterectomies, the diagnosis of postoperative intestinal obstruction was made in 17 patients, and of these, 3 required surgical relief (White et al., 1971); in another series of 225 abdominal hysterectomies, it was reported that there were no cases of intestinal obstruction. (Richardson et al. 1973) Intestinal obstruction which occurs after discharge from the hospital is apt to be treated at another institution, and therefore these figures may be low. Medical opinion, on the other hand, suggests they may be high. In the absence of better data, we assign a value of .01, diminishing with time, with a mean time of obstruction at 2.5 years. In the National Halothane Study the fitted death rate for exploratory laparotomy for patients of ages 10 to 49 (ASA risks 1, 2, and 5) was .017. Exploratory laparotomy includes all emergency surgery for intra-abdominal catastrophe, much of which carries a poorer prognosis than posthysterectomy intestinal obstruction. We therefore assign a smaller value, 0.010. For a 50-year-old woman with moderately severe hypertension the risk of emergency laparotomy is considerably greater, and we estimate this to be 0.10.

References

Bishop YMM, Mosteller F: Smoothed contingency table analysis. The National Halothane Study. Edited by JP Bunker, WH Forrest Jr., F Mosteller, et al.

National Institutes of Health, National Institute of General Medical Sciences, Bethesda, Md, 1969, pp 259–266

Bunker JP: Surgical manpower: a comparison of operations and surgeons in the United States and in England and Wales. N Engl J Med 282:135, 1970

Bunker JP, Brown BW: The physician-patient as an informed consumer of surgical services. N Engl J Med 290:1051, 1974

Cole P, Berlin JE: Prophylactic hysterectomy. Manuscript in preparation, 1976

Deane RT, Ulene A: Hysterectomy or tubal ligation for sterilization: a cost-effectiveness analysis. Inquiry, in press, 1976

Fairbairn AS, Acheson ED: The extent of organ removal in the Oxford area. J Chronic Dis 22:111, 1969

Hammond EC, Burns EL, Seidman H, et al: Detection of uterine cancer: high and low risk groups. Cancer 22:1096, 1968

MacMahon B, Worcester J: Age at menopause, United States 1960–1962. Public Health Service Publication Series 11, No. 19, National Center for Health Statistics, 1966

Moses LE: Comparison of crude and standardized anesthetic death rates. Chapter IV–2, The National Halothane Study: report of the subcommittee on the National Halothane Study. Edited by JP Bunker, WH Forrest Jr., F Mosteller, et al. Washington, DC, Government Printing Office, 1969

National Center for Health Statistics: Surgical operations in short-stay hospitals: United States, 1968, DHEW Publ. No. (HSM) 73-1762, January, 1973; Surgery in short-stay hospitals: United States, 1973, (HRA) 75–1120, Vol. 24, No. 3, Suppl., May 30, 1975

Pearson RJC, Smedby B, Berfenstam R, et al: Hospital caseloads in Liverpool, New England, and Uppsala. Lancet 2:559, 1968

Polivy J: Psychological reactions to hysterectomy. Am J Obstet Gynecol 118: 417, 1974

Richardson AC, Lyon JB, Graham EE: Abdominal hysterectomy: relationship between morbidity and surgical technique. Am J Obstet Gynecol 115:953, 1973

Shapiro S: Oral contraceptives and myocardial infarction. N Engl J Med 293:195, 1975

Smith DC, Prentice R, Thompson DJ, et al: Association of exogenous estrogen and endometrial carcinoma. N Engl J Med 293:1164, 1975

Tietze C, Pakter J, Berger GS: Mortality with legal abortion in New York City, 1970–1972. JAMA 225:507, 1973

Vayda E: A comparison of surgical rates in Canada and in England and Wales. N Engl J Med 289:1224, 1973

Weinstein MC, Stason WB: Hypertension: A Policy Perspective. Cambridge, Massachusetts, Harvard University Press, 1976

Wennberg J, Gittelsohn A: Small area variations in health care delivery. Science 182:1102, 1973

Wennberg J, Gittlesohn A: Health care delivery in Maine: I. Patterns of use of common surgical procedures. J Maine Med Assoc 66:123, 1975

White SC, Wartel LJ, Wade ME: Comparison of abdominal and vaginal hysterectomies. Obstet Gynecol 37:530, 1971

Ziel HK, Finkle WD: Increased risk of endometrial carcinoma among users of conjugated estrogens. N Engl J Med 293:1167, 1975

18

Indications for the surgical treatment of suspected acute appendicitis: a cost-effectiveness approach

Raymond Neutra

The indications for appendectomy are controversial because even after the most thorough workup, the diagnosis is often in doubt. In the face of this uncertainty, two therapeutic philosophies have arisen. The "noninterventionist" emphasizes the value of a careful clinical examination with close monitoring for a number of hours. Some say that this procedure increases diagnostic accuracy and eliminates many operations on persons with normal appendices (Medical World News, 1975, de Dombal et al., 1974). A surgeon with an "interventionist" philosophy worries about waiting too long and is willing to remove a certain proportion of normal appendices from patients with suspicious symptoms in order to avoid missing an atypical case of appendicitis (Fellig and Hanfstaengel, 1974; Jacob et al., 1975). The relative predominance of proponents of one or the other philosophy in different institutions is reflected in wide variations among hospitals in the proportion of removed appendices found to be normal at the time of pathological examination (Thomas and Mueller, 1969). It is reflected also in the large variations in appendectomy rates, which are reported among nations (Lichtner and Pflanz, 1971), or even within one state (Wennberg and Gittelsohn, 1973; Lewis, 1969). This variability has alarmed proponents of "noninterventionism," and they have suggested that surgeons who are excessively interventionist may ultimately cause a number of operative deaths greater than the appendicitis-related deaths which they are trying to avoid. Lembcke (1952) found that hospital catchment areas with high appendectomy rates had higher, not lower rates of death attributed on death certificates to appendectomy and appendicitis. He suggested that the deaths related to the removal of normal appendices might account for the excess deaths observed. Lichtner and Pflanz (1971) documented a similar phenomenon in East and West Germany as well as in Austria. These countries reported the world's highest appendectomy rates (around 6/1000 per year) and also the highest mortality related to appendicitis and appendectomy (3/100,000 per year). Data in their study from the few hospitals with tissue committees (which review the pathological status of all removed appendices) showed that 76% of appendices removed in primary appendectomies were without demonstrable abnormality as compared to 20-30% in the United States (Thomas and Mueller, 1969). These authors, like Lembcke, proposed that the higher mortality from appendectomy-appendicitis may be caused by the large number of operations on persons with normal appendices.

German surgeons have responded to this analysis by warning against the dangers of noninterventionism and by defending the status quo (Fellig and Hanfstaengl, 1974).

In the hope of clarifying the general controversy the present article presents a quantitative approach to the costs and benefits associated with the "noninterventionist" and "interventionist" management of suspected acute appendicitis. The assessment deals with lives, with postoperative disability and with economic costs. Appendectomy lends itself to this kind of analysis because the expected benefits, lives saved, and reduced disability days occur in the postoperative period and are easily quantified. The analysis has had to rely on relatively scanty data from the literature and uses many simplifying assumptions. It should be viewed, therefore, as paradigmatic rather than definitive. When more reliable information on the natural history of appendicitis is available, an analysis can be carried out whose results could be used to guide policy. In the absence of such data, the preliminary results presented here provide a tentative model and a specification of information which must be known with greater reliability. It should be noted that we are addressing the question of when to operate, not the question of whether surgery is better than a dietary preventive program as advocated by Burkitt (1972), or an antibiotic therapy as advocated by Crile and Fulton (1945), Bowers et al. (1958), and Coldrey (1959). Although these alternatives are of interest and potential importance they are not now being seriously considered by the medical profession. This chapter, therefore, does not include them but rather focuses on the controversy around surgical management itself.

AN ANALYTIC APPROACH TO SELECTING OPTIMAL INDICATIONS FOR THE SURGICAL MANAGEMENT OF SUSPECTED ACUTE APPENDICITIS

The Lembcke Hypothesis

Lichtner and Pflanz (1971) and Lembcke (1952) directed attention to the fact that areas where appendectomy rates are high may also experience high rates of death attributed to "appendicitis." They and others have hypothesized that the excess deaths are largely comprised of patients whose normal appendices were unnecessarily removed. According to this hypothesis, surgeons in areas with

Table 18-1. Probabilities of four symptoms or signs in appendicitis and NSAP* and their likelihood ratio.

	(1) Probability in appendicitis	*(2) Probability in NSAP**	*(1) ÷ (2) Likelihood ratio*
RLQ pain	0.74	0.29	2.55
Lower 1/2 pain**	0.13	0.09	1.44
Other pain	0.13	0.62	.21
Severe	0.39	0.19	2.05
Nonsevere	0.61	0.81	.75
Rebound	0.95	0.26	3.65
No rebound	0.05	0.74	.07
Tender rectal	0.43	0.16	2.69
Not tender	0.57	0.84	.68

*NSAP = nonspecific abdominal pain
**Lower ½ pain = pain in lower half of abdomen

high appendectomy rates differ from surgeons in low rate areas in that they use more relaxed indications for performing an appendectomy. To examine this hypothesis it would help to have an "appendicitis risk score" summarizing in a single number the severity of clinical findings which suggest appendicitis. It would then be possible to compare the "operating score" preferred by "interventionists," with that preferred by "noninterventionists". It was possible to develop such a score for the purposes of this paper. Patients with a score of 1 have the lowest risk, those with a score of 24 have the highest risk of appendicitis. This score is based on two symptoms (location of pain and severity of pain), and two signs (presence of right lower quadrant (RLQ) rebound tenderness and presence of rectal tenderness). Data published by Staniland et al. (1972) at Leeds provide the conditional probabilities of possessing these four characteristics among appendicitis (APP) and nonspecific abdominal pain (NSAP) patients. We have ignored other diagnoses for the moment. These probabilities are displayed in Table 18-1. Of the four findings, one takes on three values (RLQ, lower ½, other location) while the other three findings are dichotomous. This means that there are 24 possible symptom combinations ($3 \times 2 \times 2 \times 2 = 24$).

By assuming independence of symptoms (an assumption we discuss further on), it was possible to calculate the conditional probability of each of these 24 combinations among patients with appendicitis and with nonspecific abdominal pain. This was done by invoking the multiplicative law of probability for independent events. For example, in order to calculate the probability among appendicitis patients of possessing: "severe pain–right lower quadrant in location–with rebound tenderness–and rectal tenderness," the probabilities of the four findings among appendicitis patients were simply multiplied. To estimate the probability of the same combination of findings in NSAP patients, the probabilities of the four findings among NSAP patients were multiplied.

After generating the probability of the 24 combinations for appendicitis and then for NSAP, the rate of appendicitis (posterior probability) expected in each symptom combination was calculated according to Bayes Theorem (Lusted, 1968):

$$P(APP|comb_i) = \frac{P(comb_i|APP) \cdot P(APP)}{P(comb_i|APP) \cdot P(APP) + P(comb_i|NSAP)\, P(NSAP)}$$

where i goes from 1 to 24, and $comb_i$ stands for the ith combination.

The probabilities of appendicitis, P(APP), and P(NSAP) were based on data taken from de Dombal et al. (1972). These probabilities will be discussed in more detail (*vide infra*).

The 24 symptom combinations were then ordered according to the probability of appendicitis which Bayes Theorem predicted they would have. The highest rank is called rank 24 and corresponds to the combination: "RLQ, severe pain with rebound and rectal tenderness." The risk of appendicitis in patients with this symptom combination is 92%. The lowest rank, which we call rank 1, corresponds to the combination: "Other location, mild pain, without rebound, without rectal tenderness." Patients with that combination have an appendicitis rate of 0.4%. The remaining 22 combinations were filled in between these two extremes in ascending order of risk. In this manner we have created a risk score which separates the two diagnostic categories (see Table 18-2). Figure 18-1 shows the appendicitis patients (above the X axis) and the NSAP patients (distributed, for visual clarity, below the X axis). The X axis itself represents the appendicitis risk score (Fig. 18-1 and Table 18-2). It can be seen that the appendicitis patient distribution has its mode over the high risk "severe" symptoms while nonspecific abdominal pain distribution has its mode over the low risk "mild" symptoms. There is a significant area where the likelihood of appendicitis and of NSAP is about equal. This makes it difficult to select a score above which all patients should be operated.

According to the Lembcke hypothesis surgeons in high operation rate areas would be willing to perform an appendectomy on patients with mild symptoms, for example, rank 7 or above. (Rank 7 contains patients with severe lower abdominal pain and no rebound or rectal tenderness.) They would do this in order to catch the few atypical appendicitis cases in which symptoms and signs are mild. In exchange, they would be willing to operate on the many normal patients with symptoms of rank 7 or greater. As a result, the appendectomy rate would rise, and if the hypothesis is correct, the surgeons would operate on enough normal patients to cause a higher overall mortality rate. "Noninterventionist" surgeons, on the other hand, would prefer to operate only on patients with more obvious and severe symptoms, for example, at rank 13 or above. (Rank 13 contains patients with severe RLQ pain without rebound but with rectal tenderness.) They would argue that they can keep the mortality resulting from operations on normal patients low enough to counterbalance the small increase in mortality among the few atypical appendicitis patients missed. In short, noninterventionists and interventionists differ about the optimal degree of symptom severity that should be used when deciding whether or not to operate.

Table 18-2. Twenty-four possible symptom combinations are ranked as to likelihood ratio. Each combination is identified and its probability among "APP" and "NSAP" is shown.

Rank	Identity of Combination				(1) $P(comb_i \mid APP)$	(2) $P(comb_i \mid NSAP)$	(1) ÷ (2) Likelihood Ratio
24	RLQ	SEV	REB	RECT	.1179	.0023	51.26
23	L½	SEV	REB	RECT	.0207	.0007	29.57
22	RLQ	N	REB	RECT	.1844	.0097	19.01
21	RLQ	SEV	REB	N	.1563	.0120	13.03
20	L½	N	REB	RECT	.0324	.0030	10.80
19	L½	SEV	REB	N	.0275	.0037	7.43
18	RLQ	N	REB	N	.2444	.0513	4.76
17	Other	SEV	REB	RECT	.0207	.0049	4.22
16	L½	N	REB	RECT	.0429	.0159	2.70
15	Other	N	REB	N	.0324	.0209	1.55
14	Other	SEV	REB	N	.0275	.0257	1.07
13	RLQ	SEV	N	RECT	.0062	.0065	0.95
12	L½	SEV	N	RECT	.0011	.0020	0.54
11	Other	N	REB	N	.0429	.1097	0.39
10	RLQ	N	N	RECT	.0097	.0278	0.35
9	RLQ	SEV	N	N	.0082	.0343	0.24
8	L½	N	N	RECT	.0017	.0086	0.20
7	L½	SEV	N	N	.0014	.0106	.13
6	RLQ	N	N	N	.0129	.1460	.09
5	Other	SEV	N	RECT	.0011	.0140	.08
4	L½	N	N	N	.0023	.0453	.05
3	Other	N	N	RECT	.0017	.0595	.03
2	Other	SEV	N	N	.0014	.0732	.02
1	Other	N	N	N	.0023	.3122	.01

APP = appendicitis
NSAP = nonspecific abdominal pain
RLQ = pain in right lower quadrant of abdomen
L½ = pain in lower half of abdomen
SEV = severe pain
REB = rebound right lower quadrant tenderness
RECT = rectal tenderness
N = absence of above

The Approach

In order to choose such an optimal point, medical decision analysts suggest that we need to know several things (Lusted, 1968; McNeil et al., 1975; Pauker and Kassirer, 1975):

(1) The distribution of appendicitis and of NSAP patients along the risk score (illustrated by Figure 18-1)
(2) The prevalence of appendicitis and NSAP ("prior probabilities")

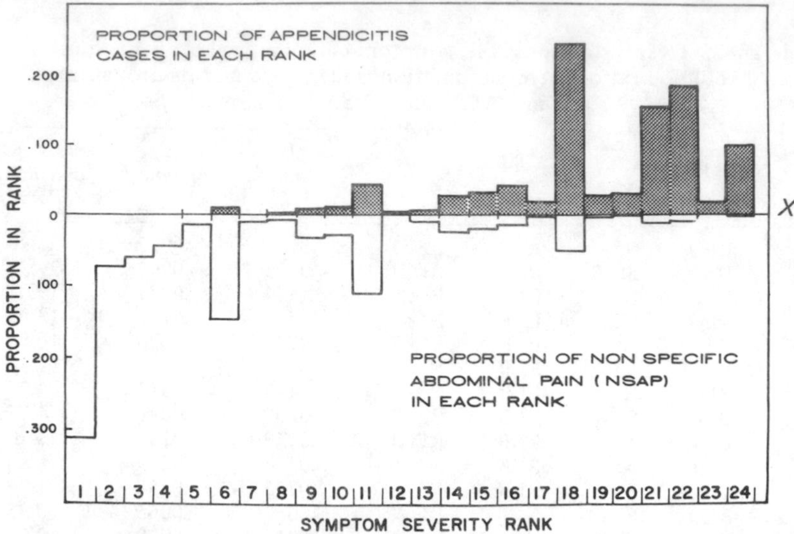

Figure 18-1. Distribution of appendicitis and NSAP patients as to appendicitis-risk score.

The figure shows two frequency distributions: that of appendicitis patients (above the X axis) and that of nonspecific abdominal pain (NSAP) patients (distributed for visual clarity, below the X axis). The X axis itself represents a symptom severity score. People with a score of 1 have the mildest symptoms. People with a score of 24 have the most severe symptoms. Although appendicitis patients have a higher mean severity than NSAP patients, there is a significant area of overlap in the two distributions. "Interventionist" surgeons might operate on patients with rank 7 or above. "Noninterventionist" surgeons might only start operating at rank 13.

(3) The costs associated with true positives, false negatives, false positives, and true negatives.

It is important to consider each of these factors carefully.

The Distribution of Cases and Non-Cases

The risk score described above is based on patients with symptoms suggestive enough to have been admitted for surgical observation at Leeds. Only the findings at the time of admission have been considered because no information about the change of symptoms over time was published. The probability of a symptom was not made conditional on the patient's age or sex, a point of importance because the difficulty of the diagnosis of appendicitis is said to vary with age and sex. The sensitivity of our conclusions to these and other simplifications will be discussed below. For now, let us accept the distribution of cases and noncases depicted in Figure 18-1 and summarized in Table 18-2.

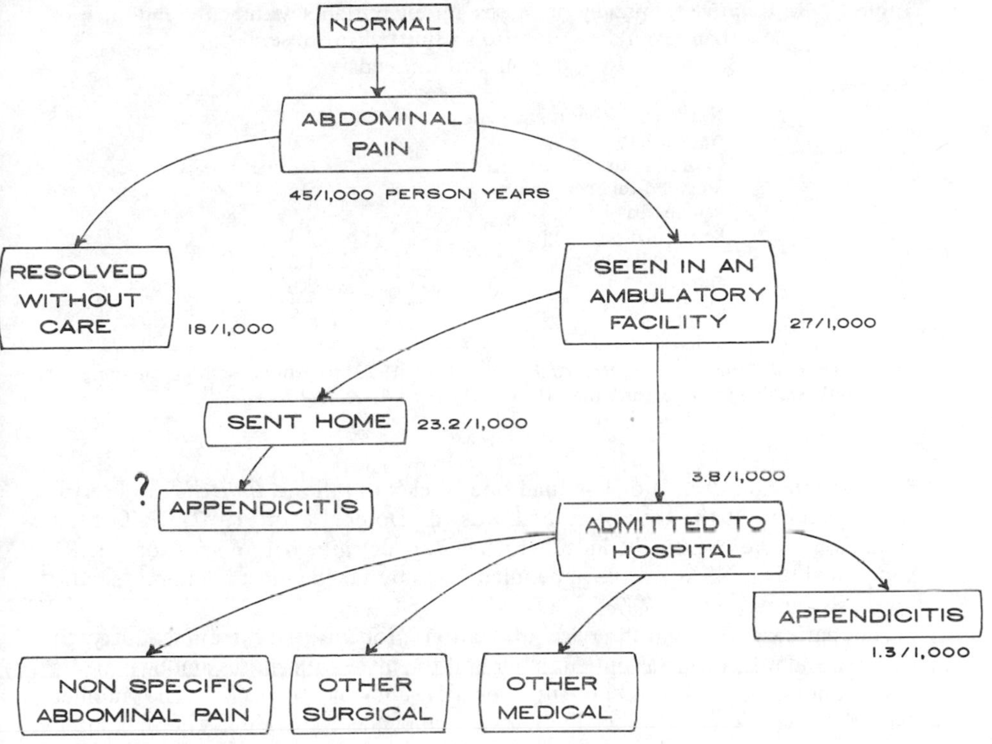

Figure 18-2. The disposition of acute abdomen in the population.
The incidence of acute abdominal pain in the population is shown in this figure. Many of the episodes receive no medical attention. Only a minority of cases is admitted to hospital. Of these one-third is caused by appendicitis.

The Prevalence of Appendicitis and NSAP

From the surgeon's point of view, the prevalences of importance are the prevalences in the office, emergency room, or on a house call where he has to make his decisions. Nonetheless, it is worthwhile first to consider the natural history of acute abdominal pain in the total population, since illness seen by the physician is very much influenced by illness in the community. Figure 18-2 presents the incidence of abdominal pain in the population and the proportion of the population seeking ambulatory and hospital care for it. The figures are adapted from Andersen et al. (1967) and Kleinman et al. (1972). The 1971 appendicitis rate is estimated by assuming that 80% (Thomas and Mueller, 1969) of the national appendectomy rate reported by the National Center for Health Statistics (1971) consists of appendicitis. The figure suggests that a good deal of filtering is taking place. Of the estimated 45/1000 episodes of acute abdomen which occur each year only 3.8/1000 population are admitted from outpatient facilities to the hospital. Table 18-3 shows the relative frequency of causes of acute abdominal

Table 18-3. Relative frequency of causes among patients with acute abdomen of less than seven days' duration admitted for observation to a surgical unit in Leeds

Nonspecific abdominal pain	49.0%
Appendicitis	28.0
Cholecystitis	8.6
Small bowel obstruction	5.6
Pancreatitis	2.6
Perforated peptic ulcer	2.3
Diverticular disease	1.3
Other	2.6
Total	100.0%

Source: From de Dombal et al., *Br Med J*, 2, pp. 9–13, 1972. Reprinted with permission of the authors, the publisher, and the editor of the *British Medical Journal*.

pain ("acute abdomen") of less than one week's duration *admitted* for observation or surgery at the University of Leeds (de Dombal et al., 1972). Half of the admissions were eventually judged to have no definite pathology (nonspecific abdominal pain, NSAP) while appendicitis was by far the most common specific diagnosis accounting for 28% of the cases.

The patterns of health service utilization probably vary from country to country and effect the absolute number and the mix of diagnoses among patients with abdominal pain who present themselves to the physician. The number presenting serves as an upper limit to the appendectomy rate. The maximum proportion of operated patients who could possibly have normal appendices would occur if all these presenting patients received an appendectomy. Thus, under the present utilization pattern American surgeons could not operate on more than 27/1000 acute abdomen "episodes" which are attended by physicians. If all these "episodes" represented separate individuals and all received appendectomies, the proportion of appendectomies resulting in the removal of normal appendices would be 95% instead of the current 15-20%. This is calculated by subtracting our estimate of the appendicitis rate (1.3/1000) from the rate of abdominal pain visits (27/1000) and expressing the difference as a percent of 27/1000. One suspects that the Germans, whose removal rate of normal appendices has been 76% (Lichtner and Pflanz, 1971), are operating on a greater proportion of patients who come under their care. Alternatively, they may see a mix of patients so much "richer" in NSAP that they cannot avoid a high rate of diagnostic error.

At any rate, for lack of any other source of data on the relative frequency of appendicitis and NSAP in an ambulatory care environment, we shall use de Dombal's probabilities among patients with symptoms suspicious enough to warrant observation in a hospital. The prevalence of appendicitis in this group can be calculated from the data in Table 18-3. It was 28/(28 + 49) or 36% and so, that of NSAP was 64%. The sensitivity of the results to assumptions about the prevalence of appendicitis is discussed below.

The Net Costs of "False Negatives" and "False Positives"

In real life, the surgeon, when faced with a case of suspected acute appendicitis, must also consider other surgical diagnoses and other medically treatable causes of abdominal pain. He cannot restrict his consideration to appendicitis and nonspecific abdominal pain, even though they are the most common diagnostic entities. Ideally, then, we should consider the penalties associated with doing an appendectomy on a patient with a medically treatable diagnosis (for example, pancreatitis) or another surgical condition (for example, a perforated peptic ulcer). Unfortunately, data are not available as to the mortality attributable to these errors, so that a simplification has been made and the task of distinguishing between appendicitis and NSAP will be the subject of our analysis. Later, we will consider the extent of the bias which has been created by this simplification.

We shall define false positives and negatives as follows: the proportion of "false positives" refers to the proportion of NSAP patients who receive an operation, the "false negatives" refer to the proportion of appendicitis patients who perforate because a needed operation was delayed or not given. An important question to be considered at this point is how many patients with symptomatic appendicitis would actually go on to perforate if they were not operated upon.

Current belief is influenced by the experiments of Wangensteen and his colleagues (1937) which suggested that appendicitis was due to an obstruction of the appendix with an inevitable rupture from intraluminal pressure, occluded circulation, and necrosis. Crile and Fulton (1945), on the other hand, propose that an inflammatory appendicitis syndrome also exists and is self-limiting. One autopsy study (Collins, 1936) purports to show that the majority of older persons show signs of severe residual scarring in the appendix, suggesting the possibility of recurrent episodic and self-limited appendicitis. In Cleveland (Green and Watkins, 1946b) some 30% of patients with symptoms of appendicitis lasting more than ten days had still not perforated at the time of operation.

Since there is no definitive study on this point, our analyses were made under each of two extreme assumptions. In the first analysis we accept Wangensteen's viewpoint and assume that 100% of unoperated patients would perforate, and only then would receive a delayed operation. In the second analysis we take an extremely optimistic view and assume that only 30% of unoperated patients would perforate but that the symptoms of the remaining 70% of unperforated patients would become sufficiently obvious that they would finally be operated upon, and that their case fatality would be that associated with the removal of an inflammed but unperforated appendix.

To be more realistic it was also necessary to recognize that a certain proportion of appendicitis patients perforate their appendices before ever reaching the hospital. This outcome cannot be prevented by the surgeon. Surgical colleagues who were consulted estimated that 80% of patients currently perforating fell into this category. The perforation rate in 23 New England hospitals (Osler Peterson, unpublished data) was 8%, so we calculated that 6.4% of appendicitis patients perforate unavoidably and have the associated case fatality. These patients perforate regardless of the indications used.

The interest in preventing perforation is motivated by the dramatic increase in case fatality which accompanies it. This increase existed both before and after the advent of blood transfusions to control septic shock, nasogastric suctioning, sophisticated electrolyte management, and perhaps antibiotics. In a series of 19,000 appendectomies between 1930 and 1940 in Cleveland (Watkins, 1942; Green and Watkins, 1946b), the case fatality for removing an inflammed appendix was 9/1000 while removal of an already perforated appendix carried with it a risk of 187/1000. They did not report the case fatality associated with "false positives," the removal of a normal appendix. During the same era, teaching hospitals reported somewhat lower figures (Lehman and Parker, 1938; Rogers and Faxon, 1942; Gilmour, 1952) but the Cleveland figures coming as they do from the community hospitals of an entire city are probably more typical of the case fatality in the country at large. By the late 1960's, case fatalities had fallen dramatically, thanks to the aforementioned therapeutic advances (Barnes et al., 1962a; 1962b). Howie (1966) in Scotland reports a case fatality for removing a normal appendix of 0.65/1000. The case fatality for removing an inflammed appendix was 1.02/1000 and for removing a perforated appendix 27/1000. These figures agree with those mentioned by other authors (Barnes et al., 1962a; Hawk, 1950) and underscore the continuing importance of perforation to appendicitis mortality. Indeed, Barnes's data (1962a) suggest that preventing perforation would eliminate 84% of appendicitis mortality. The cost of a "false negative," judging by Howie's (1966) figures, is thus over forty times greater than the cost of a "false positive." This high ratio has an important influence on our results.

It would be better to look at this problem within separate age groups. In 1970, persons over 45 accounted for more than 80% of the 1,400 deaths attributed to appendicitis in the United States (Vital Statistics of the U.S. 1970, VII, Mortality) even though less than 18% of appendicitis occurs in this age group (Pearson, 1964; Watkins, 1942). Older patients are more likely to arrive already having suffered a perforated appendix (Watkins, 1942), and their case fatality for perforated and unperforated appendicitis is about ten times higher than for persons in their twenties and thirties. These facts, plus the common impression that the clinical presentation of older patients is less obvious than that of younger patients, suggest that a definitive analysis of the appendicitis problem should be carried out separately for this age group. The lack of age-specific data on symptoms makes such an analysis impossible at this time. The sensitivity of the conclusions to this simplification is discussed below.

The excess costs of "false positives" and "false negatives" were also considered in terms of convalescence and direct hospital costs. Hospital stays for patients operated upon for perforated, inflamed, and normal appendices were obtained from unpublished data of Osler Peterson. The direct hospital costs were obtained from a publication of the American Hospital Association (1970), and convalescence information was obtained from a publication of the National Center for Health Statistics (1963). For lack of data the costs associated with "true negatives" were based on the author's estimates. Persons with NSAP who did not receive an operation were assumed to have no mortality. We assumed 10% had been hospitalized for observation, the remainder being billed only for an emer-

Table 18-4. Estimated costs of false negative, true positive, true negative, and false positive

	Delayed Operation with Perforation	*Timely Operation*
Appendicitis	Case Fatality = 27/1000 Direct Costs = \$3000 Hospital Days = 18 Convalescent Days = 61	Case Fatality = 1.02/1000 Direct Costs = \$1500 Hospital Days = 6.5 Convalescent Days = 22
	No Operation (baseline)	*Operation*
NSAP	Case Fatality = 0 Direct Costs = \$63 Hospital Days = 0.10 Convalescent Days = 3	Case Fatality = 0.65/1000 Direct Costs = \$1500 Hospital Days = 6.5 Convalescent Days = 22

gency room visit at the going Boston rate. They were assumed to convalesce for three days. The full range of costs in terms of case fatality, dollars, and convalescence is summarized in Table 18-4. It should be noted that although the monetary and convalescent costs of a "false negative" (perforation) are higher than that of a "false positive," the differential is not as striking as it is with case fatality. This, too, heavily influences our results.

How the Risk Score Dichotomy with the Minimum Deaths Was Found

Counting the option of operating upon everyone and operating upon no one, we have 25 possible divisions along the 24 rank risk scale which could be used to dichotomize the scale into "operate" and "don't operate" zones. At any one of these points the expected number of deaths can be calculated with the following formula:

Expected deaths* = (number of unavoidable perforations) (27/1000)

+

(remaining number of appendicitis patients) $P(\mathrm{OP}|\mathrm{APP})$ (1.02/1000)

+

(remaining number of appendicitis patients) $P(\overline{\mathrm{OP}}|\mathrm{APP})$ (27/1000)

*The notation here has the following interpretation: OP stands for being operated on; $\overline{\mathrm{OP}}$ stands for not being operated on; $P(\mathrm{OP}|\mathrm{APP})$ = probability of being at or above the division and thus operated among appendicitis patients; $P(\overline{\mathrm{OP}}|\mathrm{APP})$ = probability of being below the division and thus not operated among appendicitis patients, etc.

+

(number of NSAP patients) $P(\mathrm{OP}|\mathrm{NSAP})$ (0.65/1000)

+

(number of NSAP patients) $P(\mathrm{OP}|\mathrm{NSAP})$ (0)

The numbers of appendicitis patients and NSAP patients were calculated in the following way: The 1971 appendectomy rate of 1.57/1000 (National Center for Health Statistics, 1971) was applied to the U.S. 200 million population (314,000). Of these operations 80% were assumed to be appendicitis (251,200). Since de Dombal had a ratio of 64 NSAP patients to 36 appendicitis patients, the number of NSAP patients was 446,578 while the appendicitis cases numbered 251,200. However, surgical colleagues estimated that 80% of the current 8% of appendicitis patients who perforate do so unavoidably prior to hospitalization. Thus, 6.4% of the 251,200 or 16,077 persons must be counted as unavoidable perforations, while the "remaining appendicitis patients" number 235,123. Each of the 25 dichotomies has four conditional probabilities associated with it: $P(\mathrm{OP}|\mathrm{APP})$, $P(\mathrm{OP}|\mathrm{NSAP})$, $P(\overline{\mathrm{OP}}|\mathrm{APP})$ and $P(\overline{\mathrm{OP}}|\mathrm{NSAP})$. These can be calculated by accumulating the probabilities from Table 18-2. The case fatalities are those from Table 18-4.

This kind of calculation, and the analagous ones for hospital costs and convalescent days, was carried out for each and every one of the 25 possible dichotomies along the risk scale. The results are meant to represent potential yearly figures for the United States.

Results

Two analyses were carried out. The first one assumed that 100% of the nonoperated appendicitis patients would perforate. The results of this analysis are shown in Figure 18-3 and Table 18-5. The second analysis assumed that only 30% of the nonoperated appendicitis patients would perforate. These results are shown in Figure 18-4 and Table 18-6.

The top graphs in both Figures 18-3 and 18-4 show that the yearly expected number of deaths falls rapidly as perforations are prevented by operating on the patients with the most obvious symptoms. Below rank 10, however, the curve is nearly flat. Any further relaxation of indications produces minimal benefits. Although a minimum of deaths is reached at rank 4 in Figure 18-3 and rank 8 in Figure 18-4, the upswing of expected deaths is not impressive when operations are performed on patients with symptom severities below these ranks. Thus, the Lembcke hypothesis linking interventionist surgery to marked increases in appendectomy-related deaths is not supported by this analysis. Indeed, Dahm (1972) has shown that the high appendicitis mortality in East Germany, where appendectomy rates are three times the U.S. and U.K. rates, is primarily attributable to perforation, and that only 30% is attributable to excess surgery on normals. The German experience will be discussed below.

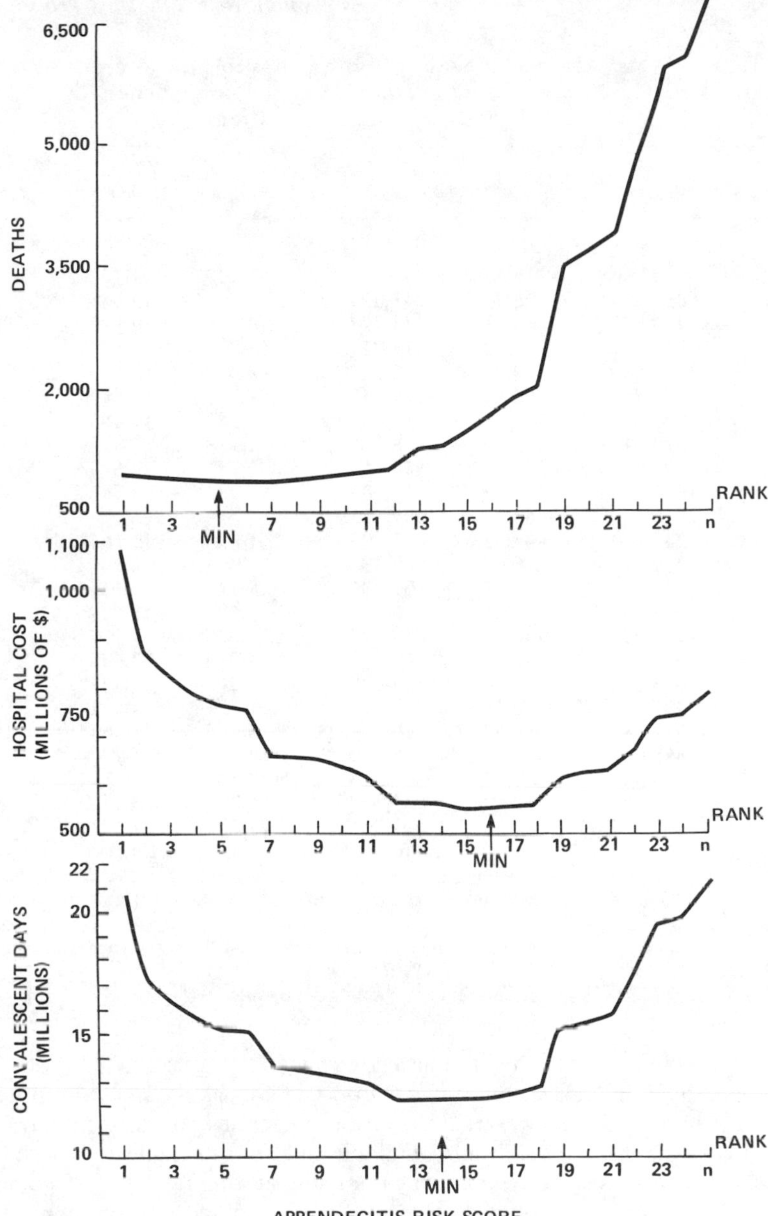

Figure 18–3. Deaths, convalescence, and costs associated with varying degrees of interventionism (100% perforation).

This figure shows the expected deaths, convalescent days, and hospital costs for every one of the possible ranks which could be used as a cutoff point between operative and nonoperative treatment *assuming that 100% of appendicitis patients not operated upon would perforate.*

The death curve is flat near its minimum which occurs when patients with mild symptoms are operated. There is a conflict between the optimum strategies for reducing deaths and for reducing convalescence and hospital costs.

Table 18-5. "Costs" associated* with each of the possible dichotomies of the risk score. A 100% perforation rate is assumed for appendicitis patients not receiving an operation.

Rank	*Total Deaths***	*Margin***	*Total Cost ($)*	*Margin*	*Total Days Lost*	*Margin*
			in 000's	in 000's	in 000's	in 000's
N***	6782	-719.17	781,734	-40,109	21,230	-1,375
24	6062.83	-126.31	741,625	-6,848	19,855	-238
23	5936.52	-1123.55	734,777	-58,763	19,617	-2,078
22	4812.97	-951.12	676,014	-47,393	17,539	-1,719
21	3861.85	-197.00	628,621	-9,479	15,820	-350
20	3664.85	-166.62	619,142	-7,286	15,470	-284
19	3498.23	-1478.22	611,856	-53,286	15,186	-2,320
18	2020.01	-125.09	558,570	-4,159	12,866	-191
17	1894.92	-257.68	554,411	-4,927	12,675	-329
16	1637.24	-191.82	549,484	1,981	12,346	-148
15	1445.42	-160.23	551,465	6,828	12,198	-34
14	1285.19	-36.01	558,293	1,998	12,164	.3
13	1249.18	-6.07	560,291	915	12,164	10
12	1243.11	-230.47	561,206	55,241	12,174	735
11	1012.64	-51.21	616,447	14,425	12,909	200
10	961.43	-40.30	630,872	19,078	13,109	291
9	921.13	-7.91	649,950	4,938	13,400	77
8	913.22	-5.74	654,888	6,312	13,477	10
7	907.48	-36.20	661,200	89,164	13,581	1,504
6	871.28	-2.61	750,364	8,566	15,084	146
5	868.67	-0.65	758,930	28,283	15,230	487
4	868.02	6.85	787,213	37,557	15,717	654
3	874.87	12.43	824,770	46,481	16,371	813
2	887.30	76.80	871,251	199,530	17,184	3,516
1	964.10		1,070,781		20,700	

*Costs are associated with a dichotomy in which the indicated rank and all ranks above it receive an operation.
**Fractional deaths have been reported since calculated costs per life saved are sensitive to these figures.
***N = no operation for any patient.

On the basis of the data used in this analysis one may conclude that a surgeon can ensure himself an acceptable mortality rate by taking an interventionist approach. He does this, however, at the cost of increasing convalescent days and hospital costs. It can be seen from the middle and bottom graphs that both convalescent days and hospital costs reach a minimum around rank 15 in Figure 18-3 and rank 18 in Figure 18-4 and then begin to increase as more normal appendices are removed. Our calculations show that the classical academic goal (Thomas and Mueller, 1969; Jacob et al., 1975) of a 15 to 20% removal rate for normal appendices is found near the minimum for morbidity. At this minimum point, 23% of the appendices removed are normal and the appendectomy rate would be 1.48/1000.* Considering only mortality is probably not reasonable. To save

*The marginal cost to save a life by moving to the minimum for *morbidity* in Figure 18-3 is about $43 million per life saved.

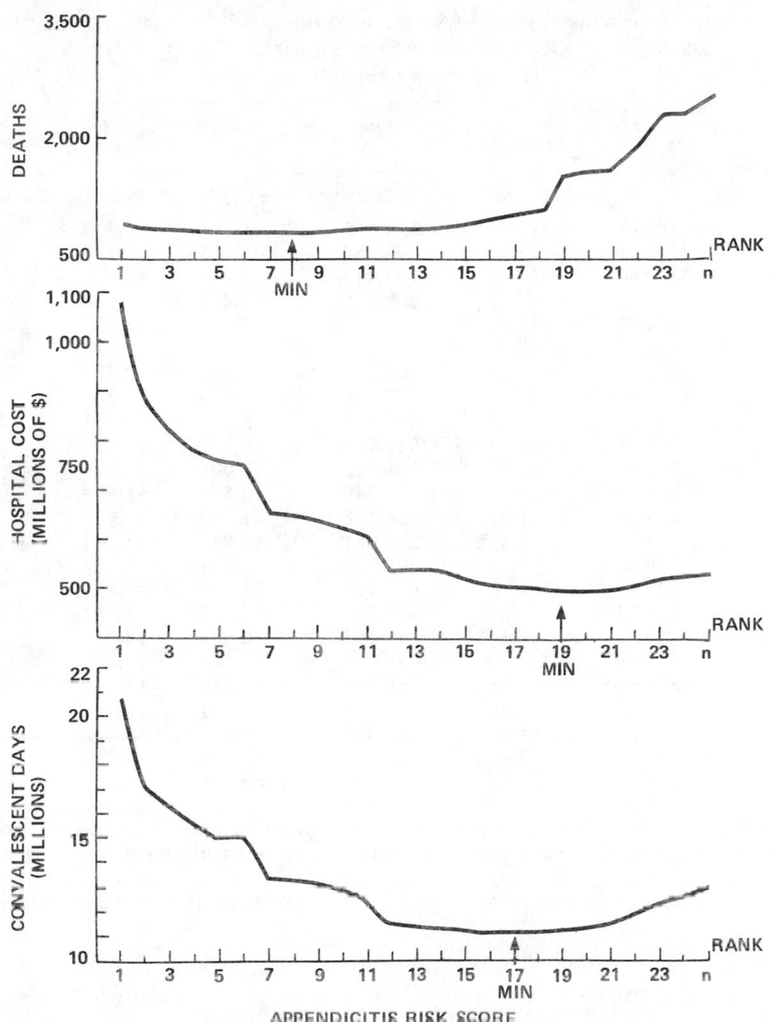

Figure 18-4. Deaths, convalescence, and costs associated with varying degrees of interventionism (30% perforation).

This figure shows the expected deaths, convalescent days, and hospital costs for every one of the possible ranks which could be used as a cutoff point between operative and nonoperative treatment *assuming that only 30% of appendicitis patients not operated upon would perforate.* The conclusions which may be drawn are similar to those in the previous figure.

one more life by shifting from rank 5 to rank 4 in Figure 18-3 and Table 18-5 one would have to perform so many operations on normal patients that the marginal cost of saving one life would be $43 million and 2,053 person-years of convalescence. The appendectomy rate in the population would be 2.4/1000 instead of 1.57/1000, and 50% of removed appendices would be histologically normal.

Table 18-6. "Costs" associated* with each of the possible dichotomies of the risk score. A 30% perforation rate is assumed for appendicitis patients not receiving an operation

Rank	*Total Deaths***	*Margin***	*Total Cost ($)*	*Margin*	*Total Days Lost*	*Margin*
			in 000's	in 000's	in 000's	in 000's
N	2505.00	-215.16	534,856	-11,004	12,927	-393
24	2290.16	-37.73	523,852	-1,735	12,534	-66
23	2252.43	-334.90	522,117	-13,239	12,468	-548
22	1917.53	-282.75	508,878	-8,813	11,920	-422
21	1634.78	-58.45	500,065	-1,481	11,498	-81
20	1576.33	-49.20	498,584	-508	11,417	-56
19	1527.13	-432.81	498,076	7,060	11,361	-292
18	1094.32	-36.51	505,136	953	11,069	-18
17	1057.81	-74.03	506,089	5,674	11,051	27
16	983.78	-53.27	511,763	9,979	11,078	121
15	930.51	-42.82	521,742	13,606	11,199	194
14	887.69	-9.47	535,348	3,530	11,393	52
13	878.22	-1.41	538,878	1,183	11,445	19
12	876.81	-46.81	540,061	65,843	11,464	1,090
11	830.00	-9.70	605,904	16,821	12,554	281
10	820.30	-5.13	622,725	21,109	12,835	359
9	815.17	-0.62	643,834	5,359	13,194	92
8	814.55	0.44	649,193	6,668	13,286	115
7	814.99	18.82	655,861	92,340	13,401	1,611
6	833.81	2.06	748,201	8,836	15,012	154
5	835.87	9.01	757,037	28,841	15,166	506
4	844.88	14.14	785,878	37,977	15,672	668
3	859.02	18.61	823,855	46,838	16,340	826
2	877.63	86.47	870,693	200,088	17,166	3,533
1	964.10		1,070,781		20,699	

*Costs are associated with a dichotomy in which the indicated rank and all ranks above it receive an operation.
**Fractional deaths have been reported since calculated costs per life saved are sensitive to these figures.

Note that regardless of the assumed extreme perforation rates in unoperated appendicitis patients (100%-30%) the same conclusions must be drawn: the death curve is flat near its minimum, the minimum occurs when patients with mild symptoms are operated upon, and there is a conflict between the optimum strategies for reducing deaths and for reducing convalescence and hospital costs.

The Sensitivity of This Analysis to the Assumptions Made

Earlier a number of assumptions were mentioned: (1) The analysis was made without separating the young from the old or (2) males from females. Other medical and surgical conditions were eliminated from the analysis. (3) The risk score was built on four findings available upon admission, thereby giving an underestimate of the true power of discrimination which a surgeon might have if he used more variables and changes in clinical findings after admission. (4) The four symptoms were assumed to be independent of each other within the two diagnostic categories; this might introduce an additional bias. (5) Finally, the prevalence of NSAP and appendicitis was taken from patients with pain of less than one week's duration admitted to one English hospital. Thus, acute abdominal conditions secondary to or associated with chronic causes of abdominal pain, such as diverticulitis or pelvic inflammatory disease in females, were excluded.

In the following paragraphs, therefore, we will explore the sensitivity of our conclusions to changes in these five assumptions. We are aided in doing this by using a formula which directly indicates the optimum dichotomy between "operate" and "don't operate." By focusing on the impact which changing assumptions have on certain components of this formula we can derive a better intuition as to how these changes would influence the position of the optimum "operating point." The formula, which has been used recently by McNeil et al. (1975), is derived in the Appendix to this chapter for the case of a continuous risk score. The general principle applies to discrete risk scores, such as our own, as well. According to this formula, the likelihood ratio pertaining to the rank bounding the optimum dichotomy is the product of the "prior odds" of NSAP and the ratio of the net cost of a "false positive" to the net cost of a "false negative." The net cost of a false positive is the cost of a false positive less the cost of a true negative. Similarly, the net cost of a false negative is the cost of a false negative less the cost of a true positive. The formula* is to be solved for the value of i that makes the two sides equal.

$$\frac{P(\text{rank}_i|\text{APP})}{P(\text{rank}_i|\text{NSAP})} = \frac{(\text{Cost}_{\text{FP}} - \text{Cost}_{\text{TN}})}{(\text{Cost}_{\text{FN}} - \text{Cost}_{\text{TP}})} \times \frac{P(\text{NSAP})}{P(\text{APP})}$$

It may be useful to develop some intuition for this formula. The term on the left is the likelihood ratio, or in Figure 18-1 the height of the appendicitis distribution at rank i divided by the height of the NSAP distribution at that rank. As we move to the left in Figure 18-1, toward milder symptoms, this term gets ever smaller. As we move to the right and the appendicitis curve gets higher and higher the term gets bigger. Thus, a small likelihood ratio pertains to a dichotomy in the zone of mild symptoms while a large likelihood ratio pertains to a dichotomy in the zone of severe symptoms.

Now consider the two terms on the right. The right-most term is the "prior odds" of being a case of NSAP. The higher the odds of NSAP, the cost term remaining equal, the bigger the likelihood ratio on the left side of the equation becomes. Thus, if the odds of NSAP were very high, one would only operate on patients with obvious symptoms. If the odds of NSAP were low (and those of appendicitis high), you would perform appendectomies even on patients with mild symptoms.

*The variable i takes on whole number values and ranges from 1 to 24. FP = false positive (removing a normal appendix); FN = false negative (allowing an appendix to perforate); TP = true positive (removing an inflammed appendix); TN = true negative (NSAP without operation)

The cost term operates in a similar manner. If we could reduce the net cost of a false negative in the denominator of this term, the term itself would become bigger and the likelihood ratio on the left would increase. Thus, if a new treatment markedly reduced the case fatality associated perforation, the cost term and the likelihood ratio would climb to a large value. That is, if perforation had little adverse effects, only severe symptoms would warrant surgery.

We can now examine the major conclusions of this paper and their sensitivity to changes in the five assumptions mentioned above.

To minimize deaths, surgeons should operate on patients with mild symptoms

Since the net cost of a false positive (.65/1000 - 0) is so much smaller than the net cost of a false negative (27/1000 - 1.02/1000) the cost term on the right side of the equation, (.65-0)/(27-1.02) is small. As a consequence, the likelihood ratio on the left hand side of the equation decreases. A small likelihood ratio implies mild symptoms.

The optimum dichotomy for preventing morbidity is found at more severe symptoms (bigger likelihood ratios) than the optimum dichotomy for mortality

The net cost of a false positive (22 days - 3 days) is not so small relative to the net cost of a false negative (61 days - 22 days) as was the case with case fatality. The cost term (22-3)/(61-22) being larger causes an increase in the likelihood ratio on the left side of the equation, indicating more severe symptoms. It should be clear from the formula that regardless of the value of the prevalences of NSAP and APP the optimum dichotomy for minimizing mortalities will always occur at milder cases than the optimum for morbidity. Similarly, assumptions of independence of symptoms, ignoring how age would affect the distributions, and using only four discriminators, all would affect the separation of the NSAP and appendicitis distributions. Regardless of the shape of these distributions however, the optimum dichotomy for mortality will still occur at milder cases than the optimum for morbidity. The particular minima which we have indicated may not be correct, but the general principle is correct insofar as we have assessed the relative net costs of "false positives" and "false negatives." Even these costs might be off by a factor of two without changing the overall conclusions.

The relative cost of false positives and negatives might be different for older people. As mentioned earlier, most deaths occur in older people. Howie (1966) presents data which allow us to assess these relative costs. The cost terms which result from his case fatality figures are as follows: Persons 30-49 years of age have a net false positive cost of (0.9/1000 - 0) and a net false negative cost of (13.8/1000 - .7/1000). The cost term is thus (0.9 - 0)/(13.8 - .7) = .069. We now compare this ratio to the same one for patients over 49 years of age. For them the net false positive cost in terms of case fatality was (4/1000 - 0) while the net false negative cost was (67.3/1000 - 5.7/1000). Their ratio was .065. The two ratios are really quite similar, so if the shape of the NSAP and Appendicitis distributions are similar for both age groups and the prevalence of appendicitis is the same, the optimum operation point would be only slightly more interventionist for older persons. But clinicians believe that there is greater overlap in the NSAP and Appendicitis distributions and that the prior odds of being an NSAP patient is probably greater for older persons. Both of these factors probably shift the optimum dichotomy back toward less interventionism. The only solution is to gather symptom, prevalence, and cost data specifically directed at this question. A similar analysis would have to be done for the two sexes, since the odds of NSAP are higher for females than for males. This shifts the optimum operating point for females towards more severe symptoms. Shepard and Zeckhauser discuss this in another chapter of the book.

By ignoring other surgical and medical conditions we have ignored the false positive and false negative costs associated with them. Most of the other conditions in de Dombal's series were surgical. A false positive for these conditions might be the inconvenience of revising an appendectomy incision to accommodate the needs of some other operative procedure. This does not seem to be great, and at any rate, many surgeons when uncertain about the diagnosis will use a midline incision to avoid that contingency. The cost of a false negative is very serious indeed for most of these surgical conditions. Thus, including other surgical conditions in the analysis would have reinforced the prescription for interventionism to save life. The inclusion of other nonsurgically treatable conditions such as pancreatitis or pelvic inflammatory disease would introduce conditions in which a false positive has definite penalties. There were no data on the magnitude of the case fatality among such patients who were explored in expectation of appendicitis. It seems unlikely that it would exceed the case fatality of those treated with the appropriate medical therapy to the degree that the case fatality for perforation exceeds the case fatality for removing a normal appendix. Nonetheless, the inclusion of such conditions is important and would shift the optimum dichotomy toward a less interventionist position along the risk score.

Finally, we should consider the appropriateness of the 24 rank risk score. It was derived assuming independence of the symptoms within the two diagnostic categories. In plain terms this means that the probability of having any one of the symptoms is not at all changed by having another. This is not the case although the intercorrelation of symptoms may not be as great as surgeons suspect. An examination of data on 2,300 appendectomy patients (Osler Peterson, unpublished data) shows only weak positive intercorrelations between the four findings used to build the 24 rank risk score. Nonetheless, this means that the degree of separation achieved in Figure 18-1 is probably an overestimate of the separation which truly could be expected on the basis of these four findings. If data were available, multivariate techniques exist to develop risk scores which take interdependence and interactions into account. On the other hand, the intuitive risk score which surgeons actually use is based on many more findings, and on changes of findings after admission to observation. As shall be seen in the next section, the false positive and true positive rates achieved by at least one surgeon—FP = .07, TP = .74—falls fairly close to operating points on the 24 rank risk score (*Medical World News*, 1975). Perhaps by coincidence, therefore, the score seems to duplicate the degree of separation achieved by some practicing surgeons.

In summary, the overall conclusions from this analysis are unlikely to be reversed when a more elaborate analysis is made on the basis of more adequate data. The optimum operating point for reducing mortality is more "interventionist" than the optimum operating point for reducing morbidity. Physicians may agree that the ideal operating point lies somewhere between these two optima but unless they can agree on the amount of convalescence equivalent to one death, there is no hope for finding one "correct" operating point upon which all parties can agree. This is an argument of values not of fact.

AN ANALYTIC APPROACH TO THE IMPLICATIONS OF CHANGING THE DEGREE OF DISCRIMINATION

Up to this point the discussion has assumed a given degree of discrimination and has focused only on changing the degree of symptom severity which warrants surgery. But there are data which suggest that surgeons can vary the degree of discrimination which they use to distinguish between appendicitis patients and those with nonspecific abdominal pain. Variations in the degree of discrimination are probably related to the completeness and reliability of the patient information gathered on admission and over time and partly due to clinical acumen in properly weighing the evidence gathered. In this article we have been restricted to symptomatic presentation on admission since this was the only kind of data available.

Issues of diagnostic performance can be represented on a "True Positive-False Positive Graph" also known as the "Receiver Operating Characteristic Graph." This term comes from the original applications to radar receivers (Lusted, 1968; McNeil et al., 1975; Peterson and Birdsall, 1953; Swets, 1973). Figure 18-5 provides an orientation. On the *Y* axis the true positive rate is shown and on the *X* axis, the corresponding false positive rate appears. In our present example, the "true positive" rate is the proportion of appendicitis patients who receive a timely operation. The "false positive" rate is the proportion of normals who are operated upon. When good patient information and good judgment have been used to achieve good discrimination, a high "true positive" rate can be achieved with a low "false positive" rate, and the coordinates will fall somewhere in the "good zone" in the upper left hand corner of the graph. If there is poor patient information, or if it is improperly assessed, poor discrimination occurs, which at its worst is no better than assigning diagnosis by the flip of a coin. In that case, the "true positives" equal the "false positives" and one has the "no-discrimination" line extending from the coordinate (0,0) to the coordinate (1,1). The zone of moderate discrimination falls between the poor and good zones.

Each dichotomy of the 24 rank severity score used in the previous analysis had an associated "true positive" and "false positive" proportion. They are shown on the dotted curve in Figure 18-6. For each of the 24 dichotomies of the score in Figure 18-1, the proportion of appendicitis patients operated in time to prevent perforation ("true positives") and the proportion of NSAP patients operated

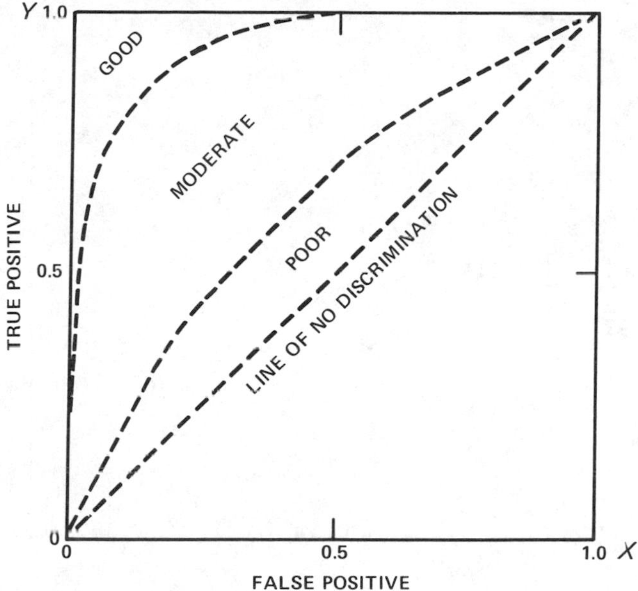

Figure 18-5. A sample true positive/false positive (ROC) graph.
The true positive/false positive graph (ROC curve) shows the true positive rate on the y axis and the corresponding false positive rate on the x axis. When good discrimination is achieved a high true positive rate is compatible with low false positive rates. Good discriminators are located in the upper left hand corner of the graph. Poor discrimination (true positive rate close to false positive rate) lies near the 45° diagonal. This diagonal represents the accuracy which would be achievable by assigning a diagnosis with the flip of a coin.

("false positives") were used to fix the coordinates of that particular point on the "true positive"/"false positive" graph. Thus, every dot on the curve corresponds to one dichotomy of the score. In the previous section, when searching for the optimum dichotomy for minimizing deaths, we are sliding along this particular curve. It seems to allow fairly good discrimination, but the literature provides examples of discrimination which are both superior and inferior to this. Recently, White (*Medical World News*, 1975) has described his experience on the pediatric surgery service at the Johns Hopkins Hospital. A few years ago, the surgeons on the pediatric service were operating at point W_1 of Figure 18-6, quite close to the no discrimination line. It was believed that the press of other responsibilities at the university hospital was interfering with patient observation and a special policy was made that any doubtful patients would be kept next to the emergency room for several hours' close observation. The results of this policy are shown at point W_2. The proportion of true positives (nonperforated appendicitis) remained the same while the false positives were reduced from 65% to 7%.

A similar experience has been described by de Dombal and his colleagues

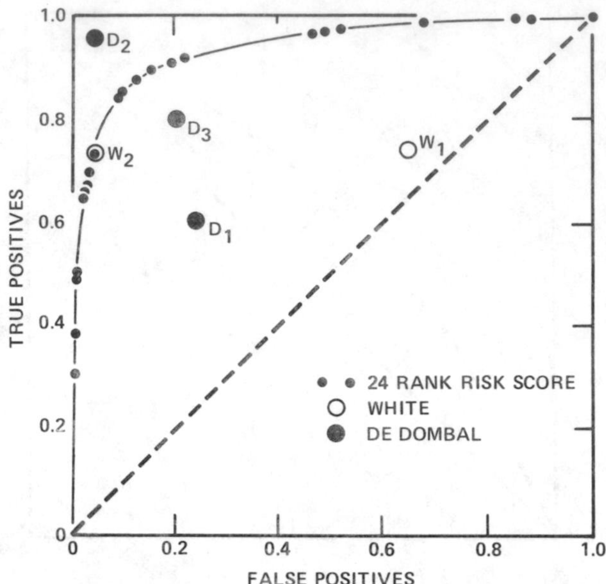

Figure 18-6. A true positive/false positive (ROC) graph for appendectomy. The family of true positive/false positive points derived from all possible dichotomies of the 24 rank severity score used in the previous analysis is shown on the dotted curve. It seems to allow fairly good discrimination. White's experience (*Medical World News*, 1975) (W_1, W_2) suggests that improved discrimination allows a decrease in normal removal rate without increasing the perforation rate. The experience of de Dombal et al. (1974) (D_1, D_2, D_3) suggests that perforation rates *and* normal removal rates can be simultaneously reduced.

(1974) in the University Hospital at Leeds. Prior to the trial which yielded the data used to create the symptom severity score in this article, they discovered that the diagnostic performance of their surgical service was located at point D_1 of Figure 18-6. The true positive rate was 60% (40% of appendicitis patients were perforated at operation) while 25% of normals received an operation.

During the trial, surgeons filled out a precodified form for symptoms whose data were fed into a computer for diagnosis. Although this diagnosis was not made available to the clinicians, they were apparently well-motivated to compete with the computer, because their performance shifted to point D_2 (96% true positives and only 7% false positives).

After the trial was over, their performance drifted back to point D_3. The authors were not sure to what they should attribute these changes. They report that the staff had not changed and that the age, sex, and symptom characteristics of patients had not changed during the three periods. Changes of motivation and changes in the data base due to a precodified form were two possible causes that they mentioned.

The removal of normal appendices is sometimes thought to be influenced by monetary considerations, but these two examples come from teaching hospitals and one comes from England. Financial motivation can probably be excluded as an explanation of deviations from ideal diagnostic performance. At these hospitals, a concerted effort at improving diagnostic acumen was the factor which made the difference. In the Johns Hopkins experience false positives were decreased without any change in the perforation rate. Perhaps most of these perforations occurred prior to hospitalization. At Leeds, the competition with a computer resulted in a simultaneous reduction of false positives *and* of perforations. Since most of the perforations were eliminated through changed diagnostic procedures, a fair number of the original perforations may have occurred in hospital. Alternatively, the criteria for pathological diagnosis may have changed. In Leeds, at least, one wonders if the usual estimate of 80% is descriptive of the proportion of perforations which occur prior to hospitalization.

Changes in the degree of discrimination can have important implications in terms of lives saved, dollars spent, and convalescent days experienced. If White's points 1 and 2 are extrapolated to the United States population (making the same assumptions as before), yearly savings of the magnitude shown in Table 18-7 can be achieved. There is a difference of 259,000 operations between the two points. Fewer operations on normal persons would reduce deaths by 169 but would reduce convalescence by about 6 million days. Hospital costs would decrease by more than a third of a billion dollars, enough to provide $687 to each of the 541,475 patients operated under the unusually interventionist strategy at W_1. This is more than enough to pay for the additional services of a doctor and/or a nurse to observe these patients in the emergency ward for a 6- to 12-hour period. An extrapolation of the de Dombal strategies shows savings, of an even greater number of lives (2,000) by reducing the perforation rate but still showing a savings in morbidity and costs as well. This is a point to be stressed. Many experienced surgeons share White's conviction that the best way to discriminate between appendicitis and nonspecific abdominal pain in patients with initially equivocal signs is to follow them carefully for a number of hours. The risk of causing additional perforations is apparently small, for the extrapolation of White's results suggest this saves lives. It saves money as well.

At this point it makes sense to reconsider the situation in German-speaking Europe. Why is their appendicitis mortality so high if the high rate of appendectomy cannot explain it? Dahm's (1972) analysis in East Germany shows that a number of adverse factors are at work. The case fatality figures which

Table 18-7. Estimated hospital cost, operations, deaths, and disability days for $White_1$ and $White_2$.

	Lives Lost	*Convalescent Days*	*Dollar Costs*	*Number of Operations*
W_1	2,142	19,000,000	920,000,000	541,000
W_2	1,973	13,000,000	548,000,000	282,000
Difference	169	6,000,000	372,000,000	259,000

she cites are slightly greater for perforated and inflammed appendices. The greater number of NSAP patients operated account for 30% of the excess deaths. The mortality for perforated appendicitis is four times greater in East Germany than it is in England and Wales. If one assumes that the appendicitis rate is the same in East Germany as it is in the United States, the proportion of appendicitis patients who perforate is a high 41%. How much of this perforation is occurring prior to hospitalization? How much of it is due to a poor degree of diagnostic discrimination? If the perforations occur prior to medical observation it may be that German surgeons are reacting to their unavoidably high perforation rate by operating on a high proportion of patients with abdominal pain. They might do better to launch a campaign to educate the public of the value of early medical examination for acute abdominal pain. The East Germans are actively investigating this problem (Dahm, personal communication).

Until a true positive/false positive analysis is made on a sample of hospitals in the United States, we cannot estimate how much room for improvement there really is at the national level. To judge by their relatively low appendectomy rates and appendicitis mortality neither the United States nor the United Kingdom has a major problem with this particular operation. Nonetheless, it seems worthwhile to study this procedure further. First of all, even within the United States there are large local variations in appendectomy rates (Thomas and Mueller, 1969; Wennberg and Gittelsohn, 1973; Lewis, 1969) which may be indicative of nonoptimum surgical policy. In areas with high appendectomy rates economic and morbidity savings may be accomplished. More important, appendectomy represents a fairly simple problem in surgical policy. If we can collect that data to provide a reasonable cost-effectiveness rationale for its management, we may be in a better position to understand elective procedures such as hysterectomy and low back surgery. The Study on Surgical Services for the United States (American College of Surgeons and American Surgical Association, 1975) has shown large variations in the rates of these procedures which give cause for concern. One suspects that they are similar to appendectomy in that relaxing the indications for performing these operations may continue to give slight benefit but at an increasing cost in dollars and morbidity.

INFORMATION NEEDED

The analysis in this article has revealed deficiencies in available information about appendicitis which could be easily remedied. This information should be collected not at isolated university hospitals but for all hospitals in a defined geographic area. The main items of interest are:

1. The relative frequency of the various causes of acute abdomen in the population, in ambulatory facilities, and in hospitals.
2. The likelihood of symptoms, signs, and laboratory results for the diagnostic categories seen in ambulatory and hospital facilities.
3. The impact of elapsing time on the risk of perforation on the one hand, and the increased accuracy due to the evolution of symptoms on the other. In

particular, the proportion of perforation which occurs prior to hospitalization (and which might respond to patient education) and the proportion which occurs while under medical supervision.

4. Case fatalities, convalescent days, and hospital costs for:
   (a) perforated appendix;
   (b) nonperforated but inflamed appendix;
   (c) normal appendix; and
   (d) other surgical or medical causes of acute abdomen which have, for lack of data, been ignored in this analysis.
5. A breakdown of the above information within age-sex categories to allow a separate analysis of the kind mentioned above for relevant subgroups of the patient population.
6. A better understanding of the processes responsible for the remarkable improvements in diagnosis reported by White and de Dombal.

With these pieces of information, an analysis of the management of suspected acute appendicitis could be carried out which would make possible definitive recommendations about the range of acceptable removal rates for normal appendices.

CONCLUSIONS

Appendectomy offers benefits which are accrued in the immediate postoperative period. These benefits can be measured in terms of reduced case fatality and reduced days of convalescence, measures which can be quantified and reliably measured. These facts make the present analysis relatively easier than analyses of surgical procedures in which the benefits are delayed in time and have to do with the quality of life. Since appendectomy lends itself to quantitative analysis it will be worthwhile to pursue it as a paradigm for other more complex procedures. Gathering the detailed information itemized above should therefore be carried out. It will allow us to corroborate the main conclusions of the present analysis which was based on data available in the literature. These conclusions are:

1. The argument about what constitutes an acceptable removal rate of histologically normal appendicies is a disagreement over values and not a disagreement over facts. To resolve the argument one would need to agree on the number of days of convalescence or the number of dollars which are equivalent to a human life.
2. All parties, however, should be able to agree that the optimal removal rate of histologically normal appendices lies somewhere between the high proportion of normal appendices one would remove to minimize death, and the lower proportion which minimizes convalescence and hospital costs.
3. Judging by the results of White and de Dombal, it is possible to increase the power of discrimination sufficiently *simultaneously* to reduce the removal rate of normal appendices while reducing the rate of perforations. This produces savings both in lives and in money.

SUMMARY

The medical literature has documented a striking geographical variability in the removal rate of histologically normal appendices, and in appendectomy rates. Physicians argue about what the ideal value of these rates should be. This chapter proposes that at least two factors contribute to this variability. The first factor is the surgeon's ability to discriminate between appendicitis and nonappendicitis patients before deciding to operate. The degree of this discrimination depends partly on the completeness of the medical information (collected on admission and over the ensuing hours) and partly on the skill with which this information is interpreted. The second source of variability, even among surgeons using the same degree of discrimination, arises from disagreement about the degree of symptom severity which warrants surgery. This chapter shows that there is a conflict between the optimum symptom severity for saving lives and the one for reducing morbidity. Continuing to relax the indications for surgery beyond those of patients with the most obvious symptoms *does* continue to save lives but at an ever diminishing rate. Unfortunately, the few lives saved by operating on patients with minimal symptoms are purchased at the great cost in convalescence and dollars associated with the removal of large numbers of normal appendices.

Published surgical experience suggests that the surgeon has a partial way out of this dilemma; namely, to increase his degree of discrimination by using very complete diagnostic information and careful clinical interpretation. Analysis of this option leads to the hypothesis that increased discrimination can reduce the removal rate of histologically normal appendices without an increase—and possibly with a decrease—in the rate of perforation. Using published statistics this chapter estimates the resultant savings in lives, convalescence, and money.

Since the benefits of different appendectomy strategies can be simply expressed in terms of case fatality rates or in days of disability, a definitive analysis of this problem is possible. To carry out such an analysis we need more detailed information than is available from the literature. Studies of acute abdominal pain are therefore proposed to generate such information from a defined region. The results of a definitive analysis could serve as an impetus for applying the same methodology to the indications for elective surgical procedures which have less easily measured or less immediate benefits.

Acknowledgments

Several surgical and policy analyst colleagues have provided significant help and important insights into the problem of the management of the acute abdomen. In particular, Dr. Benjamin Barnes read patiently through each draft and gave many valuable suggestions. Dr. William V McDermott, Jr., Dr. Francis D Moore, Emmet Keeler and Donald Shepard provided valuable criticism.

References

American College of Surgeons and American Surgical Association: Surgery in the United States: A Summary Report of the Study on Surgical Services for the United States, Baltimore, 1975, p 45 Table 20

American Hospital Association: Hospital Statistics. Chicago, Ill, 1970, p 20

Andersen R, Anderson OW: A Decade of Health Services. Chicago, University of Chicago Press, 1967, p 24 Table 8

Barnes BA, Behringer GE, Wheelock FC, et al: Analysis of factors associated with sepsis following appendectomy (1937–1959). Ann Surg 156:703, 1962a

Barnes BA, Behringer GE, Wheelock FC, et al: Treatment of appendicitis at the Massachusetts General Hospital (1937–1959). JAMA 180:122, 1962b

Bowers WF, Hughes CW, Bonilla KB: The treatment of acute appendicitis under suboptimal conditions. US Armed Forces Med J 11:1545, 1958

Burkitt DP, Walker AR, Paintor NS: Effect of dietary fibre on stools and the transit-times, and its role in the causation of disease. Lancet 2:1408, 1972

Coldrey E: Five years of conservative treatment of acute appendicitis. J Int Coll Surg 32:255, 1959

Collins DC: Mechanisms and significance of obliteration of the lumen of the vermiform appendix. Ann Surg 104:199, 1936

Crile G Jr., Fulton JR: Appendicitis with emphasis on use of penicillin. US Naval Med Bull 45:464, 1945

Dahm I: Die Appendizitis mortalitat in der DDR aus epidemiologischer Sicht. Aschv arzll Fortbild 66:514, 1972

de Dombal FT, Leaper DJ, Staniland JR, et al: Computer-aided diagnosis of acute abdominal pain. Br Med J 2:9, 1972

de Dombal FT, Leaper DJ, Horrocks JF, et al: Human and computer-aided diagnosis of abdominal pain: further report with emphasis on performance of clinicians. Br Med J 1:376, 1974

Fellig A, Hanfstaengl E: Der "informierte" patient und de Indikation zur Appendektomie. Munch Med Wochenschr 116:1321, 1974

Fitz RH: Perforating inflamation of the vermiform appendix. Trans Assoc Am Physicians 1:107, 1886

Gilmour IEW, Lowdon, AGR: Acute appendicitis. Edinburgh Med J 59:361, 1952

Green DM: Application of detection theory in psychophysics. Proc IEEE 58: 713, 1970

Green HW, Watkins RM: Appendicitis in Cleveland. Mimeographed In-house publication, p 41, Table IV, 1946a

Green HW, Watkins RM: Appendicitis in Cleveland: Final Report. Surg Gynecol Obstet 83:613, 1946b

Hawk JC Jr, Becker WF, Lehman EP: Acute appendicitis III and analysis of one thousand and three cases. Ann Surg 132:729, 1950

Howie JGR: Death from appendicitis and appendectomy: an epidemiological survey. Lancet 2:1334, 1966

Jacob ET, Bar-Nathan N, Luchtman M: Error rate factor in the management of appendicitis. Lancet 2:1032, 1975

Kleinman J, Weiss, RJ, Tanner M, et al: Emergency Medical Services in the City of Boston: Boston. Harvard Center for Community Health and Medical Care, Mimeographed, 1972, Table 27

Lehman EP, Parker WH: The Treatment of intraperitoneal abscess arising from appendicitis. Ann Surg 108:833, 1938

Lembcke P: Measuring the quality of medical care through vital statistics based on hospital service areas: 1. Comparative study of appendectomy rates. Am J. Public Health 42:276, 1952

Lewis CE: Variations in the incidence of surgery. N Engl J Med 281:880, 1969

Lichtner S, Pflanz M: Appendectomy in the Federal Republic of Germany: Epidemiology and Medical Care Patterns. Med Care 9:311, 1971

Lusted LB: Introduction to medical decision making. Springfield, Charles C Thomas, 1968

McNeil BJ, Keeler E, Adelstein SJ: Primer on certain elements of medical decision making. N Engl J Med 293:211, 1975

Medical World News: Is this appendectomy really necessary? Med World News 16:21, 1975

Metropolitan Life Insurance Company. Statistical Bulletin 35:3, 1954

National Center for Health Statistics: Length of Convalescence after Surgery 1960–1961 (DHEW Publication No 1000, Series 10, No 3). Washington, DC, Government Printing Office, 1963

National Center for Health Statistics: Surgical Operations in Short Stay Hospitals for Discharged Patients, United States, 1965 (DHEW Publication No 1000 Series A, No 7). Washington, DC, Government Printing Office, 1966, p 3, Table B

National Center for Health Statistics: Vital Statistics of the United States 1970. Volume II: Mortality. Part B (DHEW Publication No (HRA) 74–1102). Washington, DC, Government Printing Office, 1970

National Center for Health Statistics: Surgical Operations in Short Stay Hospitals, United States (DHEW Publication No (HRA) 75–1769, Series 13, No 18). Washington, DC, Government Printing Office, 1974

Pauker SG, Kassirer JP: Therapeutic decision making: a cost benefit analysis N Engl J Med 293:229, 1975

Pearson RJ: Acute appendicitis in the New Haven standard metropolitan area in 1958 and 1959. Conn Med 28:807, 1964

Peterson WW, Birdsall TG: The Theory of Signal Detectability. Ann Arbor, University of Michigan, Electronic Defense Group Tech Report 13, 1953

Rogers H, Faxon HH: A statistical study of six hundred and seventy-one cases of appendiceal peritonitis. N Engl J Med 226:707, 1942

Smith M, Wilson EA: A model of the auditory threshold and its application to the problem of the multiple observer. Psychol Monogr 67:9, 1953

Staniland JR, Ditchburn J, de Dombal FT: Clinical presentation of acute abdomen: study of 600 patients. Br Med J 3:393, 1972

Swets JA: The relative operating characteristic in psychology. A technique for isolating effects of response bias finds wide use in the study of perception and cognition. Science 182:990, 1973

Tanner WP, Swets JA: A new theory of visual detection. Ann Arbor, University of Michigan Electronic Defense Group Tech Report 18, 1953

Thomas EJ, Mueller B: Appendectomy: diagnostic criteria and hospital performance. Hosp Prac 4:72, 1969

United States Department of Health, Education, and Welfare: Monthly Vital Statistics Report (DHEW Publication No (HRA) 75–1120). Washington, DC, Government Printing Office, 1975

Verda DJ, Platt WP: The tissue committee really gets results. Mod Hosp 91:74, 1958

Wangensteen OH, Buirge RE, Dennis C, et al: Studies in the etiology of acute appendicitis. Ann Surg 106:910, 1937

Watkins RM: Appendicitis in Cleveland. JAMA 120:1026, 1942

Wennberg J, Gittelsohn A: Small area variations in health care delivery. Science 182:1102, 1973

APPENDIX

Derivation of the Formula for Finding the Likelihood Ratio at the Point of Minimum Deaths, Costs, or Days' Convalescence

The formula used for identifying the optimum dichotomy of the risk score can be written as:

$$\frac{f(x_1)}{g(x_1)} = \frac{P(\text{NSAP})}{P(\text{APP})} \cdot \frac{(\text{CFP - CTN})}{(\text{CFN - CTP})} \tag{1}$$

$f(x_1)$ = likelihood of having a score value of x_1 among cases

$g(x_1)$ = likelihood of having a score value of x_1 among non-cases

P(NSAP) = proportion of patients (prior probability) with NSAP

P(APP) = proportion of patients (prior probability) with APP

(CFP–CTN) = The cost of a False Positive (FP) which is in excess of the cost of a True Negative (TN)

(CFN–CTP) = The cost of a False Negative (FN) which is in excess of the cost of a True Positive (TP)

The derivation of this formula can be oriented to the following figure:

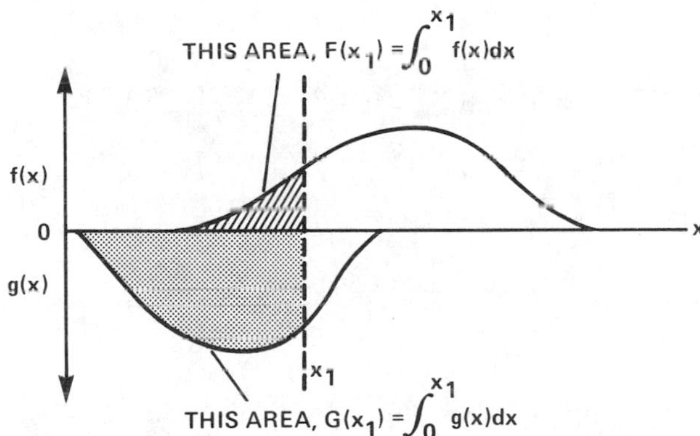

At each of the possible dichotomies along the risk score x, the total cost is expressed as:

$$\text{Total cost associated with a dichotomy at } x_1 = D(x_1) \qquad (2)$$

$$= (\text{number of patients with NSAP or APP}) \times$$

$$(\text{P(APP)}[\text{F}(x_1) \times \text{CFN} + (1 - \text{F}(x_1)) \times \text{CTP}]$$

$$+ \text{P(NSAP)}[\text{G}(x_1) \times \text{CTN} + (1 - \text{G}(x_1))\text{CEP}])$$

When cost is in terms of death, the CTP etc. are case fatalities. When cost is in terms of convalescent days, the CTP etc. are the average days of convalescence.

If the total cost has one minimum, and that minimum is not at the extremes of high risk or low risk, the slope of the cost curve ($d\,D(x)/dx$) will, by definition, be zero at that minimum.

We therefore (A) take the derivative of $D(x)$ with regard to x, (B) set it equal to zero, and (C) solve for the likelihood ratio $f(x)/g(x)$ which corresponds to the minimum $D(x)$

$$\frac{d\,D(x)}{d\,x} = P(\text{APP})\left[\frac{d\,F(x)}{d\,x}\,\text{CFN} + \left(\frac{-d\,F(x)}{d\,x}\right)\text{CTP}\right] \qquad (A)$$

$$+ \text{P(NSAP)}\left[\frac{d\,G(x)}{d\,x}\,\text{CTN} + \left(\frac{-d\,G(x)}{d\,x}\right)\text{CFP}\right]$$

but $dF(x)/dx = f(x)$, and so

$$\frac{d\,D(x)}{d\,x} = \text{P(APP)}\ [f(x)\text{CFN} - f(x)\text{CTP}] + \text{P(NSAP)}\ [g(x)\text{CTP} - g(x)\text{CFP}] \qquad (A_1)$$

$$= \text{P(APP)}\ [f(x)\ (\text{CFN} - \text{CTP})] + \text{P(NSAP)}\ [g(x)(\text{CTP}) - \text{CFP})] \qquad (A_2)$$

$$0 = \text{P(APP)}\ [f(x)\ (\text{CFN} - \text{CTP})] + \text{P(NSAP)}\ [g(x)(\text{CTP} - \text{CFP})] \qquad (B)$$

or

$$\text{P(APP)}[f(x)(\text{CFN} - \text{CTP}] = \text{P(NSAP)}\ [g(x)(\text{CFP} - \text{CTP})]$$

$$\frac{f(x)}{g(x)} = \frac{\text{P(NSAP)}}{\text{P(APP)}} \cdot \frac{(\text{CFP} - \text{CTN})}{(\text{CFN} - \text{CTP})} \qquad (C)$$

The derivation is thus completed. Note that this derivation is made for the case where the cost curve is concave, that is, where there is an "internal minimum". If the curve were convex, the point with zero slope would be a maximum, not a minimum. In the appendicitis case we know from the graph that the slope is concave.

This derivation has been carried out for the continuous case. The same formula should hold for the discrete case too. Although we need to select the nearest available discrete likelihood ratio and will often not be able to find a rank which possesses the exact likelihood ratio indicated by the formula.

19
Treatment of breast cancer

Klim McPherson
Maurice S. Fox

Breast cancer is one of the major causes of mortality in adult women, particularly among American and European women. In the United States there are approximately 90,000 new diagnoses each year, and it is estimated that seven million women now alive in America will present with the disease in their lifetime. A common treatment of early breast cancer, radical mastectomy, consists of surgical removal of the primary tumor, the breast, the axillary nodes under the arm, and the pectoral muscle. Sometimes only the affected breast is removed, an operation known as simple or complete mastectomy. Other more or less conservative procedures have been documented, as well as intermediate versions removing perhaps the axillary nodes but not the pectoral muscle. Adjuvant treatment often consists of either radiotherapy to the chest wall and the axillary nodes or, more recently, chemotherapy.

The controversy surrounding the choice of treatment has been more or less continuous since the use of mastectomy became widespread at the end of the last century. When Halsted introduced the radical operation in 1894, it represented the only reasonable possibility for effective intervention. To this day, this surgical procedure, often in conjunction with radiotherapy and/or chemotherapy, remains "accepted practice." In spite of progress in technique and advances in the quality of ancillary and adjuvant therapy, there is little evidence that these changes have been reflected in an increase in the life expectancy of patients (McKinnon, 1952). For most of this century both the death rate and the incidence of breast cancer among women have remained nearly constant at about

25–30 per 100,000 and 60–80 per 100,000 respectively (Cutler and Devesa, 1973). If such population data are reliable, it follows that the changes over the last forty or more years in the availability of therapy and its quality have had little effect on the progress or the outcome of the disease. In 1930 about 40% of those incurring the disease died of the disease, and in 1975 the same fraction still die of the disease. The population data, combined with the general observation that some patients with all the manifestations of early disease proceed relatively quickly to their death in spite of surgical intervention, while occasional individuals with undoubted malignant disease live out a normal span of life without treatment (Steckler and Martin, 1973), have kept the controversy alive. There exist justifiable doubts about the overall effectiveness of current treatment measured either in terms of "cure" or of life expectancy.

Since treatment strategy is dominated by a model of the disease process that is at best understood only in vague outline, it would seem reasonable to examine the justification of the strategy. That is not to say that these doubts necessarily carry with them the idea that current strategies of surgical intervention are without benefit or even harmful, but these possibilities cannot be ignored. The evaluation of the effectiveness of treatment has never been straightforward, largely because in breast cancer randomized trials comparing, in the extreme case, surgical treatment with the absence of treatment, have never been considered remotely ethical. The impasse created by the requirement of continuation of "accepted practice" discourages the simplest kind of investigation that would permit distinction between fact and belief on the issue of the benefit provided by surgery. Many writers have used observational data retrospectively to argue that treatment is ineffective (Jones, 1956) or, at best, limited (Park and Lees, 1951). These include comparing the survival experience of cases diagnosed early with those diagnosed apparently late in the disease process. Comparisons of contemporary groups of treated cases with (mostly) historical untreated cases have also provided some information (Bloom, 1968), but in all such studies the effects of selection and classification, as well as the confounding of variables, make it difficult to reach persuasive conclusions in either direction. What has further hindered universal acceptance of the idea that treatment is beneficial has been the failure to demonstrate significant differences, comparing treatment regimens, in many clinical trials. The clinical evidence that has accumulated demonstrates persuasively that radical mastectomy offers no greater benefit to the patient than does simple mastectomy. This being the case, what proof is there that limited surgery such as tylectomy would not offer an equal benefit to some patients? Or, for that matter, what is the evidence for surgery offering any benefit to most (Editorial, *Lancet*, 1969)?

If there are, in fact, doubts that can be justifiably raised concerning the effectiveness of surgery, then the desirability of screening to detect presumed "early" cases must be reexamined. Reservations concerning the reliability of a prognosis, based on observation of individuals whose cancer was detected after symptoms had begun to appear, applied to individuals detected in a deliberate search, compound the doubts. If deliberate search were to result in the inclusion of individuals whose histopathological signs were not precursors of the lethal disease, a study population could readily be created with improved survival characteristics that would provide a false assessment of the effectiveness of intervention.

The Disease Model

The justification for the treatment of breast cancer has rested largely on what are basically plausibility arguments concerning the underlying process of the disease (Marx, 1974). It is known that cancer cells begin to multiply in the primary site and that this growth is probably resisted to some extent by the body's immune response and perhaps by systemic regulatory processes. These responses may be more or less effective in inhibiting the spread of cancer to distant foci. It is assumed that the effectiveness of the immune response will be enhanced by the removal or destruction of as many cancer cells as possible. In principle, the aim of therapy has been and continues to be the obliteration of all the cancer cells (Urben, 1973). In cases where metastases have already developed, complete obliteration is evidently not possible with local treatment alone (Forrest et al., 1974).

The intuitive notion that the maximum purging of possibly offensive tissue is the most effective approach to the treatment of breast cancer, and of cancer in general, continues to dominate medical procedure. While it is possible that this notion is correct, there is little, if any, evidence to support it.

With such uncertainty, it is perhaps not surprising that the results of therapeutic intervention are so unpredictable and the experience so varied that doubt continues to be expressed about the appropriateness of treatment detail and investigative emphasis (Magarey, 1972). It is perhaps also not surprising that the effectiveness of treatment in altering such aspects of the disease as incidence of local recurrence, length of survival, frequency of permanent "cure," morbidity, and other aspects of quality of life has proved so problematic (Editorial, *British Medical Journal*, 1972).

The model may be so far from an adequate description of the main components of the disease process as to suggest treatment strategies that would be less than optimal. For example, if the secondary foci were to retain a "memory" of their organ of origin and were subject to organ specific growth inhibition, removal of the primary organ could result in the stimulation of growth of the secondary tumor. Partial hepatectomy results in the stimulation of cell proliferation in the remaining liver. The factor(s) responsible for the stimulation are humoral and exhibit organ specificity. The growth regulation is such that regeneration ceases when the liver regains its approximate original size. Perhaps similarly, remaining renal cells exhibit a regenerative response on removal of one of the kidneys (Butcher and Malt, 1971). Such organ-specific regulation responses could constitute a basis for re-examination of the justification of extensive surgical intervention. Consistent with this interpretation are those clinical cases of cancer that deteriorate rapidly from metastatic disease following surgical removal of the primary tumor.

A second example is the possibility that the response of the lymph nodes adjacent to the breast provides a substantial component of the immune response against the tumor itself and perhaps its secondary metastases (Fisher and Fisher, 1972). This possibility gives rise to the hypothesis that treatment of these nodes (ablation or radiation) might cripple this component of the response (Tee and Pettingale, 1974). It has also been shown that trauma, irradiation, and illness interfere with immune response to an extent which may have implications for current methods of treatment (Crile, 1973).

In fact, it seems likely that breast cancer in reality includes several biologically distinct entities. Zelen (1968) has used data from a large series of treated patients to postulate a series of (possibly) four distinct courses of the disease, some of which appear to respond to treatment while others do not. Within this general frame of reference resides the notion of biological predeterminism (Hunt, 1970), where it is argued that some breast cancers are fatal whatever treatment is offered (from the current repertoire at least) and at whatever stage they are diagnosed. At the other extreme, there are some breast cancers that may never change from a relatively benign entity into a fatal version. If such a class were to exist, those patients would suffer all of the risks and adverse effects of treatment without any benefit.

These ideas suggest that there may be characteristics of these diseases which are not now recognizable or distinguishable by existing pathological, clinical, or other means (McKinnon, 1955). Those aspects of the disease which are now thought to be implicated in prognosis do not clearly distinguish separate disease entities (Bulbrook, 1974).

Review of Clinical Trials

It is appropriate to review briefly some of the randomized clinical trials which have a bearing on the evaluation of treatment and on the understanding of the disease (Meier, 1975). Firstly, comparisons between radical mastectomy and simple mastectomy are quite crucial because of the implications on the possible role of the axillary nodes. In 1965 Kaae and Johansen published the results of a randomized comparative study of nearly 700 patients. A McWhirter simple mastectomy accompanied by radiotherapy was carried out on one half of a group of patients and an extended radical was carried out on the other half. The striking conclusion of this study is that in almost all respects, the two groups were indistinguishable, even after 10 years. This was true for patients with clinically involved nodes as well as those without evidence of nodal involvement.

A further trial (Brinkley and Haybittle, 1966) has shown an improved 5-year survival with a simple mastectomy plus radiotherapy over radical mastectomy plus radiotherapy among clinical Stage II patients. (Stage II indicates axillary node involvement as detected either clinically by palpation or by pathologic examination after all or some of these nodes have been surgically removed.) The trial also showed a significant difference in the rate of healing of the surgical wound in favor of the more modest procedure, which finally caused them to stop the trial.

Subsequent studies have substantiated these results, and we have been unable to discover a single randomized series in which radical mastectomy, with or without radiotherapy to the axilla, has shown any benefit over simple mastectomy with radiotherapy. This benefit can be assessed in terms of the proportion surviving up to 10 years, or in terms either of the incidence of local or of distant recurrence. The only systematic differences that appear concern postoperative morbidity where edema of the arm and restricted arm movement are more likely among patients with radical mastectomy (particularly when the pectoral muscles are removed). To add to these uncertainties, there is even some evidence for "a small increased mortality associated with use of local postoperative radiotherapy in early breast cancer" (Stjernswärd, 1974).

The extent to which the general results are applicable to individual patients is not known. While the evidence from clinical trials shows no difference on average between the two treatments, it remains possible that radical surgery would be better than simple mastectomy plus radiotherapy with some patients and worse with others. This has been discussed in the literature, but it remains unclear how such patients might be distinguished.

These observations have suggested to some that still more modest procedures, while reducing the degree of mutilation (Peters, 1974), would be equally beneficial. Trials have been mounted comparing lesser surgery than complete mastectomy and comparing various forms of adjuvant radiotherapy. It is argued that radical mastectomy and simple mastectomy with radiotherapy are both forms of radical treatment and therefore similar in kind. The main randomized trial including more modest surgical intervention is that reported by Atkins et al. (1972) comparing radical mastectomy with a procedure known as tylectomy (removal of the tumor and immediately surrounding tissue). Both groups received radiotherapy. In this series, patients without clinical evidence of nodal involvement (Stage I) showed no difference between the two groups in the proportion of those surviving after 10 years, although among the tylectomy group there was a higher proportion of patients with local recurrence. This observation suggests that clinical evaluation of lymph node involvement may be an effective means of determining a group of patients who will benefit in terms of life expectancy at least as much from tylectomy as they would from the more radical procedures. The benefit of the more modest procedure in improving the quality of life by reducing the functional loss and degree of disfigurement must be weighed in the balance (Asken, 1975). In contrast to the Brinkley and Haybittle study, the Stage II patients in the Atkins et al. study fared better with radical therapy.

Two important facts bear on the results of this trial which may have implications for the understanding of the disease. First, it is reported that in about 40% of total mastectomies subjected to pathological examination, cancer cells are present in parts of the affected breast distant from the primary tumor. Therefore, less than total mastectomy is likely to leave behind tumor cells which would be removed by more radical procedures. In addition, clinical evaluation of nodal involvement is known to be unreliable when contrasted with subsequent pathological examination of removed nodes (Sheridan et al., 1971). On the hypothesis that the more cancer cells removed by surgery the better, the favorable results reported concerning Stage I patients would not be expected. An alternative, which involves the role of immune response, might be that the clinical evaluation of nodal involvement by palpation is actually an assessment of the extent to which the axillary nodes are participating in the immunological response. In other words, whether the nodes actually are involved or not, if they are not clinically palpable the immune response to the tumor might still be effective. This could be a reflection of the biological nature of the tumor itself or of the capacity of a particular component of the immune response. It is possible, and perhaps likely, that clinical and pathological staging of the disease, while purporting to measure the same thing are, in fact, measuring very different aspects of the disease (Cutler, 1968).

In conformity with the widely accepted disease model, postmastectomy irradiation has been regarded as beneficial. In recent years, at least three prospectively randomized trials (Butcher et al., 1964; Kaae and Johansen, 1968; Fisher et al., 1970) have failed to demonstrate that postoperative radiotherapy results in any improvement in the 5- or 10-year survival. On the contrary, slight increases in mortality (Stjernswärd, 1974) and an increased incidence of distant metastases have been reported (Fisher et. al., 1970; Bruce, 1971). These may be the consequences of demonstrated, persisting, cell-mediated immune deficiency following postoperative irradiation (Stjernswärd et al., 1972; Meyer, 1970; Cassimi et al., 1973). In fact, Edwards et al., (1972) have reported the regression of palpable axillary lymph nodes in 75% of patients with Stage II breast cancer subjected to simple mastectomy *without* prophylactic radiotherapy. These observations suggest the prominence of the immune response in host control of malignant growth.

Recent preliminary reports suggest a benefit provided by adjuvant chemotherapy (Fisher et al., 1975; Bonadonna et al., 1976) following radical mastectomy for women with histologically demonstrated axillary node involvement. It is still too early to draw a firm conclusion concerning the effectiveness of this innovation for the particular subclass of breast cancer examined. Nevertheless, the promise offered by this approach certainly warrants close attention.

In many of the trials so far discussed, the axillary nodes have been treated by either surgery or radiotherapy and, therefore, it remains very difficult to infer the possible participatory role of these nodes in the immune response. Trials have been started (Forrest et al., 1974) comparing the responses with (a) radical mastectomy plus immediate postoperative radiotherapy for those patients with histologically confirmed involved axillary nodes and with (b) simple mastectomy and radiotherapy limited to clinically detected node involvement. For patients diagnosed as clinical Stage II this latter treatment schedule means postoperative radiotherapy to clinically involved nodes which do not regress (Edwards et al., 1972), and in Stage I patients radiotherapy if and when these nodes become clinically palpable. Another trial is under way (Murray, 1974) comparing the effects on patients with simple mastectomy of immediate radiotherapy and radiotherapy only when there are clinical signs of recurrence either in the scar or the axilla. Both trials have only reported three years' results, and it is therefore too early to detect any significant differences.

To summarize the findings of randomized trials (Table 19-1) in the treatment of breast cancer, the following appear to be the general conclusions. It must be emphasized that this is on the basis of overall results for Stage I and Stage II cancer and, therefore, in the absence of any more reliable prognostic information represents average effects which might or might not be applicable to particular individual patients.

Table 19–1. Summary of some clinical trials in treatment of breast cancer

Place, Author, Date	Comparison	Stage	Total No. Patients	% Surviving 5 Years	% Surviving 10 Years	% Free of Recurrence at 5 Years: Local	% Free of Recurrence at 5 Years: Any	Within Stage Contrasts
Copenhagen: Kaae and Johansen 1965	Extended Radical Simple + XRT	Operable	206 219	67 66	42 44	78 81	58 57	No difference in 10-yr. survival of operable cases (Stage I excluded).
Cambridge: Brinkley and Haybittle, 1966	Radical + XRT Simple + XRT	Stage II	91 113	54 66			51 58	Trial stopped because of excess of patients in group A experiencing delay in healing of wound.
London: Atkins et al. 1972	Tylectomy + XRT Radical + Partial XRT (both groups received chemotherapy)	Stages I & II	182 188	71 74	60 70	63 87		Large difference in 10-yr. survival and local recurrence favoring radical treatment among clinical Stage II.
Scotland: Hamilton et al. 1974	Radical Simple + Radical XRT	Stages I, II, & III	256 242	73 70			64 60	
U.S.A.: Fisher et al. 1970	Radical + XRT Radical + drug	Stages I & II	195 233	56 62			51 50	
Hammersmith: Burn 1974	Radical + partial XRT Simple + complete XRT	Stages I & II	92 98	72 74		91 95		
Manchester: Cole 1964	Radical + postop XRT Radical + no initial XRT	Operable	709 752	57 62	45 49			50% 5-year survival of Stage II patients in both treatment groups.
Edinburgh: Bruce 1971	Radical Simple + XRT	Operable	200 184	75 70		84 86	66 60	

XRT = X-ray therapy

1. Radical mastectomy (with radiotherapy) is equivalent in terms of survival experience to simple mastectomy plus postoperative radiotherapy. In terms of mutilation, morbidity, length of convalescence and time taken for the wound to heal, the differences are substantial.

2. For patients without clinical evidence of involved nodes, local removal of the tumor (tylectomy) plus radiotherapy appears to be equivalent in terms of survival experience to radical mastectomy (except for the higher incidence of local recurrence noted above).

3. Postoperative radiotherapy seems to offer little if any benefit and may be detrimental for some patients.

Since, in the United States for some 80% of patients presenting with breast cancer radical mastectomy is the treatment of choice (Bunker, 1970), it is evident that these conclusions are not widely agreed upon. If there were one randomized series which showed a significant advantage in terms of "cure" rate or length of survival, then presumably the radical operation could be justified on some evaluation of quantity of life against quality. However, there appears to be no such evidence. Several justifications for the persistence of the radical procedure have been offered. Firstly, it has been argued that clinical trials by others have intrinsic faults which invalidate their results (Anglem and Leber, 1972). It is further argued that when survival rates from uncontrolled studies are compared, they favor the radical operations, but considering that the criticisms of the randomized series rest on arguments of selection and inadequate randomization, this latter assertion cannot be taken seriously. Secondly, it is argued that complete resection of the axillary nodes is an essential diagnostic procedure even if not therapeutic (Moore, 1968). That must be a matter of opinion because it depends on one's perception of the disease model and the possible role of these nodes in the immune response. The value to the patient of more precise diagnosis without a corresponding therapeutic framework can also be questioned. No clear support can be gained for any particular model from the results of these clinical trials. However, the widespread practice of removal of the axillary nodes in the treatment of early breast cancer may have an adverse effect on the patient as well as interfere with further understanding of their possible role in the disease process and, therefore, with the evolution of more effective strategy of intervention.

A further reason for the persistence of the radical procedure seems to be the implicit acceptance of a disease model which postulates that cancer cells grow and spread until removed by surgery or killed with radiotherapy and/or chemotherapy. From this intuitive hypothesis follows the belief that the more surgery or radiotherapy the greater the benefit to the patient. However, such ideas require clear supporting evidence before they can form an unchallengeable basis for widespread treatment. Such a prevalent view leads inevitably to more and more radical innovations in surgical procedures and radiation despite the uncertainty of the outcome.

Crile has offered two suggestions to account for the differences between practice in the United States and elsewhere (Crile, 1973). Despite their speculative nature, both command fairly widespread acceptance, at least as possibilities. The first suggestion is based on the reputation of Halsted combined with the role that the Johns Hopkins School of Medicine played at the turn of the century in challenging the then dominant authority of the European schools. The second invokes the possible influence of fee-for-service medicine on conditioning behavior. In short, when the fee schedules for radical mastectomy are sometimes more than twice as high as those for simple mastectomy, it would be difficult to argue that this would have no effect on the decisions of some physicians, particularly where there is little evidence that simple mastectomy and radiotherapy constitute a more effective treatment. Tradition and economics might equally explain the low prevalence of radical mastectomy in Britain and elsewhere. Moreover, the escalating risk of malpractice litigation in the event of a recurrence of the disease is likely to have the effect of encouraging as much intervention as possible to guard against the possibility that any recurrence might be seen in the courts as evidence of inadequate therapeutic intervention.

SCREENING

Since many women with cancer of the breast die despite intervention, it has been argued that the intervention might have been more effective if the disease had been diagnosed sufficiently early. Here, again, the argument has been based on the plausibility of the disease model.

The recent reports of the imposing HIP Breast Cancer Screening Program (Shapiro et al., 1973) have provided the only evidence bearing on the effectiveness of screening. These reports devote a great deal of attention to "case fatality rates" among screened and unscreened women. The differences in "case fatality rates" appear to be nearly entirely confined to women over 50 years of age whose cancer was detectable by mammography and not by clinical examination.

Since the most prominent difference in mortality rate resides in the subclass of cancers detected by mammography only, the question of the reliability of detection seems justified. A number of reports have appeared documenting a substantial level of observer variability in histopathological diagnosis of cancer of the breast (MacMahon et al., 1973), lung (Feinstein et al., 1970), thyroid (Saxen et al., 1970), and melanoma (Saksela and Rintala, 1968). Saxen reports a "man-made epidemic" (a nearly tenfold increase) of carcinoma *in situ* of the uterine cervix in Finland following initiation of mass examinations. Harbitz and Haugen (1972) report a great discrepancy (nearly twentyfold) between the high frequency of prostatic carcinoma at autopsy and the occurrence of carcinoma which has been clinically manifested or caused death. In fact, among 70-year-old men, the frequency of prostate cancer in sequential autopsies may be as much as 100 times the frequency of clinically manifested disease (Cairns, 1975).

Even ignoring observer variability, is it reasonable to apply the same cytomorphological criteria of malignancy, and subsequent treatment, to lesions detected in clinically healthy people as to clinically diagnosed tumors? It seems likely that many collections of histologically characterized invasive cells either regress before they become clinically detectable or grow so slowly that they do not give rise to symptoms during the patient's lifetime. A study similar to that of Harbitz and Haugen (1972) on breast cancer at autopsy could have a substantial impact on decisions concerning the desirability of screening.

During the five years of follow-up of the HIP study, there were 40 breast cancer deaths in the study (screened plus refused screening) population of approximately 31,000 women, compared to 63 deaths in the control group of equal size. Several heterogeneities between the populations make the significance of the observed difference difficult to assess. For example, among the 11,000 women who had been offered screening and refused it, the incidence of detected breast cancer and mortality from breast cancer seems substantially lower than in the control population. If screened women are compared to the total of unscreened women, the difference in the incidence of death becomes smaller. Even if the reported difference is significant, the question of whether a more modest intervention might be as effective remains to be answered. In both groups most of the treatment was radical mastectomy, 74% in the control group and 83% in the study group, and a large fraction (more than 40%) of the patients in both groups received adjuvant radiotherapy.

The possible added risk imposed by a repetitive screening procedure *per se* should be considered. The analysis described in the BEIR report (Advisory Committee on the Biological Effects of Ionizing Radiations, 1972) suggests an absolute risk estimate of cancer of the breast per rad exposure to the breast of 8.4×10^{6} per year. Mammography involves breast x-ray exposures of 6 to 8 rads (Papaioannou, 1974). If this appraisal is correct the increased incidence of breast cancer resulting from mammography every six months or even every year would be substantial, although perhaps delayed in its appearance (as discussed in Chapter 4).

In order to justify screening, it would seem essential that the identity of malignancy detected in deliberate search be shown to coincide with malignancy detected after symptoms had begun to appear and that the treatment be limited to the minimum required to provide maximum benefit for the patient.

COSTS AND BENEFITS

The ultimate question as to whether surgical treatment of breast cancer can be justified by the benefits which it provides compared with its risks and costs remains unanswered. Breast cancer is not a unique entity, and one must regard evaluations of treatment with a degree of reservation unless it is possible to specify precisely which patients can be expected to benefit from what. However, the information available from randomized clinical trials, staging the disease as reliably as is currently possible, appears to provide a consistent picture. In the aggregate, radical mastectomy is no more effective than simple surgery in terms of survival experience, and the chances of local or distant recurrence. It does, however, cost more in dollars for surgery and hospital stay and does induce more morbidity, more mutilation, and more traumatic psychological adjustment as well as carrying a greater risk of surgical death.

Therefore, these extra costs and risks ought to be justified by some equivalent benefit. For instance, in Massachusetts in 1973 the mean fee paid for the Medicare population for simple mastectomy was $232 with a range between $100 and $500. For radical mastectomy, equivalent figures were $412 and $300 to $900. In the United States as a whole in 1972, the average length of stay after simple mastectomy was 6.0 days, and after radical it was 10.3 days (CPHA*, 1973). The costs, therefore, of surgery and hospital are about $1,500 for simple mastectomy and $2,600 for the radical procedure. With approximately 90,000 new diagnoses (Stages I and II) each year, the difference between the two extremes of all simple mastectomy and all radical mastectomy probably represents more than $100 million per year. Obviously, either extreme strategy is contrary to common sense as well as the doctrine of clinical freedom, but the figure provides an order of magnitude within which the costs lie. At the individual level, whatever gains can be expected from radical mastectomy need to be identified and quantified so that they can be compared with the known dollar costs and the known risks of morbidity and extra mutilation associated with the operation.

However, in the light of the results of clinical trials for the past thirty years, it seems unlikely that any systematic differences will emerge. It is, however, possible that a subgroup of patients exists for whom the extra expenditure and loss in some aspects of quality of life could be justified in terms of gains in others, particularly length of survival expectation. Meanwhile, randomized controlled trials have evidently failed to persuade the majority of physicians (Fisher, 1973) that most of the current practice remains difficult to justify as the most common procedure of choice. When a particular form of therapy is widely practiced, it is difficult to avoid regarding some alternative as suboptimal.

In any assessment of the cost effectiveness of future research effort, these problems of persuasiveness as well as the likely outcome of investigations of the effectiveness of screening, adjuvant therapy, and comparisons between radical and simple mastectomy need to be explicitly considered. Notwithstanding the apparent need to demonstrate benefits of a particular appraisal, for example, a therapeutic difference (or lack of) between radical and simple mastectomy, it might be appropriate to focus more attention on other aspects of treatment.

In particular, since resources for research are always limited, it could be argued that the likelihood of actually hindering progress is higher when a large proportion of those resources are spent on resolving a question whose answer seems to be a foregone conclusion. This is not to say that it is known that there is no difference (for there is bound to be some) in the aggregate effectiveness of radical versus simple mastectomy or other local intervention. Whatever difference there is will probably take an enormous clinical trial and many years to demonstrate, and even then will probably be of such magnitude that the trial will have a very limited effect on the treatment of individual patients.

CONCLUSION

Presently, for about 40% of American women diagnosed with cancer of the breast, cancer of the breast is given as the cause of death. Although such statistics are subject to ambiguity, it is clear that a large fraction of women presenting with the disease do indeed die of the disease. To at least this extent, therapeutic intervention is ineffective. The qualities of many existing programs designed to

*Commission on Professional and Hospital Activities

improve the effectiveness of treatment of breast cancer are dominated by dogmatic beliefs concerning the nature of the disease and the effectiveness of various treatment strategies.

Stoll, in his preface to the first volume of the recent series New Aspects of Breast Cancer, begins with:

"In the last 10 years a serious dilemma has faced the clinician with every breast cancer patient presenting for treatment. A highly responsible body of scientific opinion has suggested that neither surgical treatment nor radiation therapy is likely to affect the outcome of the disease in the vast majority of patients presenting. Moreover both statistical evidence from treated series of breast cancer, and analogy with immunological responses in experimental animals, have led to serious speculation that extensive surgery or radiotherapy might even accelerate the course of the disease rather than lead to cure."

The establishment, in the United States, of current "accepted practice" as a strategy for treatment of cancer of the breast does not seem to have required a demonstration of effectiveness. Radical mastectomy is so frequently the treatment of choice that it would almost seem that a tradition has been established without a clear-cut justification.

Clinical trials designed primarily to compare treatments do not necessarily permit the contrasting of competing hypotheses about the disease model (Schwartz and Lellouch, 1967). Often this is because the detailed treatment schedules are decided upon under ethical constraints which generally do not allow people to receive treatment which is less than that currently regarded as optimal. This often means that the decision about which treatment is better may be relatively straightforward after the trial is over, but implications on the understanding of the disease process is lost because of the confounding of the relevant variables (Healy and Saracci, 1971). Some trials should, perhaps, be designed to test particular explanatory hypotheses of the disease process and may, therefore, be different in kind from those designed to compare treatments. Such an approach would have to rationalize the ethical problems (Editorial, *Science*, 1974) concerned with the allocation of detailed treatment schedules. As it stands, in a situation where the effectiveness of treatment is at most fairly small, it may be possible to resist the temptation to overestimate the importance of marginal contrasts in effectiveness associated with different treatments in order to provide a basis for improvement of strategy of intervention and perhaps for a better understanding of the disease.

A more comprehensive view of the disease process must be sought in the hope of identifying more effective ways to intervene. In the meantime, we must learn how to modulate therapeutic intervention whose justification appears to reside in beliefs held both by the patient and the physician.

The transition from the circumstance in which strategy is based on belief to one in which strategy is based on fact will no doubt be difficult. The burden of proof has been shifted from the demonstration that a procedure is effective to a demonstration that a procedure provides no benefit. Proof of innocence is indeed formidable!

References

Advisory Committee on the Biological Effects of Ionizing Radiations (Report of): The Effects on Populations of Exposure to Low Levels of Ionizing Radiation. National Academy of Sciences, National Research Council, Washington, DC, 1972, p 143

Anglem TJ, Leber RE: The dubious case for conservative operation in operable cancer of the breast. Ann Surg 176:625, 1972

Asken MJ: Psychoemotional aspects of mastectomy: a review of recent literature. Am J Psychiatry 132:56, 1975

Atkins, Sir H, Hayward JL, Klugman DJ, et al: Treatment of early breast cancer: a report after ten years of a clinical trial. Br Med J 2:423, 1972

Bloom HJG: Survival of women with untreated breast cancer–past and present: Prognostic Factors in Breast Cancer. Edited by APM Forrest, PB Kunkler. Proceedings of the First Tenovus Symposium. Edinburgh, ES Livingstone, 1968

Bonadonna G, Brusamolino E, Valagussa P, et al: Combination chemotherapy as an adjuvant treatment in operable breast cancer. N Engl J Med 294:405, 1976

Brinkley D, Haybittle JL: Treatment of stage II carcinoma of the female breast. Lancet 2:291, 1966

British Medical Journal, Editorial: Treatment of early carcinoma of breast. Br Med J 2:417, 1972

Bruce Sir J: Operable cancer of the breast: a controlled clinical trial. Cancer 28: 1443, 1971

Bulbrook RD: Tests of prediction, The Treatment of Breast Cancer. Edited by Sir Hedley Atkins. Baltimore, University Park Press, 1974

Bunker JP: Surgical manpower: a comparison of operations and surgeons in the United States and in England and Wales. N Engl J Med 282:135, 1970

Burn JI: 'Early' breast cancer: the Hammersmith trial. Br J Surg 61:762, 1974

Butcher HR Jr, Seaman WP, Eckhert C, et al: An assessment of radical mastectomy and postoperative irradiation therapy in the treatment of mammary cancer. Cancer 17:480, 1964

Butcher NLR, Malt RA: Regeneration of Liver and Kidney. Boston, Little, Brown & Company, 1971, p 161

Cairns J: The cancer problem. Scientific American 233(5):64, 1975

Cassimi AB, Brunstetter FH, Kemmerer WT, et al: Cellular immune competence of breast cancer patients receiving radiotherapy. Arch Surg 107:531, 1973

Cole MP: The place of radiotherapy in the management of early breast cancer: a report of two clinical trials. Br J Surg 51:216, 1964

Commission on Professional and Hospital Activities: Length of Stay in PAS Hospitals, United States, Regional, 1972. Ann Arbor, 1973

Crile G Jr: A Biological Consideration of Treatment of Breast Cancer. Springfield, Illinois, Chas C Thomas, 1967

Crile G Jr: What Women Should Know About the Breast Cancer Controversy. New York, Macmillan Publishing Co Inc, 1973

Crile G Jr, Anglem TJ: Management of breast cancer: limited management. JAMA 230:95, 1974

Cutler SJ: The value of general survival data, Clinical Evaluation in Breast Cancer. Edited by JL Hayward and RD Bulbrook. New York, Academic Press, 1966

Cutler SJ: The prognosis of treated breast cancer, Prognostic Factors in Breast

Cancer. Edited by APM Forrest, PB Kunkler. Proceedings of the First Tenovus Symposium. Edinburgh, ES Livingstone, 1968

Cutler SJ, Devesa SS: Trends in cancer incidence and mortality in the U.S.A., Host Environment and Interactions in the Etiology of Cancer in Man. Edited by R Doll, I Vodopiza. Lyon, International Agency for Research on Cancer, 1973

Edwards MH, Baum M, Magarey CJ: Regression of axillary lymph-nodes in cancer of the breast. Br J Surg 59:776, 1972

Feinstein AR, Gelfman NA, Yesner R: Observer variability in histopathologic diagnosis of lung cancer. Am Rev Resp Dis 101:671, 1970

Fisher B: Cooperative clinical trials in primary breast cancer: a critical appraisal. Cancer 31:1271, 1973

Fisher B, Carbone P, Economou SG, et al: 1-phenylalanine mustard (L-PAM) in the management of primary breast cancer: a report of early findings. N Engl J Med 292:117, 1975

Fisher B, Fisher ER: Studies concerning the regional lymph node in cancer. II. Maintenance of immunity. Cancer 29:1496, 1972

Fisher B, Slack NH, Cavanaugh PJ, et al: Postoperative radiotherapy in the treatment of breast cancer: results of the NSABP clinical trial. Ann Surg 172: 711, 1970

Forrest APM, Roberts MM, Preece P, et al: The Cardiff-St. Mary's trial. Br J Surg 61:766, 1974

Hamilton T, Langlands AO, Prescott RJ: The treatment of operable cancer of the breast: a clinical trial in the south-east region of Scotland. Br J Surg 61:758, 1974

Harbitz TB, Haugen OA: Histology of the prostate in elderly men. Acta Path Microbiol Scand A 80:756, 1972

Healy MJR, Saracci R: Report of a symposium sponsored by the UICC on principles and practice in clinical trials. Int J Cancer 8:541, 1971

Hunt PS: Prognosis and early management in breast cancer. Med J Aust 2:544, 1970

Jones HB: Demographic consideration of the cancer problem. Trans NY Acad Sci 18:298, 1956

Kaae S, Johansen H: Simple mastectomy plus postoperative irradiation by the method of McWhirter for mammary carcinoma. Prog Clin Cancer 1:453, 1965

Kaae S, Johansen H: Simple versus radical mastectomy in primary breast cancer, Prognostic Factors in Breast Cancer. Edited by APM Forrest and PB Kunkler, Edinburgh, ES Livingstone, 1968, p 93

Lancet, Editorial: Treatment of early cancer of the breast. Lancet 2:1175, 1969

MacMahon B, Morrison AS, Ackerman LV, et al: Histological characteristics of breast cancer in Boston and Tokyo. Int J Cancer 11:338, 1973

Magarey CJ: Treatment of apparently early breast cancer. I. The dilemma. Med J Aust 2:543, 1972

Marx JL: Breast cancer research: problems and progress. Science 184:1162, 1974

McKinnon NE: Downward trend in breast-cancer mortality? Lancet 2:1086, 1952

McKinnon NE: Limitations in diagnosis and treatment of breast and other cancers: a review. Can Med Assoc J 73:614, 1955

Meier P: Statistics and medical experimentation. Biometrics 31:511, 1975

Meyer KK: Radiation-induced lymphocyte immune deficiency: a factor in the increased visceral metastasis and decreased hormonal responsiveness of breast cancer. Arch Surg 101:114, 1970

Moore FD: Discussion to: Crile G Jr. Results of simple mastectomy without irradiation in the treatment of operative stage I cancer of the breast. Ann Surg 168:330, 1968

Murray JG: Cancer research campaign breast study. Br J Surg 61:772, 1974

Papaioannou AN: The Etiology of Human Breast Cancer. Berlin, Springer-Verlag, 1974, p 167

Park WW, Lees JC: The absolute curability of cancer of breast. Surg Gynecol Obstet 93:129, 1951

Peters MV: Treatment of primary breast cancer: a radiotherapist's view. West J Med 120:343, 1974

Saksela E, Rintala A: Misdiagnosis of prepubertal malignant melanoma: Reclassification of a cancer registry material. Cancer 22:1308, 1968

Saxen E: Histological classification and its implications in the utility of registry data in epidemiological studies, Recent Results in Cancer Research. Edited by E Grundmann and E Pedersen. New York, Springer-Verlag, 1975, p 38

Saxen E, Franssila K, Hakama M: Effect of histological typing of registry material on the results of epidemiological comparison in thyroid cancer: Thyroid Cancer. UICC Monograph Series, Vol. 12. Edited by C Hedinger. Berlin-Heidelberg-New York, Springer, 1970, p 98

Schwartz D, Lellouch J: Explanatory and pragmatic attitudes in therapeutical trials. J Chron Dis 20:637, 1967

Science, Editorial: The continuing breast cancer controversy. Science 186:246, 1974

Shapiro S, Strax P, Venet L, et al: Changes in 5-year breast cancer mortality in a breast cancer screening program. 7th National Cancer Conference Proceedings. Philadelphia, Lippincott Co, 1973, p 663

Sheridan B, Fleming J, Atkinson L, et al: The effects of delay in treatment on survival rates in carcinoma of the breast. Med J Aust 1:262, 1971

Steckler RM, Martin RG: Prolonged survival in untreated breast cancer. Am J Surg 126:111, 1973

Stjernswärd J: Decreased survival related to irradiation postoperatively in early operable breast cancer. Lancet 2:1285, 1974

Stjernswärd J, Jondal M, Vanky F, et al: Lymphopenia and change in distribution of human B and T lymphocytes in peripheral blood induced by irradiation for mammary carcinoma. Lancet 1:1352, 1972

Stoll BA: Preface to Volume 1 in the series New Aspects of Breast Cancer: Host Defence in Breast Cancer. Chicago, Year Book Medical Publishers Inc, 1975

Tee DEH, Pettingale KW: Breast cancer and the immune response. Br J Surg 61: 775, 1974

Urben J: Partial mastectomy, unproven treatment for patients with potentially curable breast cancer. Clin Bull Memorial Hospital for Cancer and Allied Diseases 3:123, 1973

Zelen M: A hypothesis for the natural time history of breast cancer. Cancer Res 28:207, 1968

IV

ASSESSMENT OF COSTS, RISKS, AND BENEFITS OF NEW PROCEDURES

The continuing advance of medical science and technology has provided new and promising treatments for diseases that were regarded as hopeless only a few years ago. Indeed, we invent new treatments faster than we can assess them and—for the first time—in excess of our ability to pay for them. As a result, we are faced with ethical, economic, and professional problems of a magnitude never before encountered.

The new therapies differ from the established operations discussed in Part III in several ways. They commonly treat otherwise lethal or terminal disease. Deeply emotional issues of life, love, hope—and their potential loss—occupy the foreground, with the depletion of family resources an additional burden. The extraordinary circumstances surrounding the treatment methods force patient, physician, and family alike to ponder the quality of life that is achieved. Are isolation (hospitalization in intensive-care units), inability to speak (ventilatory support with an endotracheal tube), loss of normal capacity to swallow or empty the urinary bladder (gastric intubation or indwelling catheter), and exposure to insensitive people (as hospital staff may on occasion appear) factors we can properly weigh when choosing therapy? How can we minimize the fear and suffering experienced by the patient and his family when faced with the strange and unknown aspects of such treatment? Can society afford to ensure that the new treatments are available to all and will the resources be allocated?

The surgical treatment of end-stage renal disease and of coronary artery occlusion, analyzed in Chapters 20 by Barnes and 21 by Weinstein, Pliskin, and Stason, illustrate many of these issues. Each involves exceedingly large costs in suffering and dollars to patients and their families, and in dollars to society. The conflict between the interests of society and the individual points to the need for national planning.

An implicit, central consideration is the value of a human life. In Chapter 22 by Bendixen this issue is explicitly considered in the context of the modern intensive-care unit, where the costs of treatment for a discrete and identifiable period of time can be matched to the life expectancy of the salvaged patients. Thus, for the young patient treated for barbiturate overdosage but in previous good health, the intensive-care costs may be as low as $100 for each year of life expectancy; whereas for the middle-aged alcoholic suffering from liver and kidney failure, the intensive-care costs are estimated to be $100,000 or more for a year of additional life. Between these two extremes there is a full spectrum of patients whose lives may be saved at greater or less expense, and with greater or fewer years of life in expectation. However great the anticipated expense, the individual physician caring for such a patient has only one choice: "to make every effort, applying all available resources, until convinced that the battle has been lost." And yet, at the same time, the physician, as a member of society with special knowledge, must also participate in the decision to limit programs and facilities when the cost-benefit ratio is less favorable than for competing programs.

20

An overview of the treatment of end-stage renal disease and a consideration of some of the consequences

Benjamin A. Barnes

The current record of hemodialysis and kidney transplantation in the treatment of end-stage renal disease together with the substantial support by the federal government (Department of Health, Education and Welfare, 1974) for health care costs related to this condition raise questions concerning the possibility of developing a program to care for all medically eligible patients. The problem is complex; the therapeutic pathways for patients with end-stage renal disease shown in Fig. 20-1 suggest that there are, disregarding possible loops occasioned by secondary transplants, more than ten different therapeutic combinations to prevent or delay the lethal outcome of the disease. Within the past few years reports on the results of home and hospital dialysis and living donor and cadaveric transplants have been published, so that it is now possible to consider the implications of a simplified model like the one presented in this paper. In doing so, approximate answers may be provided for such questions as, How large will the patient population grow, What are the relative contributions to survival made by the major therapies, and What are the implications for national planning and support of costs?

SOURCE OF DATA

Two principal sources of data are the third report on dialysis and transplantation from Europe (Gurland et al., 1973) and the eleventh and twelfth reports from the ACS/NIH registry (Advisory Committee to the Renal Transplant Registry, 1973 and 1975). Other reports less extensive in numbers of patients or in dura-

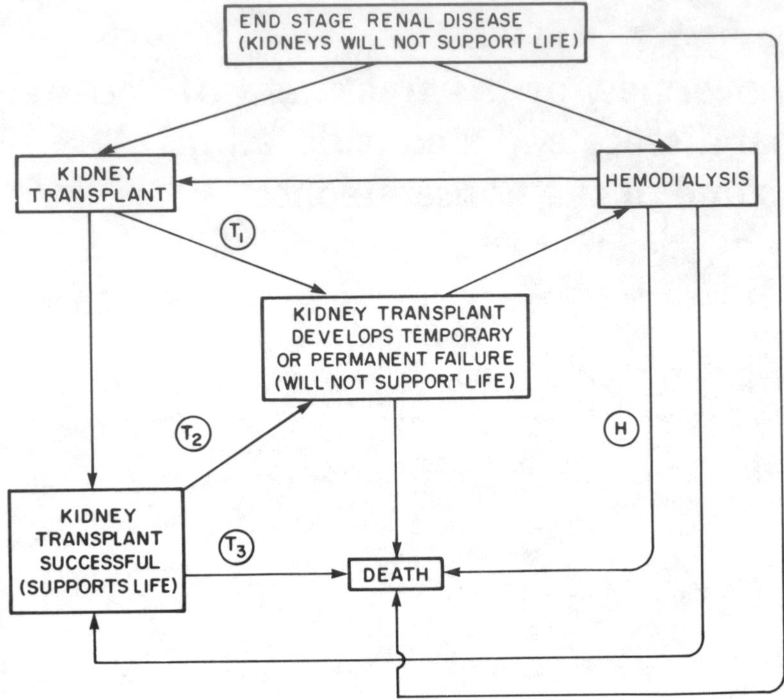

Figure 20-1. Therapeutic pathways in end-stage renal disease.
Pathways T_1, T_2, T_3, and H are considered in analysis. Recurrent loops possible by secondary transplants are not.

tion of follow-up have been consulted as well (Gross et al., 1973; Krueger, 1974; Lewis et al., 1969; Lindner et al., 1974; Lowrie et al., 1973).

MODEL

For the purposes of this paper we assume that patients with end-stage kidney disease are selected for one of four treatments: chronic home dialysis, chronic hospital dialysis, transplantation from a living donor, and transplantation from a cadaveric donor. Furthermore, it is assumed that once started on *chronic* hemodialysis a patient is not considered for transplantation and that the possibility of a second transplant may be ignored. This latter assumption is not a great departure from reality as only 10% of transplants are secondary ones (Advisory Committee to the Renal Transplant Registry, 1973; Gurland et al., 1973), and the results except for the first year of treatment do not differ greatly from chronic hemodialysis, the alternate form of therapy possible for a patient being considered for a second transplant. Data are not available giving the dates of primary and secondary transplants together with the duration of the intervening dialysis, if any. Such information would be needed for a more precise analytical treatment.

The model assigns each of the four therapies an individual mortality rate during the first year of therapy, and a lower, but constant, mortality rate in subsequent years of therapy. This corresponds to the fact that patients prone to lethal complications on dialysis are lost during the first year, succumbing to complications arising out of abnormalities in the coagulation of the blood, latent congestive heart failure, arterial occlusive disease, hepatitis, etc. Similarly, patients receiving a transplant are known to be at greater risk to immunological and/or infectious complications and technical misadventures during the first year. The major and persistent differences in survival of treatment subpopulations established during the first year of therapy have been commented on previously (Lowrie et al., 1973). The assumption that constant mortality rates prevail for at least four years after the first year of therapy is a close approximation of the actual situation as the survival data will show. After perhaps ten or more years other causes unrelated or related to the absence of normally functioning kidneys will inevitably increase the mortality rates in dialyzed or transplanted patients, but how soon this increase occurs in these groups of relatively young patients is not known at present, and the assumption that rates stay virtually constant for ten years or more may be a fair prediction since almost one-half of the recipients are under 30 years of age (Advisory Committee to the Renal Transplant Registry, 1973).

Finally, it is assumed that an annual cohort of patients is selected for treatment of end-stage renal disease each year and that this cohort is relatively constant in size. Trivial modifications of the model could allow for changes in cohort size as doubtless exist in reality as the indications for and availability of treatment for end-stage renal disease become more widely appreciated by patients and physicians. Cohort size would also be influenced by fluctuations in the population. This model by use of published data and reasonable approximations describes the cumulative effects of successive cohorts presenting for four types of therapy with characteristic mortality rates. Although "annual cohorts" are an aid in developing the model, these cohorts do not correspond to the random and continuous appearance of patients seeking therapy throughout the year. An "annual cohort" is a convenient approximation, but in fact such a step function introduces a bias into the analysis avoided by a continuous function of patient entry over time derived in the Appendix.

POPULATION KINETICS OF MODEL

P_0 = cohort size entering any one of the four therapies each year. P_0 is proportional to the total population from which patients are selected for treatment of end-stage kidney disease. Since the total population over a few years may be considered constant, P_0 is also constant for our purposes.

i = number of years

P_i = survivors of a single annual cohort, P_0, surviving under treatment by one of the four therapies through ith year.

S_i = sum of all survivors derived from i cohorts through ith year. This value will give the total number of surviving patients receiving therapy at the time of the end of the ith year of continuous operation of one of the four therapies.

$\mathscr{P}_i$ = total patient years of treatment ever given at any time to all the patients in i cohorts through ith year. This value will give the total number of patient-years of therapy received by all patients at any time through the end of the ith year of continuous operation of one of the four therapies.

$\dfrac{P_i}{P_0}$ = survivors of a single annual cohort expressed as a fraction of the original cohort size, P_0.

$\dfrac{S_i}{P_0}$ = sum of all survivors derived from i cohorts expressed as a multiple of the original cohort size.

$\dfrac{\mathscr{P}_i}{P_0}$ = total patient years of treatment ever given to all the patients in i cohorts through ith year per original cohort size.

The formulae, which are derived in the Appendix, permit a quantitative description presented here with the aid of Fig. 20-2 in which are displayed the graphs of P_i/P_0, S_i/P_0, and $\mathscr{P}_i/P_0$ with years, i, as the independent variable. These curves are plotted by means of equations (1), (2), and (3) in the Appendix. They represent respectively: the size of a treatment subpopulation of patients of initial size, 1, decreasing due to the mortality rates assumed; the size of the

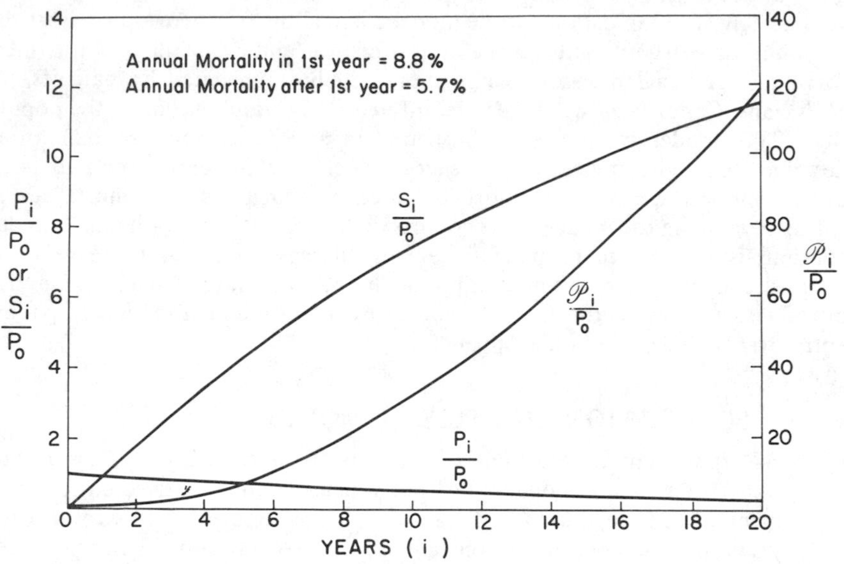

Figure 20-2. Growth curves of a treatment subpopulation.

Left-hand scale is 10× right-hand scale. Division by P_0 results in annual cohort being equal to 1 shown in the curve P_i/P_0 starting at this value and decreasing. Curve S_i/P_0 represents growth of population under treatment as successive cohorts appear. Curve $\mathscr{P}_i/P_0$ represents total patient-years of treatment given as successive cohorts appear. See text for details.

population of patients under a particular treatment increasing due to the cumulation of patients as successive annual cohorts are accepted for treatment; and the total patient-years of a particular treatment ever given to anybody in any cohort by the end of the ith year increasing for similar reason. P_i/P_0 approaches zero, S_i/P_0 continually increases but never exceeds the limit defined by equation (4), and $\mathscr{P}_i/P_0$ continually increases without limit and approaches the rate of annual increase defined by equation (4) (i.e., the limit of equation (2) and limiting slope of (3) are identical).

In Figure 20-2 the curves have been plotted using the data from Table 20-1 in regard to home dialysis. By substitution in the appropriate formulae it may be shown that for this particular treatment the total population approaches but never exceeds 17 P_0 in size. Also the maximum rate of growth per year of patient-years of treatment is 17 P_0; and, for example, 80% of these values are reached in 27 years. Similar data may be calculated for the other three forms of treatment, and by these data we appreciate the growth potential of the treatment sub-populations and the obvious influence that other forces of mortality will have in terminating the life of these subpopulations. What these disease processes are and at what point they will be of significance will only be known after clinical data over the next ten or more years have accumulated. This model and these calculations provide insight into the early implications of current therapy of end-stage renal disease, and the accurate definition of later survival must await further experience. In short, we describe the start of therapy in the absence of data to describe the ultimate effects of subsequent increasing rates of mortality.

JUSTIFICATION OF SELECTED MORTALITY RATES

In Table 20-1, to be considered below in more detail, the annual mortality rates are expressed as a fraction to avoid confusion with other data expressed as percentages in the same table. The first-year mortality rates are those published from a uniquely comprehensive and standardized source collecting patient survival and transplant function survival data for *both* dialysis and transplantation therapy (Gurland et al., 1973). It is based on 18,750 patients treated in Europe where 73% received dialysis and 27% a transplant. Other sources provide comparable data to estimate the mortality rates for the first year of therapy: 0.14 for all patients on dialysis (Krueger, 1974); 0.14 (Gross et al., 1973) and 0.12 (Lowrie et al., 1973) for home dialysis; 0.13 for hospital dialysis (Lewis et al., 1969); 0.12 (Advisory Committee to the Renal Transplant Registry, 1973 and 1975) and 0.13 (Lowrie et al., 1973) for patients receiving a transplant from a living related donor; and 0.29 (Advisory Committee to the Renal Transplant Registry, 1973 and 1975) and 0.31 (Lowrie et al., 1973) for patients receiving a transplant from a cadaveric donor. One authoritative source for dialysis mortality could not be used to establish the rate within the first year as the calculated mortality statistics start with the second year of therapy (Lindner et al., 1974).

In Table 20-1 the estimated mortality rates after the first year of therapy are mean values based on published rates for each of five years for home and hospital dialysis and for four years for the two modes of transplantation (Gurland et al.,

Table 20–1. Estimate of distribution of patients in therapy and results of therapy.

Therapy	*Dialysis 70%*		*Transplantation 30%*	
	Home	*Hospital*	*Living Donor Transplant*	*Cadaveric Donor Transplant*
Percent of All Patients on Therapy (Total = *100%*)	*20%*	*50%*	*10%*	*20%*
Time before definitive therapy				
– 6 months				During 6 months of preliminary dialysis mortality rate = 0.12 and 94% survive for transplantation
–3 months			During 3 months of preliminary dialysis loss of life uncommon	
Start of definitive therapy				
Mortality rate of 1st year	0.088	0.167	0.108	0.27
% Survival on therapy	91%	83%	89%	69% (= 0.73 × 0.94)
% Transplanted patient on dialysis			11%	19%
Mortality rate after 1st year	0.057	0.096	0.049	0.088
5th year % Survival on therapy	68%	50%	69%	48%
% Transplanted patient on dialysis			15%	18%
Number on therapy*	4.2	3.7	4.2	3.3
10th year % Survival on therapy	51%	30%	54%	29%
% Transplanted patient on dialysis			15%	18%
Number on therapy*	7.3	5.8	7.4	5.3

*Expressed as a multiple of annual cohort size selected for a particular therapy

1973). Other sources provide comparable data to estimate mean mortality rates for the second through fourth year of therapy: 0.094 for all patients on dialysis (Krueger, 1974); 0.092 for all dialysis based on 39 patients (10-year follow-up data used in calculation (Lindner et al., 1974); 0.11 for home dialysis based on 736 patients (Gross et al., 1973); 0.09 for hospital dialysis based on 302 patients (Lewis et al., 1969); 0.072 for patients receiving a transplant from a living related donor (Advisory Committee to the Renal Transplant Registry, 1973 and 1975); and 0.13 for patients receiving a transplant from a cadaveric donor (Advisory Committee to the Renal Transplant Registry, 1973 and 1975). From another source calculation of data presented graphically provides estimates of annual mortality rates between the first and fifth year as 0.05 for home dialysis, 0.04 for recipients of a transplant from a living donor, and 0.06 for recipients with a cadaveric kidney transplant (Lowrie et al., 1973). From these available sources it may be noted that trends in mortality rates over time were somewhat variable; and therefore, the mean values from one source (Gurland et al., 1973) seem as satisfactory as any. Future data may permit a degree of precision not possible at present.

The European source (Gurland et al., 1973), because of its size among other features, was favored in choosing data for dialysis mortality. The mortality data from this same source for transplantation are slightly better than those published by the ACS/NIH registry weighted heavily by experience from the United States, where the criteria for acceptance into a transplantation program may be less restrictive than in Europe. The data cited from different sources are not in complete agreement with the mortality data in Table 20-1, but they are sufficiently close to warrant confidence in the broad application of the data in Table 20-1. Other circumstances in different communities may be readily considered by the substitution of more appropriate mortality rates.

In Table 20-1 the mortality rates based on published data for the first four or five years of therapy have been used to estimate survival at the end of the tenth year as well as the increase in number on therapy. However, since the mortality rates will probably rise as other forces for mortality express themselves in this population lacking their own functional kidneys, the estimated percent survival and increase in number on therapy at the end of the tenth year should be regarded as maximal values.

RESULTS

In Table 20-1 italicized percentages at the top refer to the initial partition of *all* patients treated for end-stage kidney disease into treatment groups. The remaining percentages, not in italics, in the table designate a proportion of patients *within* a treatment group that is surviving including survival on dialysis after a transplant has failed. These percentages are calculated on the basis that the original number of patients selected for any one treatment equals 100%.

The partition of the annual cohort of patients into four modes of therapy is somewhat different from European practices as currently reported (Gurland et al., 1973). The distribution in Table 20-1 for the United States represents an estimate based on impressions of physicians active in dialysis and transplantation and on data presented at government hearings (Subcommittee on Oversight, 1975). This partition will vary in different communities where certain modes of therapy are not available and where local interests and skills will favor a particular therapy. The National Dialysis Register reported that 25% of patients on hemodialysis in 1975 were treated in their homes and that the percentage is declining because payment mechanisms and reimbursement processes have made hospital dialysis more attractive (Subcommittee on Oversight, 1975). However, as these artificial constraints are eliminated, home dialysis will tend to increase in relation to hospital dialysis, and transplantation therapy will tend to increase in relationship to all forms of dialysis.

Patients receiving a transplant generally have a preliminary period of hospital dialysis in preparation for transplantation as the decision for a particular mode of therapy and the selection of a suitable donor often require months to complete. Also, prior to transplantation a period of dialysis is generally needed to reverse the morbid changes of the uremic state in preparation for the operation and for intensive immunosuppressive therapy in the postoperative period. Loss of life is uncommon in the typical three-month waiting period for a living donor and is considered insignificant in Table 20-1. However, recipients of cadaveric donor transplants often wait six months or longer because of the difficulties in obtaining a compatible donor when the recipient is sensitized by prior exposure to HL-A antigens through pregnancy or multiple whole blood transfusions. Because of the length of the waiting period and because, in individual cases, recipients of cadaveric organs are frequently selected for this type of transplant in view of an associated disease such as diabetes mellitus or advanced cardiovascular pathology, allowance must be made for death occurring while on preliminary dialysis.

There are no national data on the distribution of waiting times for a cadaveric transplant, and these vary considerably from one community to another depending on the numbers of sensitized patients in the recipient pool, the minimum criteria for HL-A compatibility observed by a transplantation center for an acceptable match, and the availability of cadaveric organs for transplantation. In Table 20-1 a typical waiting time of six months has been assigned during which a dialysis mortality rate between those of home and hospital dialysis has been assumed to be operative. This waiting time is close to that of 5.6 months noted in 1972 for a large sample from the total pool of recipients for cadaveric kidneys in the United States (Opelz and Terasaki, 1974). Mortality during this interval is attributed to the therapy of cadaveric kidney transplantation.

Turning to the lower portion of Table 20-1 the two rows immediately below the line give the mortality rate and survival on therapy of the first year. Beneath the percent survival at the end of the first year for patients having received a transplant, two percentages, 11% and 19%, represent those patients returned to dialysis because of the functional failure of the transplants. These two percentages are a subset of the survivors and are derived from the European experience (Gurland et al., 1973). If the data from the ACS/NIH registry were used, the percentages would be 14% and 20% (Advisory Committee to the Renal Transplant Registry, 1973). In both reports these figures are derived by subtracting from the reported patient survival the transplant function survival to obtain that proportion of patients surviving on dialysis. An unknown number, possibly half, of these patients become candidates for secondary transplants. Slightly more than 80% of all the patients accepted for treatment of end-stage renal disease survive the first year and enter a phase where the mortality rates are significantly lower. As noted above, for a first approximation these rates may be regarded as relatively constant for each mode of therapy, at least through the fifth year of therapy.

The next horizontal block of data in Table 20-1 displays the percentages surviving at five years calculated with the constant mortality rates tabulated, and they are similar to those reported in other sources: 61% for home dialysis at 4.5 years (Gross et al., 1973), 58% for hospital dialysis at 5 years (Lewis et al., 1969), 65% for living donor transplants (Advisory Committee to the Renal Transplant Registry, 1973), and 41% for cadaveric donor transplants (Advisory Committee to the Renal Transplant Registry, 1973). The increase in numbers on therapy at the end of five years is expressed as a factor of the original subpopulation size selected for one of the four treatments and is calculated by equation (2) in the Appendix. Given the constraints of the model certain characteristics of these four treatment subpopulations may be defined. As seen from equation (1) there will be derived from each annual cohort a small, decreasing, annual increment to the total number under treatment, S_i/P_0.

From equation (4) it may be calculated that the size of the subpopulations under treatment will never exceed $16P_0$ for home dialysis, $9P_0$ for hospital dialysis, $19P_0$ for living donor transplant, and $9P_0$ for cadaveric donor transplant. Are these considerable expansions achieved within a few years or are they delayed so that other forces of mortality prevail to limit the subpopulation sizes? The latter is clearly the case as may be appreciated by use of equation (5) to calculate that in these four subpopulations, respectively, 50% of maximum size would be achieved in 12, 7, 14, and 7 years given the constant mortality rates. Thus in the long run other factors will intervene to increase the mortality rates and limit the subpopulation sizes. However, within the five-year period during which data are available on mortality the growth of the treatment subpopulations by a factor of 3.3 to 4.2 is virtually assured if health care resources are available to all who fulfill existing medical indications for therapy.

As noted above, using the European (Gurland et al., 1973) and ACS/NIH (Advisory Committee to the Renal Transplant Registry, 1973) registry data the difference in each report between patient survival and transplant function survival gives the proportion of patients in whom a transplant has failed and who are surviving on dialysis or possibly on a secondary transplant. This difference is relatively constant and is calculated for Table 20-1 from the European data in the second through fifth year as 15% and 18% for the two groups of transplant patients. Comparable calculations based on the ACS/NIH data are slightly lower being 11% and 14% for living donor transplants and cadaveric transplants respectively. It may seem inconsistent that this group of patients on dialysis following failure of a transplant should remain relatively constant in size over time when the functional survival of transplants is decreasing. Presumably the entry into the dialysis group post-transplant is approximately balanced by the mortality of dialysis (a value not known for this specific group of patients) and the incidence of secondary kidney transplantation. These are the only ways a patient may be removed from dialysis after failure of a transplant. Approximately a little more than half of this group of patients surviving a transplant failure will ultimately be selected for a secondary transplantation and are not considered further in this paper. Those that remain on chronic dialysis, in home or hospital, representing 7 to 8% of all the transplanted patients are an additional treatment group for dialysis facilities in addition to those patients originally selected for dialysis.

In the last horizontal block of data in Table 20-1 the tabulated results are calculated on the basis of a five-year extrapolation through the tenth year of therapy. Although we have seen that the use of constant mortality rates throughout the second through fifth year of therapy provides estimates of survival tolerably close to reported experience, extrapolation through the tenth year currently lacks this confirmation. The purpose of the calculation is to predict what will happen by the end of the tenth year *in the absence* of additional, significant mortality factors. In younger patients where additional factors of any weight may not materialize over a ten-year period the predicted survivals and increase in number on therapy may prove to be accurate estimates. Conversely, in older patients it would not be surprising to find observed mortality rates greater than those in Table 20-1 with a consequent decline in survival and with observed numbers on therapy less than those predicted at ten years. Because of the obvious uncertainties as to the value of future mortality rates, extension of these arguments beyond ten years has not been attempted.

DISCUSSION

The implications of Table 20-1 may be considered first in regard to the numbers of patients to be treated for end stage renal disease, second in regard to the cost per surviving patient at the end of the fifth year of treatment, and third in regard to the cost for the United States. These three topics will be discussed in relation to the four modes of therapy considered in this paper.

In Europe the number of new patients per million of population selected in 1972 for treatment of end-stage renal disease has been recorded (Gurland et al., 1973) and representative values are: 43 in Denmark (highest), 33 in Switzerland, 30 in Sweden, 21 in France, 19 in the United Kingdom, and 15 in Europe as a whole. The more affluent countries of western Europe have had in recent years a rapid increase in the numbers of new patients treated until the proportion entering treatment annually is approximately 40 patients per million. Size of the annual cohort of patients fluctuates approaching or exceeding this value in several countries. From this example in a part of the world where the distribution of health care has been accelerated by state or national planning and where the incidence of end-stage renal disease, diagnosis, and standards of treatment are similar to the United States, it appears that this country may need to make provision for the care of about 40 new patients per year per million of population in the implementation of P.L. 92-603.

Thus for the United States with a total population of 212 million in 1974 the numbers of new patients qualifying for therapy is estimated to be over 8,400 each year. The estimate of 10,000 each year has been given (Subcommittee on Oversight, 1975), but we use the lower figure in the following discussion. Following the partition expressed in Table 20-1 in italicized percentages 5,900 new patients would be eligible for dialysis and 2,500 for kidney transplantation. Ignoring the length of time needed to expand existing facilities to provide for their treatment, the entry into the system of five annual cohorts of this size would at the end of the fifth year result in the following numbers of patients cumulated in the four treatment categories: 7,100 on home dialysis, 16,000 on hospital dialysis, 3,500 with a successful or failed kidney transplant from a living donor, and 5,500 with a similar kidney transplant from a cadaveric donor. With constant mortality rates the total number of patients on therapy at the end of the tenth year would be 52,000. In 1975 it was estimated that 20,000 patients were on dialysis in the United States (Subcommittee on Oversight, 1975), and in 1973 it was estimated that 4,900 patients were alive following kidney transplantation (Advisory Committee to the Renal Transplant Registry, 1973). The need for planning and support to enlarge current facilities for the treatment of end-stage renal disease is obvious.

National surveys estimate the cost of a successful transplant to be $15,000 for the first year including the hospitalization for the operation and $1,500 in succeeding years for drug items and doctor visits. The American Hospital Association estimates the cost of home dialysis to be $6,000 per year including rental of the machine and of hospital dialysis to be $30,000 per year (Subcommittee on Oversight, 1975). For home dialysis, additional training and other start up costs amount to $2,000 during the first year.

The above data are summarized in the following tabulation of medical care costs to be used in this analysis:

Annual medical care costs

Treatment of End-Stage Renal Disease		*Year of Therapy*	
		1st year	*After 1st year*
Dialysis	home	$ 8,000	$ 6,000
	hospital	30,000	30,000
Transplantation–	living donor	15,000	1,500
	cadaveric donor	15,000	1,500

By means of equation (2) in the Appendix the total number of patient-years of therapy for a *single* cohort for *i* years of therapy may be calculated. Using the above estimates and allowing for the greater cost during the first year of therapy except for hospital dialysis, the total medical care costs for a *single* annual cohort on a particular treatment through the fifth year may be computed. When these costs are divided by the proportion of the patients surviving through five years as tabulated in Table 20-1 (expressed as a fraction rather than a percentage), the costs per survivor appear as follows:

Total medical care costs through five years per survivor

Treatment of End-Stage Renal Disease		*Cost*	*Cost Discounted 5% Annually*
Dialysis–	home	$ 40,000	$ 31,000
	hospital	220,000	170,000
Transplantation–	living donor	28,000	22,000
	cadaveric donor	34,000	27,000

Because hemodialysis entails considerable ongoing annual expenses in contrast to transplantation, discounting the yearly costs at a 5% rate decreases their present worth in relation to transplantation costs. Dialysis in a hospital appears $50,000 less expensive per survivor at five years by this adjustment. These data are relevant to the question: How much must be spent in support of a method of health care to obtain one survivor after five years of therapy? This is one of several ways to view health care costs, and hospital dialysis appears roughly five to eight times as costly per survivor as other treatments without a corresponding improvement in patient survival. If there were a corresponding improvement of significance; another justification for hospital dialysis would be established in addition to the usual indications for this therapy. However, none now exists; and these data give impetus to the support of less expensive home dialysis as well as transplantation.

From the data presented in Table 20-1 estimating the size of treatment subpopulations at five and ten years together with the costs of treatment in 1975 dollars, it is possible to estimate the cost of treatment during the fifth year and during the tenth year granted an annual cohort of 8,400 patients, the constraints of the model, and estimated mortality rates. The estimated cost during the tenth year is probably a maximum limit in view of the anticipated increase in mortality rates over those in Table 20-1 for the sixth through tenth years. If the mortality rates do not change appreciably, 52,000 patients will be in treatment at the end of the tenth year. These annual costs of treatment are estimated by means of equation (3) in the Appendix as follows:

Estimated cost of treatment with an annual cohort of 8,400 patients

Treatment of End-Stage Renal Disease		*Year of Therapy*		
		1st year	*5th year*	*10th year*
Dialysis–	home	$ 13 million	$ 32 million	$ 65 million
	hospital	115	310	600
Transplantation–	living donor	12	14	18
	cadaveric donor	22	25	30
	Totals	$162 million	$381 million	$713 million

If the annual cohort is over 10,000, then 60,000 patients will be in treatment at the end of the tenth year at a cost during that year of over $800 million. In the Appendix the influence of discounting survival is considered although the assumptions involved currently make this refinement of secondary interest.

These estimates may be compared to the total amount of personal health care expenditures in the United States in 1973 of $80 billion and to the total per capita national expenditure for health services and supplies in 1973 of $430 (United States Department of Commerce, 1975). During this year the gross national product exceeded $1,200 billion. Cost-benefit analysis of the treatment of end-stage kidney disease is necessary but not easy for reasons well expressed in the Gottschalk report of 1967 quoted here:

"The difficulty of putting a value on human life, apart from livelihood, is well known. Of equal difficulty would be the measurement of the benefit due to a reduction in orphanhood, in terms commensurate with the other benefits and cost. Finally, and perhaps most important, is the conclusion reached by the Committee that, in the absence of overwhelming costs (as reflected by an appreciable fraction of the GNP), treatment for end-stage renal disease should be made available to all persons qualified to receive it from a medical standpoint. The reasons for this decision are the irreversibility of the decision not to do so, as far as an individual is concerned; the existence for the first time of a technology capable of prolonging the lives of persons otherwise doomed to an early death; the relative youth of these persons; the prospects of further improvements in technology; and the fact that the patients are known and identifiable, not members of a statistical distribution, enhances the community's interest in doing something in their behalf" (Gottschalk, 1967).

Because of the expected increase in mortality rates five to ten years after initiating therapy, the changes in the age distribution of the population of the United States, the hoped for improvements in dialysis and transplantation therapy, the inevitable modification of indications for therapy, the effects of preventative programs, the possible major redistribution of patients among the four modalities of treatment, the unpredictable circumstances of those patients maintained on dialysis or given a second kidney transplant following failure of the initial one (a group deliberately ignored in this analysis), and because of other less significant factors, the estimates calculated in Table 20-1 particularly in the tenth year, must be viewed with some reservations. They give increased understanding of the dimensions of the whole problem and provide information relevant to future planning. As additional facts become available the basic model and methods of calculation may be appropriately modified.

SUMMARY

Available data on the results of hemodialysis therapy and renal transplantation permit the construction of a model of end-stage renal disease treatment in terms of patient survival. From this model extrapolations through ten years of therapy are tentatively presented together with estimates of the total number of patients on therapy and annual costs of care in the United States. The model indicates that 52,000 to 60,000 patients will be in treatment at the end of the tenth year at an annual cost of $700 to 800 million.

APPENDIX

P_0 = (see page 327)

P_i = (see page 327)

k = annual mortality rate of first year of therapy assumed to be constant throughout first year.

m = annual mortality rate after first year of therapy. Published reports (see above) are not in agreement as to whether m tends to increase or decrease over time, and as a first approximation it is assumed to be constant for purposes of this paper.

a = $1 - k$ = annual survival rate during first year of therapy.

b = $1 - m$ = annual survival rate after first year of therapy.

S_i = (see page 327)

$\mathcal{P}_i$ = (see page 328)

In Table 20-2 an iterative calculation is set forth to derive an expression for P_i for whole year intervals. In the second column the population at risk at the start of each year derived from a single cohort is given with P_0 for the first year. Each year the population derived from a single cohort is decreased by the number of deaths noted in the third column. By subtraction the fourth column gives the population alive at the end of the year. This value is simplified algebraically and carried forward as the population at risk at the start of the next year in the second column.

Table 20–2.

Year	*Population at Risk at at Start of Year*	*Deaths during Year*	*Population Alive at End of Year*
1	P_0	P_0k	$P_1 = P_0 - P_0k = P_0a$
2	$P_0(1-k) = P_0a$	P_0am	$P_2 = P_0a - P_0am = P_0ab$
3	$P_0a(1-m) = P_0ab$	P_0abm	$P_3 = P_0ab^2$
4	P_0ab^2	......	....
	.	.	.
	.	.	.
	.	.	.
i	P_0ab^{i-2}	$P_0ab^{i-2}m$	$P_i = P_0ab^{i-1}$

It is convenient to deal with the fraction of survivors, P_i/P_0; and converting to a continuous function where i may assume any value equal to or greater than 1 we have

$$\frac{P_i}{P_0} = ab^{i-1}, \text{ where } i \geqslant 1. \tag{1}$$

This equation describes our model where P_0 patients enter the system at the start of each year although in reality patients would be uniformly distributed over the year of entry. This apparent departure from reality is of no consequence as may be shown by considering cohorts of patients entering over a time interval of a fraction of a year such as a day or less. The same formulations would result, and the uniform entry situation implies a continuous function. The annual cohort is followed by similar cohorts of P_0 patients, and we now derive an expression to determine the total number of surviving patients, S_i, receiving therapy at any point in time, ith year, taking into account the accumulation of surviving patients under therapy for different lengths of time occasioned by i successive cohorts.

Since the model has a function discontinuous at $i = 1$, because of the change in mortality, the expression for S_i will be the sum of two integrals. The integral over the years where $i \geqslant 1$ comes directly from equation (1), and where $i \leqslant 1$ the integral is *mutatis mutandis* the equivalent as follows:

$$S_i = \int_0^1 P_0 a^x \, dx + \int_1^i P_0 \, ab^{x-1} dx, \text{ where } i \geqslant 1,$$

$$= P_0 \left[\frac{1}{\ln a} a^x \right]_0^1 + P_0 \left[\frac{a}{\ln b} b^{x-1} \right]_1^i,$$

and

$$\frac{S_i}{P_0} = \frac{a-1}{\ln a} + \frac{a}{\ln b} (b^{i-1} - 1). \tag{2}$$

The expression for $\mathscr{P}_i$, the total number of patient-years of therapy received by all patients at any time through the ith year of continuous operation of one of the four therapies, follows from the integration of equation (2) over time:

$${}_i = P_0 \left[\int_0^1 \frac{a-1}{\ln a} dx + \int_1^i \frac{a}{\ln b} (b^{x-1} - 1) \, dx \right]$$

$$= P_0 \left[\frac{a-1}{\ln a} x \right]_0^1 + P_0 \left[\frac{a}{\ln b} \left(\frac{b^{x-1}}{\ln b} - x \right) \right]_1^i$$

$$\frac{S_i}{P_0} = \frac{a-1}{\ln a} + \frac{a}{\ln b}\left(\frac{b^{i-1}-1}{\ln b} - i + 1\right) \tag{3}$$

$$\lim_{i\to\infty} \frac{S_i}{P_0} = \frac{a-1}{\ln a} - \frac{a}{\ln b}, \tag{4}$$

which defines the maximum size that will be attained by the subpopulation of patients under any one of the four treatments provided the mortality rate remains constant after the first year.

$$\frac{S_i}{\left(\lim\limits_{i\to\infty} S_i\right)} = R = \frac{\dfrac{a-1}{\ln a} + \dfrac{a}{\ln b}(b^{i-1} - 1)}{\dfrac{a-1}{\ln a} - \dfrac{a}{\ln b}}$$ from equations (2) and (4), and

$$i = 1 + \frac{\ln\left[(R-1)\left(\dfrac{a-1}{a}\cdot\dfrac{\ln b}{\ln a} - 1\right)\right]}{\ln b}, \tag{5}$$

which defines the number of years, i, that must elapse before the population of treated patients reaches a fraction, R, of its maximum or equilibrium size.

Discounting years of survival on the basis of time preference for early rather than late benefits of survival provides another means of comparing the four treatments. The assumptions involved are difficult to defend from all criticism, and the analysis is presented primarily as a model (Shepard, 1976). In the following tabulation total costs in dollars, unadjusted for survival and discounted at 5% annually, and survival in years discounted at 10% annually, because of the known preference for youth over old age, are displayed with their ratio giving a different evaluation of the cost of survival at the end of five years:

Total medical care costs and survivals through five years per survivor

Treatment of End-Stage Renal Disease		*(A) Cost Discounted 5% Annually*	*(B) Survival Discounted 10% Annually*	*Cost per Survivor through Five Years A/B*
Dialysis–	home	$21,000	0.42 yr	$ 50,000
	hospital	86,000	0.31	280,000
Transplantation–	living donor	15,000	0.43	35,000
	cadaveric donor	13,000	0.30	43,000

From these data hospital dialysis through five years appears eight times as costly as a successful living donor transplant. On the basis of total costs discounted 5%

annually alone the factor unfavorable to hospital dialysis is 6. Considering survivals discounted 10% annually alone the factor is only 1.4 because the differential in costs is of greater weight. As a means of comparison between treatments the ratio of total dollar costs computed at some reasonable discount rate (here 5%) to total years of survival also discounted (arbitrarily here 10%) is an index that may be applied to advantage in other cost-benefit analysis.

Acknowledgement

The author is most grateful for the review of the mathematics provided by Dr. Frederick Mosteller.

References

Advisory Committee to the Renal Transplant Registry: The 11th Report of the Human Renal Transplant Registry. JAMA 226:1197, 1973

Advisory Committee to the Renal Transplant Registry: The 12th Report of the Human Renal Transplant Registry. JAMA 233:787, 1975

Gottschalk CW, Chairman: Report of Committee on Chronic Kidney Disease to the Bureau of the Budget. Government Printing Office, 1967

Gross JB, Keane WF, McDonald AK: Survival and rehabilitation of patients on home dialysis. Ann Intern Med 78:341, 1973

Gurland HJ, Brunner FP, Dehn HV, et al: Combined report on regular dialysis and transplantation in Europe, III, 1972. Proc Eur Dial Transplant Assoc 10:17, 1973

Krueger KK: Report on the National Dialysis Registry. Proc Annual Contractors Conference of the Artificial Kidney Program, 7th Conf: 197, 1974

Lewis EJ, Foster DM, de la Puente J, et al: Survival data for the patients undergoing chronic intermittent hemodialysis. Ann Intern Med 70:311, 1969

Lindner A, Charra B, Sherrard DJ, et al: Accelerated atherosclerosis in prolonged maintenance hemodialysis. N Engl J Med 290:697, 1974

Lowrie EG, Lazarus JM, Mocelin AJ, et al: Survival of patients undergoing chronic hemodialysis and renal transplantation. N Engl J. Med 288:863, 1973

Opelz G, Terasaki PI: National utilization of cadaver kidneys for transplantation. JAMA 228:1260, 1974

Shepard DS: Personal communication, 1976

Subcommittee on Oversight of the Committee on Ways and Means, House of Representatives, June 24 and July 30 and October 22, 1975 Washington, D.C., Government Printing Office

United States Department of Commerce. Statistical Abstract of the United States: 1974 (95th edition) Washington, D.C., Government Printing Office, 1975

United States Department of Health, Education, and Welfare. Office of Policy Development and Planning. Final Policies P.L. 92-603, Section 2991. End-stage renal disease program of Medicare, April 1974

21

Coronary artery bypass surgery: decision and policy analysis

Milton C. Weinstein
Joseph S. Pliskin
William B. Stason

1. INTRODUCTION

Coronary artery bypass graft surgery (CABG) is the primary surgical approach to the treatment of coronary artery disease. Estimates indicate that more than 30,000 such procedures are being performed yearly in the United States (Mundth and Austen, 1975). Despite its widespread use, medical experts hold widely varying opinions in regard to its appropriate applications. The lack of compelling data, as might be derived from controlled studies, is one major reason for this. Several cooperative studies currently in progress in this country and abroad may help resolve some of the questions of proper indications and efficacy.

But even if clinical trials yield valid and conclusive data on mortality and morbidity for surgery and its alternative, medical management, decisions as to which patients should receive surgery would still rest on difficult judgments regarding the relative values attached to length of life and quality of life for the individual patient. Moreover, there would remain the societal issue of whether it is worth spending the resources necessary to achieve whatever incremental health benefits may accrue to the patient treated surgically.

Decision analysis provides a systematic approach to complex medical decision problems that involve multiple decision variables, a variety of possible outcomes

The research for this chapter was supported in part by grants to the Center for the Analysis of Health Practices from the Robert Wood Johnson Foundation, the Commonwealth Fund, and the Edna McConnell Clark Foundation.

and substantial uncertainty (Raiffa, 1968; Forst, 1971; Schwartz et al., 1973). It addresses these complexities explicitly, and enables one to proceed from consideration of component elements of the problem to the development of a composite model for decision making. Though physicians use a similar process informally in their daily decision making they usually do it implicitly, and often inconsistently. Formalization of the decision-making process has considerable potential to improve the quality of care provided, especially in complex situations. Flexibility for revision as new knowledge becomes available, and for expression of individual patient preferences, further enhances the value of the technique.

In this paper, decision analysis is used to consider the decision whether or not to offer coronary artery bypass surgery to each of five hypothetical patients. First, a structural framework is developed that permits the decision maker (e.g., patient, physician, surgeon, or health planner) to incorporate his or her own subjective assessments as well as the best objective data available in reaching this decision. Next, probability assessments obtained from a cardiologist (WBS) are used to derive decision rules for each of the five patients considered individually. Finally, society's problem of resource allocation under scarcity is addressed by relating the expected magnitude of health benefits from surgery in each case to the resource costs required. In addition to providing insights into the issues raised by coronary bypass surgery, this analysis also illustrates the use of decision analysis as a technique for evaluating clinical procedures.

2. DEFINITION OF PATIENT CHARACTERISTICS

In deciding whether to operate, the physician takes into consideration a number of relevant characteristics of the patient. These include (1) personal characteristics, (2) medical characteristics including medical history, symptoms, and clinical signs, (3) information obtained from coronary angiography, and (4) preferences of the patient.

Table 21-1 lists the set of patient characteristics that have been included in the analysis. The choice of variables is based on several sources (McNeer et al., 1974; Cannom et al., 1974), and on the criterion that each variable should significantly influence the choice between surgical and medical management.

Personal characteristics considered are age and sex. Medical characteristics include the levels of angina and heart failure, and the history of myocardial infarction. Angina and congestive heart failure are classified according to the degree of exertion required to precipitate symptoms according to the New York Heart Association (NYHA) classifications (Appendix A). Angina is further classified by its stability. Only documented myocardial infarctions are considered, and the distinction is made between a relatively recent event (six months or less), and a relatively distant event (more than six months).

Coronary angiography yields vital information on the number of arteries occluded and their operability, and on left ventricular function. For purposes of this analysis, occlusion is arbitrarily defined as 70% or more obstruction. This cutoff point is often used in the literature (McNeer et al., 1974). Distinctions

Table 21–1. Patient characteristics.

Personal Characteristics
- Age: 40, 50, 60
- Sex: M, F

Medical Characteristics
- Angina:
  - A_0: No angina
  - A_1: NYHA angina class[a] I or II, stable
  - A_2: NYHA angina class[a] III or IV, stable
  - A_3: Unstable
- Congestive Heart Failure:
  - H_0: Absence of symptoms
  - H_1: Moderate CHF (NYHA functional class[b] I or II)
  - H_2: Severe CHF (NYHA functional class[b] III or IV)
- History of Myocardial Infarction:
  - M_0: No prior MI
  - M_1: MI, at least six months prior
  - M_2: MI, within six months

Data Obtained from Angiography
- Number of arteries occluded (more than 70%) and operability:
  - R_0: None
  - R_1: One
    - R_{11}: Operable
    - R_{10}: Not operable
  - R_2: Two
    - R_{22}: Both operable
    - R_{21}: One operable
    - R_{20}: Neither operable
  - R_3: Three
    - R_{33}: All operable
    - R_{32}: Two operable
    - R_{31}: One operable
    - R_{30}: None operable
- Ejection Fraction:
  - E_0: More than 45%
  - E_1: Between 35 and 45%
  - E_2: Less than 35%

Preference Characteristics
- Preference for activity:
  - Relatively active
  - Relatively sedentary
- Attitude toward risk on survival
- Relative preference for present and future life years

[a]The New York Heart Association angina scale is given in Appendix A.
[b]The New York Heart Association functional classification is given in Appendix A.

among the specific arteries (left anterior descending, left circumflex, right) are not made. Occlusion of the left main coronary artery is not considered because it is generally acknowledged that surgery is the treatment of choice for such patients. Moreover, distinctions as to the nature of the occlusion (diffuse vs. local, for example) are not made, except to the extent that this determines operability. A patient with two-vessel disease may have two, one, or no operable

Table 21–2. Five hypothetical patients and their characteristics.

Patient 1:	1. 50-year-old male
	2. NYHA class I or II stable angina (A_1)
	Moderate congestive heart failure (H_1)
	MI more than six months prior (M_1)
	3. One-vessel disease, operable (R_{11})
	Ejection fraction between 35% and 45% (E_1)
Patient 2:	1. 60-year-old male
	2. NYHA class I or II stable angina (A_1)
	No congestive heart failure (H_0)
	No previous MI (M_0)
	3. Two-vessel disease, both operable (R_{22})
	Ejection fraction greater than 45% (E_0)
Patient 3:	1. 50-year-old male
	2. NYHA class III or IV stable angina (A_2)
	Severe congestive heart failure (H_2)
	MI more than six months prior (M_1)
	3. Three-vessel disease, all operable (R_{33})
	Ejection fraction less than 35% (E_2)
Patient 4:	1. 50-year-old male
	2. No angina (A_0)
	No congestive heart failure (H_0)
	MI more than six months prior (M_1)
	3. Two-vessel disease, both operable (R_{22})
	Ejection fraction greater than 45% (E_0)
Patient 5:	1. 40-year-old male
	2. NYHA class III or IV stable angina (A_2)
	No congestive heart failure (H_0)
	No previous MI (M_0)
	3. One-vessel disease, operable (R_{11})
	Ejection fraction greater than 45% (E_0)

(bypassable) vessels. Ventriculogram results, as a reflection of left ventricular function, are expressed by the ejection fraction for cardiac output, divided into three categories: greater than 45%, between 35 and 45%, and less than 35% (McNeer et al., 1974). A higher ejection fraction indicates better cardiac function, and is associated with a better prognosis.

Based on these characteristics, five hypothetical patients typifying a range of cases were constructed in order to provide a clinical framework for the analysis. They are intended to be illustrative of the spectrum of cases that might present as surgical candidates, but not necessarily to be representative of all such patients. The profiles of these patients, in terms of the characteristics in Table 21-1, are given in Table 21-2. Only male patients are considered, since they represent a substantial majority of those with coronary disease who are considered candidates for surgery (McNeer et al., 1974; Cannom et al., 1974). It is assumed that none of these patients has other diseases (e.g., renal, pulmonary, or neoplastic) or other cardiac abnormalities (e.g., valvular lesions, cardiomyopathy, aneurysm) that might either enhance surgical risk or shorten life expectancy. This is not meant to imply that such patients should be excluded from consideration for surgery, but merely simplifies the analysis. Similarly, the nuances that define an individual case are ignored.

In each case, the analysis was done once assuming that the patient's preferences reflect an active lifestyle, and again assuming that the patient is relatively sedentary. The effect of this variable is to alter the trade-off between length of life and quality of life in a sense to be defined subsequently.

3. BASIC DECISION TREE

In analyses of this kind, it is usually best to begin with a relatively simple decision tree, going back and introducing complexities only as needed to capture essential aspects of the problem. This process led to the decision tree used in the analysis shown in Figure 21-1.

The first decision point (Ⓐ) represents the choice between surgery and medical management. Following that decision, the outcomes unfold, including the immediate results of surgery (Ⓑ), and long-term survival and quality of life (Ⓒ and Ⓓ). A possible extension of the decision tree to permit consideration of the prior decision to catheterize the patient is described in section 9.

3.1 Decision to Operate (Ⓐ in Figure 21-1)

The results of coronary angiography join the set of personal and medical characteristics as data available in making the focal decision of whether or not to operate. It is assumed that at the time of the decision the patient has already been observed for some time, so that delay to observe further changes in these characteristics over time serves no useful purpose.*

In addition, two rather restrictive assumptions are invoked: (1) if medical management is chosen, then future angiography and surgery are ruled out, and the patient will continue on medication indefinitely; and (2) if the surgery route is followed, any subsequent angiography or surgery is ruled out. The first assumption is the more restrictive and may result in underestimation of the expected value of the medical-management strategy. This strategy is clearly dominated by one that does allow future reconsideration of surgery.** However, the assumption that the patient has been observed for a significant length of time does mitigate the limitations imposed by this assumption. Conversely, the second assumption results in underestimation of the value of the surgical strategy, but only to a minor degree since relatively few patients are subjected to a second bypass operation. In effect, the present analysis assumes that the effects of these two assumptions cancel each other and hence can be neglected.

A third assumption is that medical management consists of the best available medication(s) for the individual patient. This assumption permits the focus to remain on the comparison between surgery and medical management without

*This assumption would not apply to emergency patients with unstable angina or myocardial infarction, but no such patients are included in the set of cases considered here.

**An ideal model would include strategies involving an infinite cycle of decision points, thus permitting reconsideration of the therapeutic decision at future points in time. The structure of such a model is discussed in section 9.

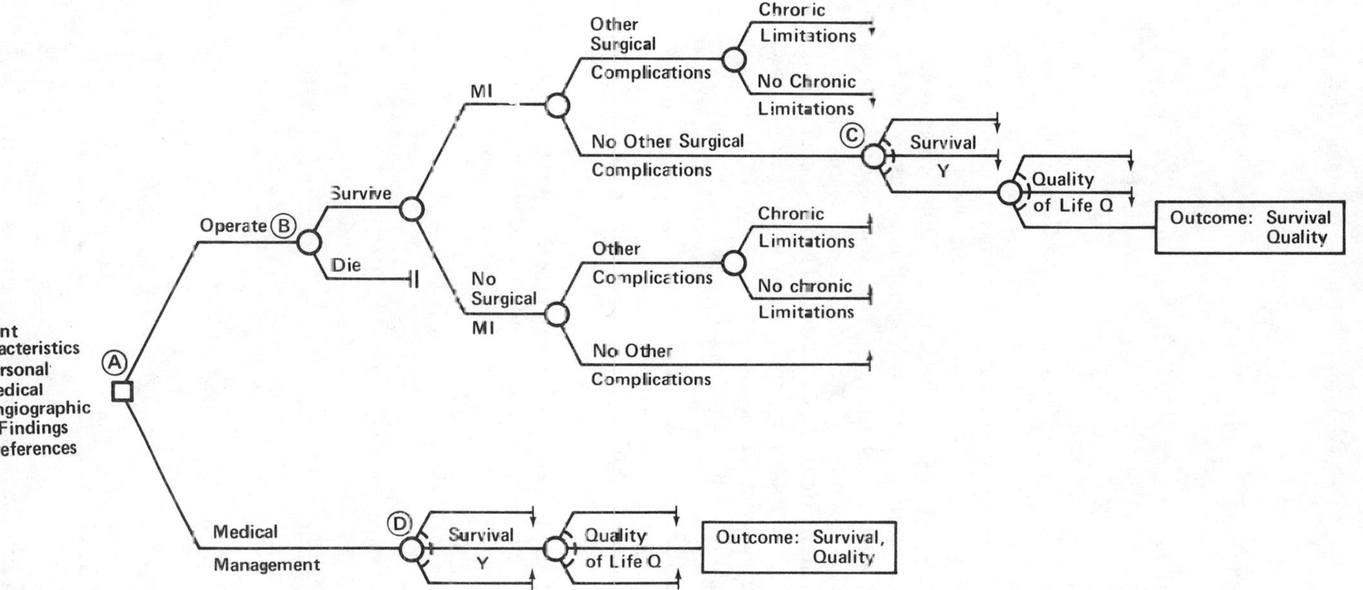

Figure 21-1. Basic decision tree for coronary artery bypass surgery.

This decision-flow diagram, or decision tree, indicates the sequence of possible outcomes following the decision whether or not to operate on a patient with a given set of characteristics. It is assumed that the results of angiography are known.

Key: □ denotes decision point.
○ denotes chance point (i.e., a point at which uncertainty is resolved).
An arrow (↑ or ↓) indicates that the branching structure beyond that point is similar to that found at the prototypical node in the direction of the arrow.
A double bar (||) indicates a terminal branch.
Dotted curved lines at a chance point ( ) indicate a range of possible outcomes, the branches shown being only representative of that range.

considering the subsidiary problem of selecting an optimal medical regimen and ensuring adherence to it.

3.2 Surgical Mortality and Complications (Ⓑ in Figure 21-1)

Following surgery, the patient may or may not survive. Immediate surgical mortality is distinguished from subsequent mortality and is defined as death occurring within 30 days.

Possible surgical complications include: myocardial infarction, pulmonary embolism, stroke, renal failure, infection, postoperative hemorrhage, post-pericardiotomy syndrome, and hepatitis. Myocardial infarction is given special attention due to its relatively high frequency and its particular importance in predicting long-term outcomes of coronary artery disease. Stroke is also given special attention, with two possible nonfatal long-term outcomes considered: complete recovery, and chronic limitations due to residual paralysis or mental defects. Other major complications have been aggregated, and chronic limitations due to them ignored. For example, acute renal failure occurring post-operatively may develop into chronic renal failure, but this is a rare occurrence. Surgical complications, like surgical mortality, are defined as events occurring within 30 days of surgery. The decision tree shows the unfolding of these morbid and mortal complications following Ⓑ in Figure 21-1.

3.3 Long-Term Outcomes Following Surgery and Medical Management (Ⓒ and Ⓓ in Figure 21-1)

The valued outcomes are length of life and quality of life. The latter is affected by the degree of angina and by other symptoms or limitation of activity. Trade-offs may be possible; that is, quality of life may be improved at the expense of some years of life. If so, then it is important to face this trade-off explicitly. The

Table 21-3. Outcome variables included in the analysis.

Years of life following treatment decision (Y)
Angina, year 1 (A_0, A_1 or A_2)[a]
Angina, years 2-5 (A_0, A_1, or A_2)
Angina, years 6-Y (A_0, A_1, or A_2)
Bed disability due to surgical complications[b]
No disability
Disability
Chronic limitation due to stroke[c]
No chronic limitation
Chronic limitation

[a]See Table 21-1.
[b]Due to all complications. Bed disability is assumed to occur in the first year following surgery except for stroke, which may result in chronic lifetime limitation of activity.
[c]Chronic limitation due to other surgical complications are not considered.

utility analysis described in section 5 is designed to incorporate the patient's preferences in making that trade-off.

The particular outcome measures used in the analysis are shown in Table 21-3. Survival is measured in years. Quality of life is measured in terms of the severity of angina and the presence or absence of acute and chronic disability resulting from the complications of surgery. Ideally, both would be measured in continuous time. To simplify the analysis, however, arbitrary time periods following the therapeutic decision are used, namely: the first year, years two through five, and the rest of the life of the patient. Postoperative bed disability is assessed as either absent, if no complications occurred, or present if complications occurred. Chronic limitations due to stroke are noted as present or absent.

Outcomes subsequent to surgery and medical management follow points Ⓒ and Ⓓ, respectively, in Figure 21-1.

4. ASSESSMENT OF PROBABILITIES

Based on the structure of the decision problem (Figure 21-1), probability estimates for each of the five patients were obtained. The detailed list of estimates is given in Appendix B, and relates to three groups of events: immediate sequelae of surgery (including a 30-day survival and complications), long-term outcomes following surgery, and long-term events following medical management. These estimates are intended to represent national averages across all types of institutions that perform coronary artery surgery.

Data in the form required are not often reported in the literature. Perhaps this analysis will prompt clinical studies to compile data of this type and, possibly, will stimulate the development of decision-oriented data banks. In the meantime, estimates represent the best "guesses" of one of the authors (WBS) and are derived from the fragmentary data available in the literature, supplemented by subjective judgments.

The analysis would obviously be strengthened both by the addition of further objective clinical data and by consideration of the opinions of a broad spectrum of cardiologists and cardiac surgeons. It is hoped that this analysis will be replicated in different settings to improve confidence in the results obtained and to increase the extent to which they can be generalized.

Survival curves were assessed by the following method. For each patient, for both surgery and medical management, survival probabilities were assessed at 1 year, 2 years, and 5 years. Survival following year one was assumed to be approximated by the Weibull probability distribution, under which the annual probability of survival may vary with age. Mathematically, the probability of living at least y years is given by

$$\text{Prob}\,(Y \geqslant y) = e^{-uy^a},\ y > 0.$$

When $a = 1$, this is the well-known exponential distribution. Since mortality rates increase with age, a value of $a > 1$ is anticipated. For each patient case and treatment option, the parameters u and a were estimated from the assessments of 2-year and 5-year survival.* A check on the reasonableness of the resulting survival curves was obtained by computing the implied life expectancy.

Estimates of other probabilities were obtained as point assessments.

5. OUTCOME EVALUATION AND UTILITY ANALYSIS

To arrive at decisions based on the probability distributions for the several outcomes, the decision maker must apply his own preferences to value alternative combinations of these attributes. In the present context, the preferences may be those of the patient, the physician, or some combination of the two. In principle, the values attached to the outcomes might have been left unspecified, permitting each individual decision maker to use his own preferences to weigh them against each other. To demonstrate how variations in preferences might affect the optimal decision regarding coronary bypass surgery, a range of preferences was analyzed, corresponding to those of a relatively active patient, who attaches a high cost to limitation of activity, and those of a relatively sedentary patient, who is less affected by limitation of activity.

The outcomes of interest include:

1. length of life,
2. level of angina,
3. bed disability following surgery, if applicable, and
4. chronic limitation of activity due to postoperative stroke, if applicable.

A fifth attribute—cost—was incorporated by methods described in section 10.

To combine these several attributes into a single quantitative measure reflecting preferences, the method of multiattributed utility functions was employed (Raiffa, 1969).** The nature of this approach is illustrated by a simple hypothetical example. Suppose that for a given type of patient, surgery offers a 90% chance of survival, with a life expectancy of 20 years if the patient survives. The life expectancy for this patient would thus be $.9 \times 20 = 18$ years. Suppose surgery also promises a lifetime of no angina. Medical management for this patient yields a life expectancy of 20 years (two years more than surgery) but promises a lifetime of Class II angina. Whether surgery or medical management is optimal depends on subjective preferences. First of all, life expectancy may not adequately reflect the patient's or the physician's, preferences for survival, since the 10% chance of immediate death in surgery may reduce the patient's certainty equivalent*** by more than the implied two years. More important, the

*A more sophisticated approach would elicit several survival assessments (e.g., 1-year, 2-year, 5-year, 10-year), and perform a least squares fit to the data in the equation

$$\ell n(-\ell n\, P_y) = \ell n\, \mathrm{u} + a \cdot \ell n(y) + \text{error},$$

where P_y is the rate of y-year survival. This was not done, however, in the present study.

**See Chapter 1 (Pliskin and Taylor) for background on utility theory and its application to medical decisions under uncertainty.

***In this context, the certainty equivalent is that length of life that the decision maker would accept for certain in exchange for the gamble on survival. See Chapter 1 (Pliskin and Taylor) for further discussion of this concept.

trade-off between length of life and quality of life must be evaluated. A question that might be asked of the patient or physician is: "What fraction of your remaining expected years would you give up in order to eliminate the angina?" If the answer were less than 10%, medical management would be preferred; otherwise, surgery would be the better choice.

Utility functions were constructed to quantify the outcomes and assign them numerical values. Parameters of the function (i.e., its weights) may describe such characteristics of preferences as degree of risk aversion with respect to length of life, valuation of present relative to future life years, and willingness to trade length of life for quality of life.

The arguments of the utility function are the remaining life years Y, and a vector describing the quality of life in each year $\mathbf{Q}$. The quality of life measure was obtained by combining the three quality-related attributes (angina, bed disability, chronic limitation) into a single attribute, as follows. In the absence of bed disability and chronic limitation, levels A_0 (no angina) and A_2 were arbitrarily assigned utility values of 1 and 0, respectively. The intermediate level A_1 was assigned a utility value between 0 and 1 reflecting preferences regarding activity (see Appendix C). The utility value was modified by chronic limitation due to stroke, which was assumed to lower the utility for quality $\mathbf{Q}$ by some percentage P_1, and by the disability associated with surgical convalescence which was assumed to lower the utility for quality in the first year by some percentage P_2 ($P_2 < P_1$) if complications occur, and by a lesser percentage P_3 ($P_3 < P_2$) if complications do not occur. Outcomes are thus described in terms of:

Length of life (Y),
Quality level in the first year (Q_1),
Quality level in the next four years (Q_{2-5}), and
Quality level in the remaining years (Q_{6+}).

The quality measures were then combined into a single quality index $\bar{Q}$, by averaging the utilities in each period and weighting them by the lengths of the periods.

The form of the final utility function $u(Y,\bar{Q})$ was based on several additional assumptions. First, the assumption of mutual utility independence between length of life and quality was invoked (see Appendix C). This says that choices between survival curves, given equal quality of life, do not depend upon the underlying quality,* and that choices between lotteries on quality, given equal survival, do not depend on the length of life. Next, it was assumed that life expectancy completely describes the patient's (or physician's) preferences for survival. Finally, it was assumed that a patient destined to live Y years with class III or IV angina (A_2) will be willing to sacrifice a proportion P of that life so that he may live (1-P) times Y years with no angina at all (A_0). Thus, the parameter P incorporates preferences for activity levels and reflects the basic trade-off between survival and quality of life.

*This assumption is behaviorally plausible in the present context; it would be less so if the quality of life could become "worse than death." New methods of utility analysis are being developed to allow for that possibility (Fishburn and Keeney, 1975).

Together, these assumptions imply (Pliskin et al., 1976) a utility function of the form

$$u(Y,\bar{Q}) = (1-P)Y + PY\bar{Q}.$$

This is the form used in the analysis. For a relatively active patient, the weight P was arbitrarily given the value of 0.3; for a relatively sedentary patient, the weight P was given the lower value of 0.2 reflecting more emphasis on life years relative to angina level.

It is usually the case that one cannot attach any meaning to expected utility values per se, but only use them as preference indices to rank order the various alternatives. However, the utility function used in this analysis has been so constructed that expected utility values represent quality-adjusted life expectancy. This is so because the utility measure is simply life years, deflated by a factor reflecting the quality level and the extent to which quality is valued. If quality is optimal ($\bar{Q} = 1$), or if quality is not valued at all ($P = 0$), then the utility function simplifies to life years alone.

6. DETERMINATION OF OPTIMAL THERAPY

The decision analysis was performed for the five hypothetical patients whose characteristics are described in Table 21-2. For each patient it was done twice, once assuming the patient's preferences reflect an active lifestyle and again assuming the patient is relatively sedentary.

Optimal treatment was determined by using the subjective probability assessments (Appendix B) for each chance point in the decision tree (Fig. 21-1) and by maximizing expected utility.

7. RESULTS OF THE DECISION ANALYSIS

Expected utility, or quality-adjusted life expectancy, is presented in Table 21-4 for each of the five patients by treatment modality and preference pattern (sedentary or active). For example, a relatively sedentary patient 1 can expect an average of 12.7 quality-adjusted life years if he undergoes bypass surgery, and 13.5 years if he is managed medically. An active Patient 1 can expect 12.3 years with surgery and 12.5 years with medical management, somewhat less than his sedentary counterpart. For all patients, the adjusted life expectancy is higher for the sedentary preference pattern because diminutions of quality are treated as relatively less costly compared to survival.

The results of the decision analysis are compared in Table 21-4 to the prior judgments about optimal therapy expressed by one of the authors (WBS). These comparisons provide insight into factors affecting current decision-making in the treatment of coronary artery disease. The results for each patient are evaluated as follows:

Patient 1: The prior probability that surgery would be optimal for this patient had been assessed at 0.5 if he had an active lifestyle, but only 0.3 if he had a sedentary lifestyle. The estimated quality-adjusted life expectancies following

Table 21-4. Results for five hypothetical patients[a].

Patient	Treatment	Expected Utility[b] Active[c] Patient	Difference	Expected Utility[b] Sedentary[d] Patient	Difference	Prior Probability of Optimality[e]	
						Active	Sedentary
1	Surgery	12.3	−0.2	12.7	−0.8	.5	.3
	Medical	12.5		13.5		.5	.7
2	Surgery	12.6	0.4	12.9	−0.1	.7	.3
	Medical	12.2		13.0		.3	.7
3	Surgery	1.2	0.4	1.2	0.3	.05	.05
	Medical	0.8		0.9		.95	.95
4	Surgery	13.4	0.3	13.7	0.3	.10	.10
	Medical	13.1		13.4		.90	.90
5	Surgery	15.2	8.5	15.6	8.1	.80	.80
	Medical	6.7		7.5		.20	.20

[a]See Table 21–2 for description of characteristics.
[b]Quality-adjusted life expectancy. See section 5 for method of derivation.
[c]Assumes a willingness to trade 30% of life expectancy for relief from NYHA class III or IV angina.
[d]Assumes a willingness to trade 20% of life expectancy for relief from NYHA class III or IV angina.
[e]Subjective judgment, prior to the study, that the corresponding therapy would be optimal.

surgery and medical management are almost identical for an active patient, but favor medical management for a sedentary patient. In this case, the results of the analysis are in complete agreement with prior judgment.

Patient 2: Prior judgment indicated a 0.7 chance of operating on an active patient and a 0.3 chance of operating on a sedentary one of this type. The results of the analysis support the direction of the prior judgment but the utility values are too close to confirm any significant difference.

Patient 3: In this case a striking difference between the results of the analysis and prior judgment is evident, the former favoring surgery and the latter strongly favoring medical management. One explanation for this discrepancy is that because Patient 3 is such a poor risk and has so little to gain from either treatment modality (a life expectancy of 1.2 years at best), the strong tendency is to avoid the radical approach, surgery, with its high immediate mortality, pain, and suffering. Moreover, coronary artery bypass surgery is expensive, and given the small net benefit of surgery, its relative cost-effectiveness for such patients is poor (see section 10). This particular example suggests that resource costs may enter clinical decisions, though perhaps not as often as desirable from a social point of view.

Patient 4: For either an active or sedentary patient of this type, the results indicate near equal benefits from surgery and medical management. Prior judgment, however, strongly favored medical management regardless of the patient's preferences for activity. Explanation of this discrepancy may lie in the fact that this patient has no angina, so that the incentive provided by the well-demonstrated ability of surgery to achieve pain relief is absent. In addition, cost-effectiveness considerations may be involved. If the two alternatives offer equal benefits, then costs would be considered and would dictate against the more expensive approach.

Patient 5: The results showing that surgery offers more than double the adjusted life expectancy attainable with medical management are in complete concurrence with the prior judgment that surgery would be the optimal treatment for this patient.

Sensitivity analyses were performed to determine the extent to which changes in the probability assessments entering the analysis would affect the results. The parameter having the single most important effect was the estimate for surgical mortality, while the probabilities of postsurgical myocardial infarction and chronic limitation due to surgical complications had almost no effect. As expected, the direction of the results was sensitive to the probability assessments for those patients whose decision between surgery and medical management was close, and not at all sensitive for patients for whom the decision was clear-cut. For the former, however, a switch in the optimal strategy is predicated on only small changes in utility.

The decisions most sensitive to the probability assessments were those for Patients 1 (active) and 2 (sedentary). If the surgical mortality rates for these patients are less than 3.4% and 4.0%, respectively, then surgery becomes preferred. However, the results for the sedentary counterpart of Patient 1 continue to favor medical management even if surgical mortality were zero, and the rate of surgical death would have to exceed 8% before medical management would be indicated for an active Patient 2.

The results for Patients 3 and 4 were insensitive to changes in surgical mortality. In order to change the optimal decision to medical management, surgical mortality would have to be over 6% for Patient 4 and well over 60% for Patient 3.

Due to the overwhelming margin between surgery and medical management for Patient 5, the results were not sensitive to realistic changes in any of the probabilities.

8. ISSUES RAISED BY THE DECISION ANALYSIS FOR CORONARY ARTERY BYPASS SURGERY

There has been much criticism of the extensive use of CABG surgery in the absence of data from controlled trials that CABG surgery prolongs life or relieves pain. However, the lack of data, particularly those relating to the more distant future, does not imply complete ignorance, nor does it mitigate the need to make therapeutic decisions. Subjective assessments based on the best information available formed an integral part of this analysis as they do, in fact, in most medical decisions.

Medical management was believed *a priori* to be the preferred treatment for Patients 3 and 4 but the analysis suggested that surgery is more beneficial. In a related study (Pliskin et al., 1975), such discrepancies were even more striking, again indicating surgery for patients initially believed to be better off when managed medically. Based on the judgments of cardiologists participating in both of these studies, it may be that not enough surgery is being performed, rather than the widely believed converse!

There are many possible explanations for the discrepancies between the prior judgments of physicians and the decision rules implied by the analysis. One important factor is that the physician, when faced with suggestive but inconclusive evidence supporting surgery, tends to emphasize, and perhaps overemphasize, the use of therapeutic modalities with which he is familiar and comfortable. Hence, he persists in medical management until the weight of evidence favoring surgery becomes sufficiently strong to cause him to change. He discounts the importance of outcomes associated with "soft" probabilistic judgments.

A second factor may be physician conservatism with regard to immediate surgical death. The fear of losing a patient on the operating table may override the prospect of preventing future death or pain, possibly because a surgical death can be attributed directly to the current decision. Stated another way, there may be a strong sense of responsibility for an immediate death which is absent when death occurs sometime in the future. While physicians may accept quality-adjusted longevity as a valid criterion for decision making, actual physician behavior may also reflect these other concerns.

A third possible explanation for the discrepancy between actual practice and the decision rules implied by this analysis is that fear of malpractice suits, which are much easier to prosecute in the case of immediate death, may lead to the practice of "defensive medicine" which results in aversion to the more radical modality, surgery.

Finally, consideration of cost may enter into the decision-making process, as discussed in the preceding section in connection with Patients 3 and 4.

An important aspect of the analysis is its quantitative approach to evaluating quality of life and some of the trade-offs between life years and quality of life. How much longevity a patient is willing to forego for an improvement in quality of life is a highly personal matter, but should not be ignored. Because longer life and improved quality are sometimes conflicting objectives, any decision to operate or not will implicitly assume some trade-off between the two. This analysis has attempted to make this trade-off explicit, and it was assumed that the relative preferences of active patients are different from those of sedentary ones. In one patient (number 2), this difference affected the decision. Because medical practice tends to place the major burden of decision making in the physician's hands, the physician may welcome techniques to take patient preferences into account. Decision analysis is one method of helping to focus on this consideration in making responsible judgments.

9. EXTENSIONS OF THE ANALYSIS

Several extensions of the analysis are possible to permit systematic consideration of other aspects of the coronary artery bypass decision problem. Among these are: (1) the prior decision whether to perform coronary angiography on a patient with a given history, symptoms and signs, (2) the modified decision problem in which the possibility of postponing the decision to operate pending further developments is recognized, and (3) the societal problem of resource allocation in which the cost of surgery formally enters into the analysis. The first two are discussed briefly here, to indicate how such analyses or reanalyses might be structured. The third—society's resource allocation problem—is developed in section 10.

9.1 The Decision to Perform Coronary Angiography on a Patient

Figure 21-2 shows an extension of the decision tree of Figure 21-1 in which the initial decision to perform angiography is considered explicitly. In this case, the patient presents with personal and medical characteristics, but without angiographic data. The initial decision (Ⓐ′ in Figure 21-2) is whether to perform angiography.

If angiography is elected, then its results become known. As in Figure 21-1, these results include the number of obstructed and operable coronary arteries, and the ejection fraction as a measure of left ventricular function. Note also that death is a possible outcome of angiography. Following angiography, the decision tree is identical to Figure 21-1.

If angiography is not elected (Ⓔ), the tree resembles that following the postangiography decision not to operate (Ⓓ), except that the probabilities are those for patients with unspecified arteriographic or ventriculographic data.*

9.2 Sequential Analysis

In the main analysis, it was assumed that a decision not to operate is irrevocable. In reality, it is desirable and routine to permit the option to reconsider this decision pending changes in the patient's condition.

To conceptualize this, a dynamic adaptive model might be used as shown in Figure 21-3. The branch following angiography remains the same (it is still assumed that once the angiogram is in hand the decision will not be reconsidered), but the medical-management branch would allow reconsideration. For simplicity it is assumed in the figure that reconsideration is permitted at one-year intervals. Thus, if the patient survives the year, the patient's characteristics including age, current angina level, current MI status, and current heart-function status are reassessed. The decision at this point reverts back to the initial decision point with the new characteristics. The survival and quality of life during the year are noted and enter into the final outcome evaluation for the patient.

10. SOCIETY'S PROBLEM: COST VERSUS BENEFIT

Decision analysis may indicate that for some classes of individuals coronary bypass surgery is preferable to medical management (i.e., yields a higher quality-

*Mathematically, the probabilities are marginal probabilities with respect to the angiographic and ventriculographic variables, but conditional with respect to the personal and medical variables.

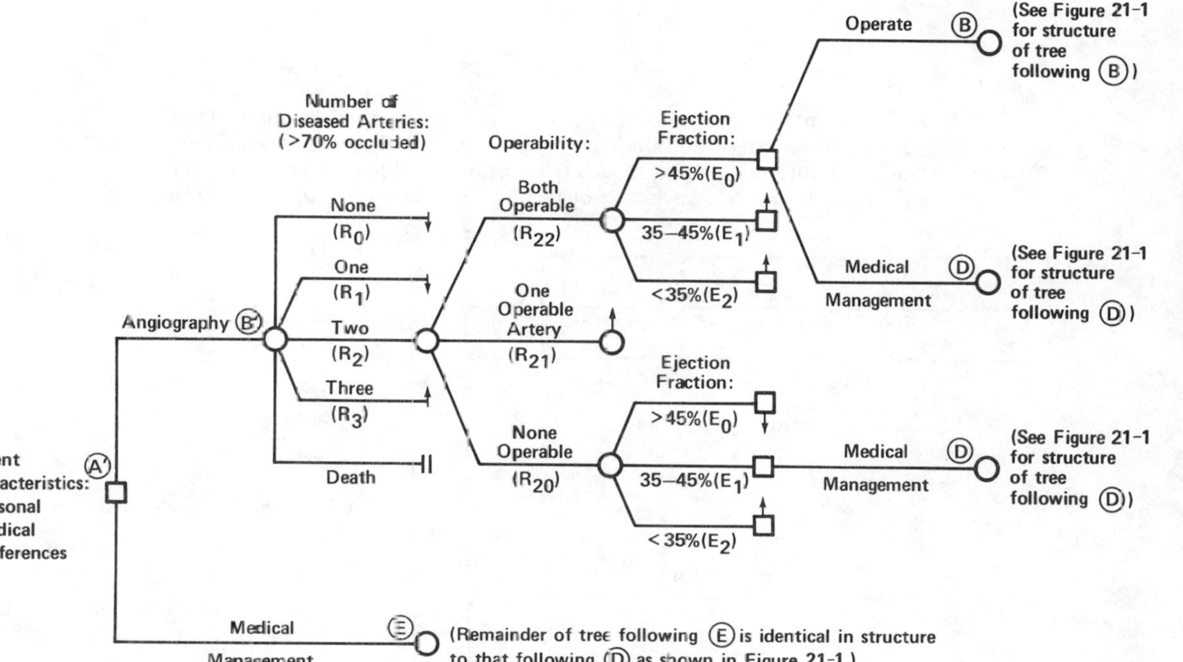

Figure 21-2. Extended decision tree for angiography and possible coronary artery bypass surgery.

This decision-flow diagram indicates the sequence of events beginning with the decision whether or not to give angiography to a patient with a given set of characteristics. Following the results of angiography, the decision is made whether to operate.

Key: See Figure 12-1.

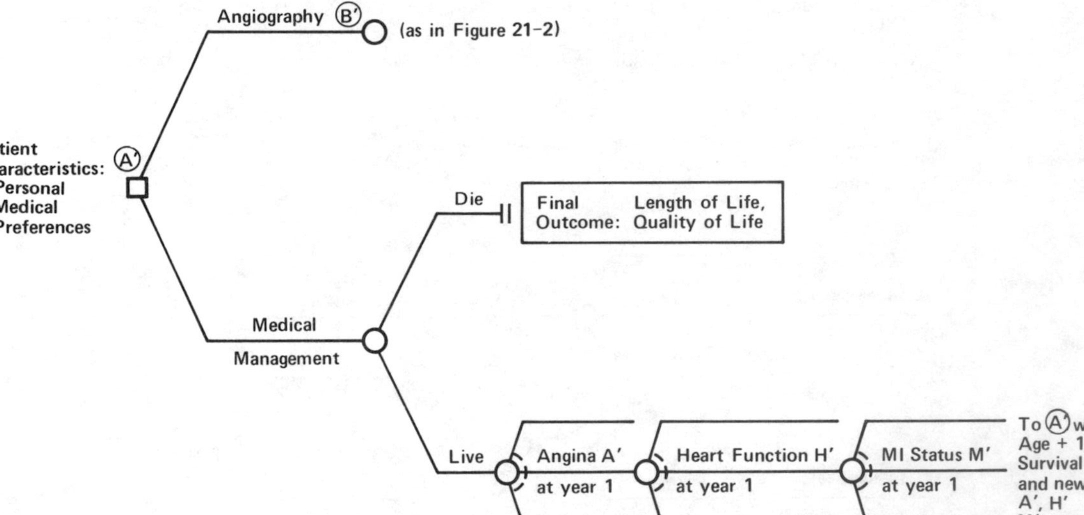

Figure 21-3. Adaptive sequential decision model.

This decision-flow diagram reflects the possibility for periodic reconsideration of the decision whether or not to give angiography. After each year of medical management the patient is reevaluated in light of his new condition.

Key: See Figure 21-1.

adjusted life expectancy). The difference may be substantial for some classes; for others it may be small. Since each operation performed involves the expenditure of resources not required by medical management, we in society should consider whether, individually or collectively, we are willing to forgo alternative uses of the resources expended in order to obtain the expected benefits of coronary artery bypass surgery. From the point of view of society, is the expenditure of limited health care resources on coronary bypass surgery an efficient way to prolong life and improve its quality?

If each individual had to pay for his or her own operation, the forgone consumption would be the patient's own, and, if the patient were well informed as to the probabilities of outcome (or well advised by a physician), then the cost-benefit problem would be an individual one. The patient's own preferences for improved health as opposed to alternative forms of consumption would automatically be taken into account, just as individual preferences are taken into account through the marketplace for food, clothing, shelter, and other commodities.

For many reasons, such markets no longer exist. Since demand for medical care depends on the onset of disease and is therefore subject to great uncertainty, individuals find it in their interest to pool their risks through insurance. If insurance is unrestricted, however, individuals pay nothing when the opportunity to receive medical care arises. The result is excessive medical care relative to patient's preferences, and high premiums. Deductibles and coinsurance reduce these incentives, but they also diminish the advantages of risk sharing.

Since responsibility for efficient allocation of health resources cannot be left to the marketplace, cost-effectiveness determinations are required to guide resource allocation (Weinstein and Stason, 1976). Two basic principles apply:

(1) Under conditions of limited resources for health care, priorities for alternative uses of these resources should be based on the amount of health benefits produced per dollar spent. This principle applies both to allocation within a categorical health problem such as coronary heart disease and to trade-offs among expenditures on different areas of health care.

(2) For decisions in which the amount of health resources may be increased at the expense of nonhealth programs or private consumption (i.e., from taxes or premiums), any decision implies some dollar valuation of additional health benefits. For example, a decision to increase the national health expenditure on coronary bypass surgery would reflect the value judgment that it is worth more to spend a certain amount of money to reduce anginal pain or save one year of life than to produce other goods or services that people value (e.g., police protection, education, or private consumption).

The denominator of the cost-effectiveness ratio used in the present analysis is the difference between the values of the utility function for surgery and medical management. This difference is, in effect, the incremental expected number of quality-adjusted life years purchased. The numerator of the ratio is the incremental cost of surgery, which is assumed to be $10,000 or $15,000, a range suggested by a preliminary study of cases at a local hospital. At higher rates of surgery, scarcities of such resources as operating facilities, blood for transfusion, or adequately trained surgical teams may increase this cost or limit the avail-

Table 21-5. Cost per year of increased quality-adjusted life expectancy for five hypothetical patients[a]

Patient Number	Cost = $10,000		Cost = $15,000	
	Active	*Sedentary*	*Active*	*Sedentary*
1	Undefined[b]	Undefined[b]	Undefined[b]	Undefined[b]
2	$25,000	Undefined[b]	$37,500	Undefined[b]
3	27,000	$35,700	40,500	$53,600
4	31,300	35,700	46,900	53,600
5	1,170	1,230	1,760	1,840

[a]See Table 21-2.
[b]Negative net benefit from surgery.

ability of surgery. Alternatively, higher rates might lower costs by increasing the efficiency of surgical teams and ensuring fuller utilization of existing facilities. For the purposes of this analysis, however, it is assumed that neither scarcity nor economies of scale will cause the average cost to deviate from the range chosen. It is further assumed that the lifetime costs of long-term follow-up and medication following surgery are comparable to those for medical management, so that these cancel out of the net cost calculation.

10.1 Cost-Effectiveness Results

The differences between the expected utilities for surgery and medical management (Table 21-4) represent the incremental number of expected quality-adjusted life years afforded by surgery as compared to medical management. Except for Patient 1, for whom surgery appears to be inferior to medical management, and Patient 5, for whom surgery appears to be substantially superior, the estimated marginal benefits of surgery are all less than one quality-adjusted year. This indicates that for Patients 2, 3, and 4, the decision between surgery and medical management is a very close one.

Table 21-5 presents the cost-benefit results, based on the benefits from Table 21-4 and assuming an incremental cost of surgery of either $10,000 or $15,000. For those patients for whom the analysis indicates surgery should be performed, the cost per year of quality-adjusted life saved ranges mainly from $25,000 to $36,000 if the cost of surgery is $10,000 and from $38,000 to $54,000 if the cost is $15,000. For Patient 5, however, the cost per year of life saved is between $1,200 and $1,800.

Tables 21-6 and 21-7 interpret the cost and benefit data in somewhat different terms. Table 21-6 presents the data from the viewpoint of the individual citizen.* The premium each American adult male would have to pay each year

*The incidence rates of 0.2% and 0.3% in Tables 21-6 and 21-7 were derived as follows. The prevalence of angina pectoris in adult males is estimated at 3.8% (NCHS, 1965). Assuming an average duration of angina of 10 years, this suggests an incidence of 3.8 per 1,000. If half of these cases are operated upon, the incidence of CABG surgery in Coronary Heart Disease would be about 2 per 1,000. If 90% were operated upon (Wechsler and Sabiston,

Table 21-6. Average increase in quality-adjusted life expectancy and annual "premium" for coronary bypass surgery for adult males in the United States.

	Annual Health Insurance Premium		
Annual Incidence of Operable CHD	*Cost = $10,000*		*Cost = $15,000*
0.2%	$20/year		$30/year
0.3%	$30/year		$45/year
	Average Annual Benefit Per Capita[a] (quality-adjusted life days)		
Annual Incidence of Operable CHD	*Utility Benefit[b] = 0.5 years*	*Utility Benefit[b] = 1.0 years*	*Utility Benefit[b] = 5.0 years[c]*
0.2%	0.37 life days/year	0.73 life days/year	3.7 life days/year
0.3%	0.55 life days/year	1.10 life days/year	5.5 life days/year

[a]Expected quality-adjusted days of life saved for each year an average male has access to coronary bypass surgery.
[b]Expected benefit per operation.
[c]Upper-bound value.

would range from $20 to $45 depending on the incidence of operable cases and the cost of surgery. Table 21-6 also shows, from the individual point of view, what that premium would purchase, in quality-adjusted life expectancy terms, assuming that the average benefit of surgery over all patient types is either 0.5 years (as suggested by Table 21-4 for Patients 2, 3, and 4) or 1.0 years (a liberal estimate giving more weight to Patient 5), or 5.0 years (an upper bound estimate giving substantial weight to Patient 5 and other strong candidates for surgery not represented by the cases selected). Thus, for example, if surgery costs $15,000, the benefit is 1.0 years, and the incidence of operable CHD is 0.2%, then a premium of $30 would purchase, on average, three-quarters of one quality-adjusted life day per year.

Table 21-7 presents the same data in aggregate national terms for the adult male population. Thus, while CABG may cost from $1.3 to $3.0 billion per year, it may save from 65,000 to 200,000 years of quality-adjusted life each year.

10.2 Discussion

The data in Table 21-5, giving the estimated cost of saving a year of quality-adjusted life, suggest that for most patients with coronary disease, coronary artery bypass surgery is *not* a particularly efficient use of scarce health resources. A notable exception is Patient 5, who represents the classical candidate for surgery: a young man with a strong heart and severe angina.

1974), the incidence would be about 3.5 per 1,000. The incidence rates were independently derived by noting that 700,000 new cases of CHD occur each year, by assuming that 450,000 are males, and that half (or 225,000) manifest themselves as angina rather than as myocardial infarction or sudden death (NCHS, 1965). Of the population of 65 million adult males, this represents an incidence of 3.5 per 1,000, which approximates the 3.8 per 1,000 derived above.

Table 21-7. Total national health benefit and cost for coronary bypass surgery for adult males in the United States.

	Total National Cost	
Annual Incidence of Operable CHD	*Cost = $10,000*	*Cost = $15,000*
0.2%	$1.3 billion/year	$2.0 billion/year
0.3%	$2.0 billion/year	$3.0 billion/year

	Total National Benefit[a] *(quality-adjusted life years)*		
Annual Incidence of Operable CHD	*Utility Benefit*[b] *= 0.5 years*	*Utility Benefit*[b] *= 1.0 years*	*Utility Benefit*[b] *= 5.0 years*[c]
0.2%	67,000 life years/year	133,000 life years/year	670,000 life years/year
0.3%	100,000 life years/year	200,000 life years/year	1,000,000 life years/year

[a]Expected quality-adjusted years of life saved obtained by providing coronary bypass surgery to all males with incident operable coronary disease.
[b]Expected benefit per operation.
[c]Upper-bound value.

A number of criteria for evaluating the economic value of a year of life saved has been proposed (Weisbrod, 1961; Schelling, 1968; Acton, 1973). Among these are variants of (1) the earnings, or human capital, approach in which the annual productive capacity of an individual is taken as proxy for the value of a year of his or her life; and (2) the willingness-to-pay approach, in which the value of a year of one's life is taken to be the amount the individual would pay to save it. According to either criterion, the range of values derived by this analysis is above the acceptable range for all but Patient 5. Average annual earnings are well under $20,000, and Acton's survey of willingness to pay found similar values (Acton, 1973). Furthermore, these figures compare unfavorably to estimates of the cost-effectiveness of other competing health programs such as high blood pressure control (Weinstein and Stason, 1976). If future benefits are discounted, as they should be for economic reasons (Weinstein and Stason, 1976), then the cost-effectiveness ratio is increased still further.

Therefore, it may be concluded that for virtually all categories of patients, resources may be used more productively if applied elsewhere. Thus, considerations of cost-benefit can reverse the optimal decision made from a purely medical viewpoint.

It is useful to view both benefit and cost from the individual point of view, since it is individuals, through insurance premiums or taxes, who ultimately purchase the health benefits. As Table 21-6 suggests, $20 to $45 a year would purchase for each adult male the availability of a procedure that would extend each year of life by an expected number of 0.37 to 5.5 days or improve the expected quality of life by an equivalently valued amount. On a national level (Table 21-7), from $1.5 to $3.0 billion per year would purchase from 67,000 to

1,000,000 years of life per year for males. In themselves, these figures can be misleading, since we may be intimidated by their sheer magnitudes, but when interpreted in terms of cost-effectiveness they do suggest that unless something approaching our upper-bound estimate of benefit holds, CABG may be cost-ineffective even though it may be the superior treatment for most patients.

11. CONCLUSIONS

The strength of any conclusions drawn from this analysis is limited by the validity of, and generalizations that can be derived from, the subjective data used. Nevertheless, the results do reveal some surprises and provide some insights.

From the point of view of the clinical decision for the individual patient, the analysis led to conclusions counter to prior clinical judgment in the direction of favoring surgical intervention. It was found that surgery was the optimal course of action for almost all patient types considered. To be sure, bias creeps into both the subjective assessments entering the analysis and the prior clinical judgment, but because the decision-analytic method decomposes the problem into its component parts and forces one to be explicit in each subjective judgment, it may well result in a more objective decision.

From the point of view of society's resource allocation, however, coronary bypass surgery appears less attractive. Indeed, the cost per year of life saved (adjusting for changes in quality of life) clearly exceeds levels generally available elsewhere in the health sector (Weinstein and Stason, 1976), and those based on considerations of earnings or willingness to pay. Thus, coronary bypass surgery may be a perfect example of what has been referred to as the dilemma of the medical "commons" (Hiatt, 1975). What is optimal medical care for the individual patient may not be optimal when we, as society collectively, consider what it is costing us.

APPENDIX A. NEW YORK HEART ASSOCIATION CLASSIFICATIONS FOR ANGINA PECTORIS AND CONGESTIVE HEART FAILURE[a]

Angina Pectoris

Class I: Patients with cardiac disease but without resulting limitation of physical activity. Ordinary physical activity does not cause undue anginal pain.

Class II: Patients with cardiac disease resulting in slight limitation of physical activity. They are comfortable at rest. Ordinary physical activity results in anginal pain.

Class III: Patients with cardiac disease resulting in marked limitation of physical activity. They are comfortable at rest. Less than ordinary physical activity causes anginal pain.

[a]*Source:* New York Heart Association (1964)

Class IV: Patients with cardiac disease resulting in inability to carry on any physical activity without discomfort. Symptoms of anginal pain may be present even at rest. If any physical activity is undertaken, symptoms are increased.

Congestive Heart Failure

Class I: Patients with cardiac disease but without resulting limitation of physical activity. Ordinary physical activity does not cause undue fatigue, palpitation, or dyspnea.
Class II: Patients with cardiac disease resulting in slight limitation of physical activity. They are comfortable at rest. Ordinary physical activity results in fatigue, palpitation, or dyspnea.
Class III: Patients with cardiac disease resulting in marked limitation of physical activity. They are comfortable at rest. Less than ordinary physical activity causes fatigue, palpitation, or dyspnea.
Class IV: Patients with cardiac disease resulting in inability to carry out any physical activity without discomfort. Symptoms of cardiac insufficiency may be present even at rest. If any physical activity is undertaken, symptoms are increased.

APPENDIX B. PROBABILITIES ASSESSED

A. *Immediate Sequelae Following Surgery* (node Ⓑ in Figure 21-1)

1. *Surgical mortality:* The probability of death within 30 days of surgery.
2. *Nonfatal myocardial infarction:* The probability of an MI within 30 days of surgery, given that the patient survived 30 days.
3. *Other major complications:* The probabilities of other major complications (stroke; others including acute renal failure, severe pulmonary embolism, hemorrhage, and infection) conditional on whether or not an MI occurred in the postoperative period.
4. *Chronic severe limitation due to stroke:* The probability, given a postoperative stroke, that chronic severe limitation will ensue.

	Patient Number				
Probability of	*1*	*2*	*3*	*4*	*5*
1. Surgical Mortality	.05	.05	.50	.04	.03
2. Nonfatal MI	.05	.10	.20	.10	.05
3. Major Complications					
Given no MI	.010	.010	.03	.010	.010
Given MI	.015	.015	.05	.015	.015
4. Chronic Limitation Given Major Complication	.20	.20	.30	.20	.20

B. *Long-Term Outcomes Following Surgery* (node Ⓒ in Figure 21-1)

1. *Angina level in year 1:* The probabilities that the patient will have angina levels A_0, A_1, or A_2 in the first year following surgery, conditional on whether or not an MI occurred in the postoperative period.
2. *Survival following surgery:* The survival curve following surgery, conditional on the occurrence or nonoccurrence of a postoperative MI and on the level of angina in year 1.
3. *Angina level in years 2-5:* The probabilities of each level of angina in years 2-5, conditional on the level of angina in the first year.
4. *Angina level in years 6 and beyond:* The probabilities of each level of angina in years 6 and beyond, conditional on the level of angina in years 2-5.

With Surgery, Probability of	*Patient Number*				
	1	*2*	*3*	*4*	*5*
1. Angina, Year 1					
Given No MI					
A_0	.85	.80	.70	.95	.70
A_1	.12	.18	.05	.04	.25
A_2	.03	.02	.25	.01	.05
Given MI					
A_0	.85	.80	.70	.95	.70
A_1	.12	.18	.05	.04	.25
A_2	.03	.02	.25	.01	.05

	Patient Number														
	1			*2*			*3*			*4*			*5*		
	Angina, Year 1			*Angina, Year 1*			*Angina, Year 1*			*Angina, Year 1*			*Angina, Year 1*		
With Surgery, Probability of	A_0	A_1	A_2	A_0	A_1	A_2	A_0	A_1	A_2	A_0	A_1	A_2	A_0	A_1	A_2
2. Survival															
Year 1															
No MI	.95	.93	.82	.96	.94	.90	.70	.60	.50	.97	.95	.90	.97	.97	.94
MI	.92	.90	.75	.95	.93	.88	.60	.55	.40	.95	.94	.88	.96	.96	.93
Year 2 (Given Year 1)[a]															
No MI	.97	.95	.90	.97	.95	.92	.80	.75	.60	.97	.96	.92	.98	.98	.95
MI	.96	.95	.90	.96	.95	.92	.75	.70	.60	.96	.95	.91	.98	.98	.95
Year 5 (Given Year 1)															
No MI	.85	.78	.63	.85	.78	.69	.39	.30	.12	.85	.82	.69	.89	.89	.78
MI	.82	.78	.63	.82	.78	.69	.30	.23	.12	.82	.80	.66	.89	.89	.78
3. Angina, Years 2–5															
A_0	.74	.10	.10	.80	.05	.02	.70	.20	.05	.80	.05	.05	.70	.05	.05
A_1	.20	.60	.20	.15	.80	.18	.05	.50	.05	.15	.80	.15	.20	.80	.10
A_2	.06	.30	.70	.05	.15	.80	.25	.30	.90	.05	.15	.80	.10	.15	.85
4. Angina, Years 6+	*Angina, Yr 2-5*			*Angina, Yr 2-5*			*Angina, Yr 2-5*			*Angina, Yr 2-5*			*Angina, Yr 2-5*		
	A_0	A_1	A_2	A_0	A_1	A_2	A_0	A_1	A_2	A_0	A_1	A_2	A_{06}	A_1	A_2
A_0	.60	.05	.02	.70	.05	.02	.70	.10	.05	.80	.05	.03	.85	.05	.05
A_1	.30	.60	.10	.25	.80	.13	.05	.60	.05	.15	.80	.12	.10	.85	.10
A_2	.10	.35	.88	.05	.15	.85	.25	.30	.90	.05	.15	.85	.05	.10	.85

[a]Originally, it was planned to assess survival before assessing angina in year 1, but practical experience indicated that it is easier to first assess levels of angina following surgery and conditional on that, survival.

C. *Outcomes with Medical Management* (node Ⓓ in Figure 21-1)
   1. *Survival.*
   2. *Angina level in years 2-5* (angina in year 1 is given by current angina level).
   3. *Angina level in years 6 and beyond* (conditional upon angina in years 2-5).

With Medical Management, Probability of	*Patient Number* 1	2	3	4	5
1. Survival					
Year 1	.97	.96	.50	.96	.92
Year 2 (given Yr 1)	.97	.96	.60	.96	.92
Year 5 (given Yr 1)	.85	.82	.12	.82	.69
2. Angina, Yrs 2-5					
A_0	.10	.05	.05	.70	.05
A_1	.60	.80	.05	.25	.10
A_2	.30	.15	.90	.05	.85

3. Angina, Years 6+	*Angina, Yrs 2-5* (Patient 1)			*Angina, Yrs 2-5* (Patient 2)			*Angina, Yrs 2-5* (Patient 3)			*Angina, Yrs 2-5* (Patient 4)			*Angina, Yrs 2-5* (Patient 5)		
	A_0	A_1	A_2	A_0	A_1	A_2	A_0	A_1	A_2	A_0	A_1	A_2	A_0	A_1	A_2
A_0	.60	.05	.02	.70	.05	.02	.70	.10	.05	.80	.05	.03	.85	.05	.05
A_1	.30	.60	.10	.25	.80	.13	.05	.60	.05	.15	.80	.12	.10	.85	.10
A_2	.10	.35	.88	.05	.15	.85	.25	.30	.90	.05	.15	.85	.05	.10	.85

APPENDIX C. UTILITY ANALYSIS

First, it is assumed that length of life (i.e., survival or remaining life years) is *utility independent* of quality of life. This means that preference for lotteries over length of life (Y) with the vector of quality attributes (**Q**) held at a fixed level $\mathbf{Q}_0$ are identical, regardless of the amount of $\mathbf{Q}_0$. In other words, the choice between two survival curves (or lotteries on length of life) does not depend on the level of angina. This is a reasonable assumption as long as quality cannot become "worse than death."

The following numerical example illustrates the meaning of utility independence. Consider a 50-50 lottery between living 10 years with class I or II angina (A_1) and 2 years with Class I or II angina. This lottery is usually written

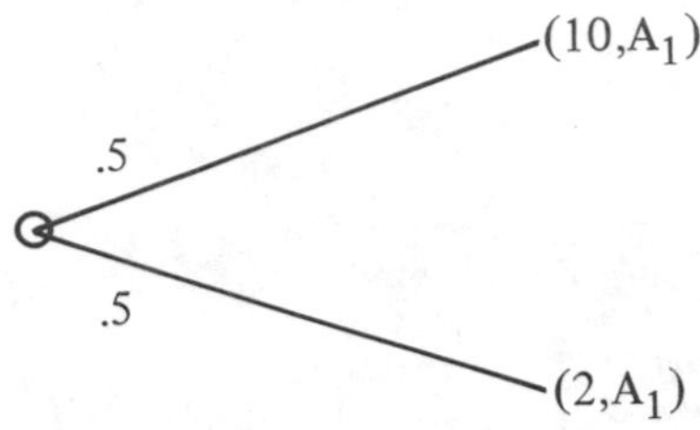

Assume that for a given patient (or other decision maker) the certainty equivalent for this lottery is $(5,A_1)$, (i.e., the patient is indifferent between living 5 years with angina A_1 for certain and participating in the above lottery). Now suppose the common quality level is changed to A_0 (no angina) or A_2 (class III or IV angina). If life years are utility independent of quality, then the certainty equivalent must be $(5,A_0)$ or $(5,A_2)$, respectively. If, for any lottery of the form given above (i.e., with a fixed level of quality), the certainty-equivalent length of life depends only on the survival possibilities and not on the (common) quality level, then utility independence is verified.

Second, it is assumed that quality of life is utility independent of life years. This means that the choice between two lotteries on quality of life with fixed length of life does not depend on the specific length of life involved. This should hold for all possible lengths of life and any combination of quality levels.

These two assumptions were not invoked arbitrarily. In another clinical setting, kidney dialysis and transplantation, these assumptions afforded a realistic expression of the considered preferences of one clinician (Pliskin and Beck, 1976). They were also accepted by several physicians in informal interviews referring to the specific context of coronary bypass surgery.

Together, these two assumptions (mutual utility independence) imply (Raiffa, 1969) that the utility function is of the form

$$u(Y,\mathbf{Q}) = af(Y) + bg(\mathbf{Q}) + (1-a-b)f(Y)g(\mathbf{Q}). \tag{1}$$

The forms of $f(Y)$ and $g(\mathbf{Q})$ were derived from some further assumptions. The function $f(Y)$ was taken to be simply Y, so that life expectancy serves as a summary index of a survival curve. The function $g(Q)$ was derived by first defining functions $g_1(Q_1)$, $g_{2\text{-}5}$ $(2_{2\text{-}5})$ and $g_{6+}(Q_{6+})$ for each of the three arbitrary periods of life. The value of $g_i(Q_i)$ was equal to unity for angina level A_0 and to zero for angina level A_2. The value π for the intermediate level A_1 is such that the lottery

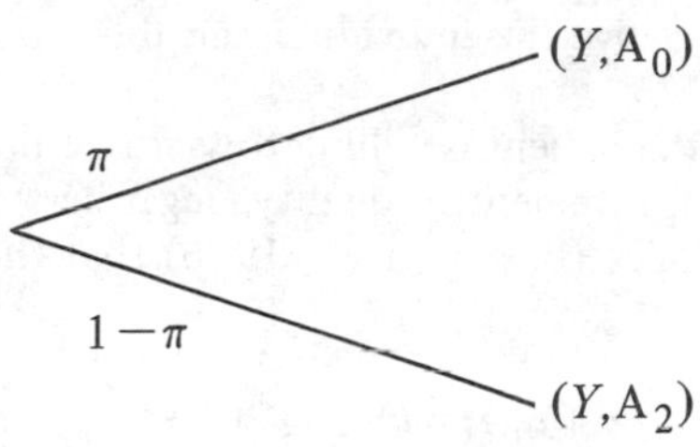

is considered indifferent to a certainty of (Y,A_1). In the analysis, $\pi = .95$ for a sedentary patient, and $\pi = .80$ for an active patient. The aggregate function $g(Q)$ is defined as the weighted average of utility for quality of life over the lifetime of Y years, as follows:

$$\frac{1}{Y}\,[\min(1, Y)g_1(Q_1) + \min(4, \max(Y-1,0))g_{2\text{-}5}(Q_{2\text{-}5}) + \max(Y-5,0)g_{6+}(Q_{6+})]\,,$$

where min and max denote the minimum and maximum of the subsequent pairs of expressions. The first term is quality in the first year, the second term is quality in years two through five and the third term is quality in years six and beyond, each being weighted by the proportion of life falling into the corresponding period.

The weights a and b in the utility function (1) were derived as follows.

If the patient (or decision maker) were indifferent between the two lotteries

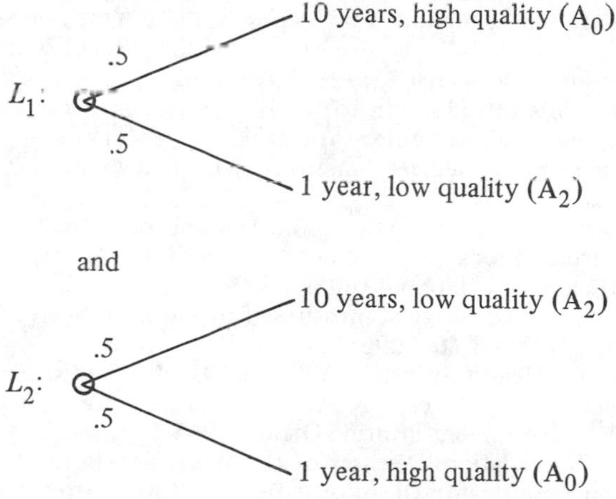

then $a + b = 1$, and therefore, u(Y,Q) would be purely additive (Raiffa, 1969). If this were the case, it would be said that *marginality* held between life years and quality (i.e., only the marginal probability distributions mattered). However, our experience has demonstrated that most people tend to prefer L_1 over L_2. This implies (Raiffa, 1969) that $a + b < 1$. The constants a and b will depend heavily on the individual's preferences for activity, the value of b being larger relative to a the more active the individual and the more the individual values relief from pain.

The assumption that the patient is willing to sacrifice the same proportion P of life years for a given improvement in quality, regardless of the number of years involved (see text), implies (Pliskin et al., 1976) that the utility function is of the form

$$u(Y,Q) = (1-P)Y + PY\bar{Q},$$

where $\bar{Q}$ is the weighted average of quality over the lifetime. This is equivalent to the original formulation (equation 1) in which $a = 1-P$ and $b = 0$. Thus, when $P = 1$, $a = b = 0$ and quality is valued as highly as life itself. In the analysis, $P =$ 0.3 for a sedentary patient, and $P = 0.2$ for an active patient.

Acknowledgments

The authors wish to thank Mr. Matthew Farber for his able assistance in data processing and computer programming, and also Drs. Peter Braun, Peter Cohn, Robert Johnson, and John Lamberti. Finally, we wish to thank the Editors for their thoughtful reviews and helpful suggestions.

References

Acton J: Evaluating Public Programs to Save Lives: The Case of Heart Attacks. R-950-RC. Santa Monica, California, Rand Corporation, 1973

Cannom DS, Miller DC, Shumway NE, et al.: The long-term follow-up of patients undergoing saphenous vein bypass surgery. Circulation 49:77, 1974

Fishburn PC, Keeney RL: Generalized utility independence and some implications. Operations Research 23:928, 1975

Forst BE: A Doctor's Introduction to Decision Analysis. Professional Paper No. 82. Arlington, Virginia, Center for Naval Analyses, 1971

Hiatt HH: Protecting the medical commons: Who is responsible? N Engl J Med 293:235, 1975

McNeer JF, Starmer CF, Bartel AG, et al.: The nature of treatment selection in coronary artery disease: Experience with medical and surgical treatment of chronic disease. Circulation 49:606, 1974

Mundth ED, Austen WG: Surgical measures for coronary heart disease (third of three parts). N Engl J Med 293:124, 1975

National Center for Health Statistics. Vital and Health Statistics, Series 11, No. 10, Coronary Heart Disease in Adults, United States—1960–1962. Washington, DC, Government Printing Office, 1965

New York Heart Association. Diseases of the Heart and Blood Vessels: Nomenclature and Criteria for Diagnoses. Boston, Little, Brown and Co., 1964

Pliskin JS, Beck CH, Jr: A health index for patient selection: A value function approach—with application to chronic renal failure patients. Management Science 22:1009, 1976

Pliskin JS, Shepard DS, Weinstein MC: Utility Functions for Life Years and Health Status. Working Paper. Center for the Analysis of Health Practices, Harvard School of Public Health, 1976

Pliskin JS, Stason WB, Weinstein MC, et al.: Coronary Artery Bypass Surgery: Analyses of Clinical Decision-Making, Resource Allocation, and Priorities for Clinical Investigation. Working Paper. Center for the Analysis of Health Practices, Harvard School of Public Health, 1975

Raiffa H: Decision Analysis: Introductory Lectures on Choice Under Uncertainty. Reading, Massachusetts, Addison-Wesley, 1968

Raiffa H: Preferences for Multiattributed Alternatives. RM- 5868- DOT/RC. Rand Corporation, Santa Monica, California, 1969

Schelling TC: The Life You Save May Be Your Own, Problems in Public Expenditure Analysis. Edited By S Chase. Washington, DC, The Brookings Institution, 1968

Schwartz WB, Gorry GA, Kassirer JP, et al.: Decision analysis and clinical judgment. Am J Med 55:459, 1973

Wechsler AS, Sabiston DC, Jr: The Effectiveness of Coronary Bypass Grafts in Managing Myocardial Ischemia, Controversy in Internal Medicine II. Edited by FJ Ingelfinger, RV Ebert, M Finland, AS Relman. Philadelphia, WB Saunders, 1974

Weinstein MC, Stason WB: Hypertension: A Policy Perspective. Cambridge, Massachusetts, Harvard University Press, 1976

Weisbrod BC: Economics of Public Health, Philadelphia, University of Pennsylvania Press, 1961

22

The cost of intensive care

Henrik H. Bendixen

Today most patients in respiratory failure survive. Twenty years ago the great majority died. We now treat many more patients with respiratory failure than in the past, mostly in intensive care units. Twenty years ago such units were almost unknown. Now virtually every acute care hospital has at least one intensive care unit.

Despite the lives saved and the almost explosive growth of these units, they have remained under constant scrutiny and criticism. In view of the high cost of this care, such scrutiny is reasonable. With the intensive use of manpower, technology, laboratory tests, blood products, and other resources, the cost is inevitably high. Even when the patient survives, it is natural to ask if the same result could have been achieved at less cost. When the patient dies, critics are quick to suggest a misuse of resources in a hopeless cause.

Many physicians have been critical of intensive care units, in part because they claim such a large share of a hospital's resources, in part because the intensive care unit, with its own medical staff, departs from the classic "one patient to one physician" relationship.

Intensive care has been called dehumanizing, even when successful. When the patient dies in the face of maximum therapeutic effort, questions are raised about infringement upon the dignity of dying. In a review of the National Health Service of Great Britain, Cochrane (1972) urged examination of the effectiveness and efficiency of medical care. When discussing heroic efforts for the hopelessly ill, he quoted Agatha in T.S. Eliot's *The Family Reunion* who also wanted action,

> Not for the good that it will do
> But that nothing may be left undone
> On the margin of the impossible.

In answering our critics we often take recourse to the anecdote, knowing that no one will question the application of intensive care for three months to the patient with polyradiculitis: say a young girl, or a mother of small children. This is a reversible disease. The paralysis will recede if the patient can be kept alive during the course of the disease. This requires artificial breathing combined with meticulous nursing care and nutrition to avoid superimposed infection and other hazards. With this disease we succeed most of the time and are almost never questioned when embarking on such treatment. The weight of emotion, when combined with the available data, makes it "unthinkable" not to use all available resources in a maximum effort to save these lives.

From the recent past I remember two patients vividly: both were men over seventy years of age with severe tetanus, both requiring the use of curare more or less continuously for a month (to prevent the muscle contractions and convulsions); and both needing mechanical respiration for more than a month. In view of the known high mortality of the disease and the advanced age of the patients, was it a poor use of costly resources to undertake the treatment? As it happens, both men were treated, and both survived and had complete recoveries.

At regular intervals we provide expensive treatment of patients with severe alcoholic liver cirrhosis. Many of these patients die during the hospital stay or shortly thereafter. We continue to question whether this expenditure of resources is justified. Since no one has given a good answer, we continue the expenditure.

Whatever emotional views we have, hard data are lacking, certainly in the form of the controlled clinical trial and established cost-benefit ratio. Since the polio epidemics of the 1950s, I have wished to know what we are doing and how well. A desire to carry out statistical analysis sounds easy to satisfy, but the progress has been slow. Our first such effort (Bendixen et al., 1965) (see Table 22-1) subdivided our patient population into "homemade" categories and looked at survival overall and by category. At that time we did not look at outcome in any way other than as survival, and long-term follow-up was done only sporadically. We were aware of the high cost of this care but made no attempt at systematic quantification.

By necessity intensive care units are small, and disease or patient categories many. In order to allow valid comparisons, data must be collected over a long period of time or from many units, with all the inherent difficulty and high cost. My hope in undertaking an examination of the cost of intensive care was to find out how much the cost-benefit ratio varies from one patient category to another by examining actual patient data, including outcome and cost information. The published information was insufficient for this purpose. Therefore, my examination is presented in a "model system" for which I make no stronger claim than that it is plausible and consistent with what data we have.

Table 22–1. Patients requiring respirator support for more than twenty-fours,* treated in the Respiratory Unit of the Massachusetts General Hospital between Oct. 1, 1961 and Dec. 31, 1964.

Category	*% Survivors*	*Mean age in years*	*Number of patients*	*Number of survivors*
Abdominal surgery	37	63	57	21
Cardiopulmonary bypass	52	46	52†	27
Drug ingestion	90	36	41	37
Neurosurgery	56	38	36	20
Miscellaneous	58	47	36	21
Thoracic and abdominal aortic aneurysms	45	65	33	15
Neuromuscular diseases‡	66	50	29	19
Flail chest injuries	75	42	24	18
Thoracic surgery	36	54	22	8
Chronic lung disease	68	63	19	13
Thymectomy for myasthenia gravis	100	29	18	18

*The average duration of stay in the Respiratory Unit was twelve days.
†Includes 11.2% of all patients undergoing open heart surgery at the hospital from Oct. 1, 1961, to Dec. 31, 1964.
‡Excludes thymectomy for myasthenia gravis.
(Adapted from: H.H. Bendixen, et al., *Respiratory Care.* C.V. Mosby Company Publishers, St. Louis, 1965.)

THE MODEL EXERCISE

The aim of the model study is to examine patient costs and benefits by disease groups for the purpose of arriving at the dollar cost of achieving survival. Since longevity generally is considered a benefit, we shall extend the model exercise to view the cost in relation to predicted remaining life span. For the purpose of calculating the intensive care cost, C, of making one patient live one year after discharge, the following equation is used:

$$C = \frac{\text{cost per day} \times \text{duration of stay}}{\text{survival fraction} \times \text{predicted remaining life span}} \tag{1}$$

where the numerator gives the total cost in dollars; where in the denominator the survival fraction gives the fraction of the total number of patients in the disease group who survived the hospitalization (they survived the acute trauma or illness); and where the predicted remaining life span gives the number of years that the average survivor may be expected to live once discharged from the hospital.

Clearly, the in-hospital cost given in the numerator does not represent the total cost of an illness, nor is it supposed to. As one examines the various groups, it becomes apparent that costs, other than intensive care costs, whether these are alternative or additional costs, are lowest in those groups of patients that have the most favorable cost-benefit relation; while in those groups in which the cost of making one patient survive one year is very high, the additional or alternative costs are also very high. Enoch Powell (1966) referred to this phenomenon as a multiplier effect, the expensive treatments preserving lives which will demand further expensive treatment.

We simply wish to examine the cost of the critical and expensive effort at a crucial time in the course of the illness. The assumption is made that the "credit" for survival belongs to the intensive care unit; and also that the alternative to intensive care is demise. I recognize that the care alternative to intensive care also carries a definite cost. Strictly speaking, we should examine the difference in cost between intensive care and its alternative. The latter is highly variable, and I have chosen to ignore it. In this study the main point is to reveal the variation of intensive care cost from one patient group to another.

This approach assumes not only that survival is a benefit, but also that survival value is a multiple of survival time; i.e., that two years of survival has twice the value of one year of survival. In time, we shall have to consider also the quality of life after survival of critical illness or trauma and express such quality in quantitative terms. We need both objective data, such as ability to return to work, and subjective data, such as a rating of the quality of life by the survivor himself (see Chapter 10 for further discussion of subjective data and long-term follow-up of quality of life). We turn now to examples.

THE PATIENT WITH BARBITURATE OVERDOSE

The patient with a barbiturate overdose (or similar fairly simple drug overdose) has the following characteristics: short hospital stay and relatively low cost per day, because comparatively few laboratory tests and blood products are needed. The in-hospital survival is very high. In fact, it is rather unusual for the barbiturate overdose patient not to survive as long as brain damage has not occurred prior to arrival at the hospital. The predicted remaining life span is considerable, because the typical patient is young and because recurrence of attempted suicide is not excessive. We are concerned with the patient with an overdose sufficient to stop spontaneous breathing. In this patient, the alternative to intensive care with respirator support is prompt demise. In this case, the in-hospital cost of nonintensive care would be very low.

In Figure 22-1a we present data and a calculation for the patient with barbiturate overdose. I should point out that we have no firm data on remaining life span. It is easy enough to find tables giving predictions of remaining life span for any given age group, but it is difficult to know the extent to which the recovery from illness or trauma is complete. Generally speaking, the data seem the most reliable for the groups with the most favorable cost-benefit relation. We observe that something less than $100 worth of intensive care buys a year of life for one patient. Figure 22-1b shows the effect of varying the factors in the equation, the point being that it takes large changes in the denominator to change cost by a factor of ten.

Figure 22–1a. Barbiturate overdose.

Hospital Cost per Day	$600
Length of Stay	4 days
Survival	95%
Life Span Remaining	30 years

Hospital Cost per Year Saved

$$\frac{600 \times 4}{30 \times .95} = \$84 \text{ per year}$$

In this figure, as in Figures 22–2, 3, 4, and 5, the hospital cost per day has been rounded off to the nearest $100 and the survival and life span to the next lower multiple of 5. The respective numbers are entered into Equation (1) to give the estimated dollar cost per additional year of life following the episode of intensive care.

THE PATIENT WITH POLYRADICULITIS

This patient is also relatively young, but the duration of treatment is a few months instead of a few days. The cost per day is low, because of the modest need for laboratory work, blood, and blood products. The survival is very high and the degree of recovery very good indeed, resulting in a long predicted remaining life span. The data are given in Figure 22–2, and we observe that the expenditure of more than $100 but less than $1000 will buy a year of life for one patient.

THE PATIENT WITH MULTIPLE TRAUMA

This patient is typically on the young side of middle age, although the age distribution varies somewhat from hospital to hospital. The hospital stay is of variable duration, but the average is long. The cost per day is high because of the need for many laboratory tests and blood products. The in-hospital survival may vary from one intensive care unit to another, depending on the type of trauma which predominates as well as other patient characteristics, but it is consistently better than 50%. In this category, the long-term survival (life span remaining) prediction is particularly soft. Figure 22-3 gives data showing that providing one year of life for one patient requires the expenditure of more than $1000, but less than $10,000.

THE PATIENT WITH ABDOMINAL CATASTROPHE

Nearly everyone reporting on survival in the intensive care unit will refer with dismay to a group of patients with a survival which year after year remains poor

Figure 22–1b. Barbiturate overdose.

$$\frac{600 \times 4}{30 \times .95} = \$84 \text{ per year}$$

Variations

cost per day

$$\frac{400 \times 4}{30 \times .95} = \$56 \text{ per year} \qquad \frac{800 \times 4}{30 \times .95} = \$112 \text{ per Year}$$

Length of Stay

$$\frac{600 \times 3}{30 \times .95} = \$63 \text{ per Year} \qquad \frac{600 \times 6}{30 \times .95} = \$126 \text{ per Year}$$

Survival

$$\frac{600 \times 4}{30 \times .98} = \$82 \text{ per Year} \qquad \frac{600 \times 4}{30 \times .5} = \$160 \text{ per Year}$$

Longevity

$$\frac{600 \times 4}{40 \times .95} = \$63 \text{ per Year} \qquad \frac{600 \times 4}{20 \times .95} = \$126 \text{ per Year}$$

Extremes

low cost

$$\frac{400 \times 3}{40 \times .98} = \$32 \text{ per Year}$$

high cost

$$\frac{800 \times 6}{20 \times .5} = \$480 \text{ per Year}$$

At the top of the figure is shown the cost equation from Figure 1a. Under "variations" is shown the effect of changing one factor at a time. The point to be made is that each factor may be varied substantially without driving the cost per additional year of life above $1000.

despite all efforts and while improvements are made in other areas. Perhaps unfairly, we refer to this patient category as "postoperative." What we are referring to is a very small group of patients, among large numbers of postoperative patients, who have or contract an abdominal catastrophe (for example a perforated viscus or gastrointestinal bleeding), who are usually old and otherwise debilitated, who have or contract an infection, or who are nutritionally depleted, bordering on starvation. In this small group, often admitted to the intensive care unit as a desperate last effort, the hospital cost per day is high, the stay is relatively long,

Figure 22-2. Polyradiculitis.

Hospital Cost per Day	$300
Length of Stay	60 days
Survival	95%
Life Span Remaining	30 years

Hospital Cost per Year Saved

$$\frac{300 \times 60}{30 \times .95} = \$632 \text{ per Year}$$

Figure 22-3. Multiple trauma.

Hospital Cost per Day	$1000
Length of Stay	60 days
Survival	65%
Life Span Remaining	15 years

Hospital Cost per Year Saved

$$\frac{1000 \times 60}{15 \times .65} = \$6153 \text{ per year}$$

the survival poor, and longevity among survivors short. The calculation is presented in Fig. 22-4; not surprisingly it requires the expenditure of more than $10,000 but less than $100,000 to buy one year of life for one patient.

THE PATIENT WITH HEPATO-RENAL FAILURE

It is likely that the patient with hepatic failure, associated with varying degrees of renal failure, is near the extreme in contrast between in-hospital cost and outcome. The typical patient is a man in or just past middle age, whose hepatic cirrhosis (on the basis of alcohol overuse) is far advanced and complicated by failure of the kidneys in addition to the liver failure. His hospital stay is often long and the price per day very high because of many laboratory tests and a high usage of plasma and other blood products. The in-hospital survival is poor and the remaining life span disappointingly short. Figure 22-5 shows the startling

Figure 22-4. Abdominal catastrophe.

Hospital Cost per Day	$1200
Length of Stay	30 days
Survival	20%
Life Span Remaining	3 years

Hospital Cost per Year Saved

$$\frac{1200 \times 30}{3 \times .2} = \$60{,}000 \text{ per year}$$

Figure 22-5. Hepato-renal failure.

Hospital Cost per Day	$1200
Length of Stay	30 days
Survival	20%
Life Span Remaining	1 year

Hospital Cost per Year Saved

$$\frac{1200 \times 30}{1 \times .2} = \$180{,}000 \text{ per year}$$

proposition that it may require the expenditure of something in excess of $100,000 to buy one year of life for one patient. Freely admitting that one is calling for a value judgment, one may ask also about the quality of that year.

COMPARISON OF COSTS

In order to examine cost differences among patients in greater detail, Table 22-2 and Fig. 22-6 were constructed. The factors in the numerator of equation (1) (i.e., cost per day and duration of stay) appear less powerful than those in the denominator (survival fraction and life span remaining) in determining the dollar cost of making one patient live one year. In Table 22-2 and Fig. 22-6 the numerator is held constant at an intermediate cost per hospital stay of $7200 (12 days at $600 per day). This allows the graphical display in Fig. 22-6 of the influence of survival fraction (or per cent mortality) and predicted life span remaining.

Table 22–2. Hypothetical dollar costs of intensive care per year of survival.

Estimated years of post-hospital survival		*100*	*50*	*25*	*12.5*	*6.25*	*3.125*	*1.5625*	*.7813*
Mortality %	Survival								
0	1.0	72	144	288	576	1152	2304	4608	9215
50	0.5	144	288	576	1152	2304	4608	9215	18430
75	0.25	288	576	1152	2304	4608	9215	18430	36800
87.5	0.125	576	1152	2304	4608	9215	18430	36800	73723
93.75	0.0625	1152	2304	4608	9215	18430	36800	73723	147446
96.875	0.03125	2304	4608	9215	18430	36800	73723	147446	294893
98.4375	0.015625	4608	9215	18430	36800	73723	147446	294893	589786
99.2187	0.007813	9215	18430	36800	73723	147446	294893	589786	1179444

The less influential factors in the numerator of equation (1) are held constant as \$600 cost per day × 12 days' duration of stay = \$7200. This allows examination of the influence of the factors in the denominator: survival fraction (or per cent mortality) and predicted remaining life span. The table gives the numbers used to plot the graphs in Figure 22–6. The values in the table were chosen to allow easy calculation and interpolation. Sample calculation:

$$\frac{7200}{1.0 \times 100} = \$72/\text{year} \qquad (1)$$

The entries indicate the estimated dollar cost (for one episode of intensive care) per year of post-hospital survival.

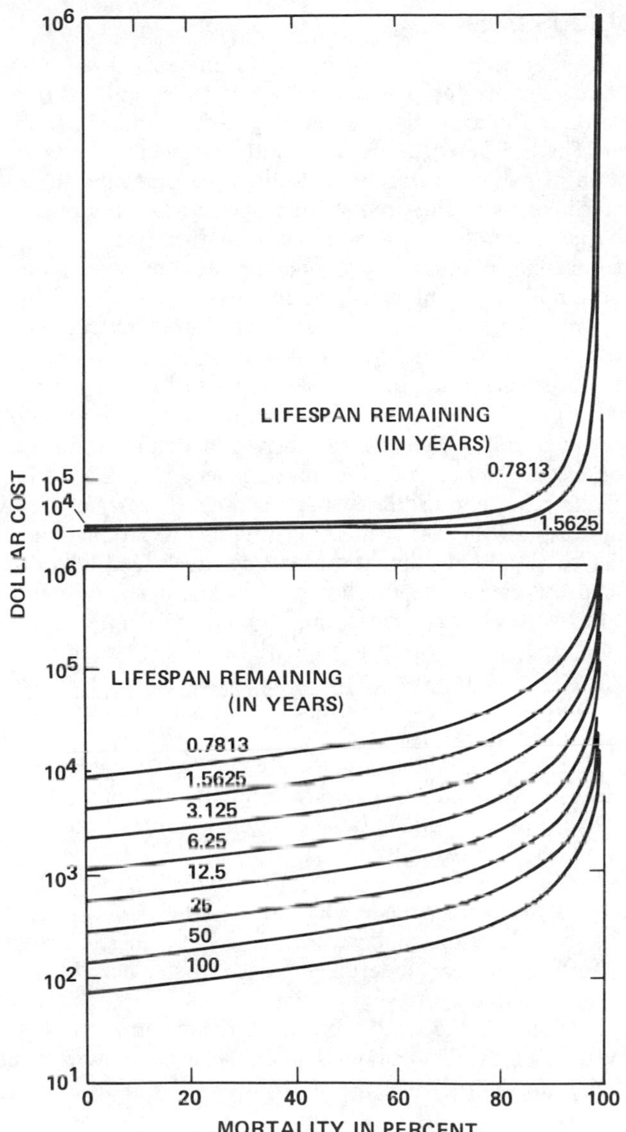

Figure 22-6.
The graphs are constructed using numbers obtained from Table 22-2. In both graphs the dollar cost (for this episode of intensive care) of buying one year of life (of the life span remaining) is on the vertical axis; and the per cent mortality is on the horizontal axis. In the graphs are isopleths representing the various values for life span remaining. Notice that in the upper graph only two isopleths for remaining life span have been plotted because the scale does not allow sufficient separation. Such separation becomes possible in the semilog plot in the lower graph.

DISCUSSION

The model exercise shows that the cost (for one episode of intensive care) of buying one year of life for one patient varies tremendously from one patient group to another. The examples chosen vary a thousandfold from one extreme to the other. These differences are the result of viewing hospital cost in relation to the fraction of patients surviving as well as the predicted life span remaining for the average survivor. The product of a low survival fraction and a short remaining life span accounts for the poor cost-benefit ratios.

The model exercise permits an examination of what varying one or more factors may accomplish. As an example, it would appear that an extra day of hospital stay, in order that the patient with barbiturate overdose may be seen by a psychiatrist, will change the cost-benefit ratio only trivially. And if the risk of recurrence of suicide attempt in fact is reduced by psychiatric attention, the small added cost of the extra day of stay (duration of stay varies only linearly!) may be more than outweighed by an increase in predicted life span remaining.

The use of the semilog scale in the lower panel of Fig. 22-6 allows separation of the isopleths representing life span remaining. The scale used in the upper panel of Fig. 22-6, on the other hand, is intended to produce the visual impression that the total patient population may be subdivided into three parts: one within the narrow area along the horizontal axis; a second within the narrow area along the vertical axis; and a third in the border territory between the horizontal and the vertical axis. Most patient groups, when expressed in this way, may be found in the horizontal area, which may be looked upon as the area of the favorable cost-benefit ratio. By contrast, the vertical area represents unfavorable cost-benefit ratios.

Even though the horizontal area is the area of the favorable cost-benefit ratio, waste here is not precluded and may give accountants and auditors a field day. Philosophically, however, the horizontal area is representative of the patient care efforts which, clearly, must be carried out. It is the task of accountants and auditors to help us do as economically as possible that which we all agree must be done. By contrast, the vertical area is the area representing such unfavorable cost-benefit ratios that we are obliged to question whether such patient-care efforts should be undertaken in the first place. Such efforts are as questionable intellectually as they are financially. It may be unavoidable that, occasionally, the cost-benefit ratio for an individual may be found in the unfavorable (vertical) area. What policy makers need to know is whether identifiable classes or groups of patients are found consistently in the areas of unfavorable cost-benefit ratios.

Among the assumptions used in the model exercises, the most questionable may well be that the alternative to intensive care is demise. The assumption certainly is valid in the case of a substantial barbiturate overdose; and here the cost-benefit ratio is highly favorable. At the other end of the spectrum, in dealing with a patient with hepatorenal failure, it is difficult to prove that survival is better after intensive care than after nonintensive care. Thus, it appears that the more favorable the cost-benefit ratio, the more valid the assumption (analogous, perhaps, to the observation that the cost of application of effective technology is very moderate compared with the cost of using what Thomas (1971) calls "nontechnology" or "halfway technology.")

We should ask when to undertake the heroic effort and for how long. We can predict reasonably well what will happen to 100 patients. For the individual patient we may offer probabilities but never certainty. Because we cannot be certain, the individual physician caring for the individual patient must press on, using all resources available to him, until he is at "the margin of the impossible."

When we think about how far to carry the heroic effort, we need to consider also what our patients want (and their relatives; and "public opinion"). It seems to be the healthy philosopher who is concerned about the "dignity of dying," while patients who survive the heroic effort—at least those with their faculties intact—are almost uniformly pleased with the fact of survival. They may be critical of details in management and personnel (Badger, 1974), but very few would have preferred to die, and the families of patients dying in intensive care units are almost uniformly grateful for the efforts made (Morgan et al., 1973). In my own experience, it is unusual for the patient or his relatives *not* to wish for an all-out effort against unfavorable odds.

In other areas we find a similar strong public opinion in support of the all-out effort categorically applied. What goes into a rescue attempt at sea is enormous in time, resources, and cost; often on "the margin of the impossible." And an airline captain may be fired for not going to the nearest airport promptly when one passenger displays symptoms of what could be a heart attack, at a cost to the airline of thousands of dollars, in addition to inconvenience to many. Such is, apparently, the public opinion on the kind of effort they expect.

I submit that we have worried too much about the heroic effort, perhaps because we have been intimidated by critics. The patient does not want his physician to do what is good for mankind; or for someone's budget. The patient wants his physician to do what is good for *him*, the patient. When responsible for serving and caring for the individual patient, the physician is obliged to make every effort, applying all available resources, until convinced that the battle has been lost; i.e., until he has identified the margin of the impossible for that patient. On the other hand, the physician must not *fail* to identify this margin, to recognize brain death when demonstrably present, and to discontinue "life" support after brain death.

The individual physician, in his efforts to save the individual patient, cannot, and cannot be expected to, consider the allocation of resources. Society and its government, on the other hand, must accept this responsibility, and indeed, the physician, wearing a different hat, must advise society and participate in the decision to limit investments in programs such as intensive care units if the cost-benefit ratio is less favorable than for competing programs—a theme which is developed in Chapter 2 and one which recurs throughout this book.

SUMMARY AND CONCLUSION

Conventional analyses hold intensive care to be expensive. The model exercise has demonstrated a thousandfold difference in cost, from one extreme to the other among intensive care unit patient groups, when cost is expressed as the dollar cost of making one surviving patient live for one year. Intensive care cost is highly variable, and much of that care shows a highly favorable cost-benefit ratio.

References

Badger TL: The physician-patient in the recovery and intensive care units. Arch Surg 109:359, 1974

Bendixen HH, Egbert LD, Hedley-Whyte J, et al: Respiratory Care. St. Louis: CV Mosby Company Publishers, 1965

Cochrane AL: Effectiveness and Efficiency. The Nuffield Provincial Hospitals Trust. Abingdon: Burgess & Son Ltd, 1972

Morgan A, Daly C, Murawski BJ: Dollar and human costs of intensive care. J Surg Res 14:441, 1973

Powell JE: A New Look at Medicine and Politics. London: Pitman Medical Publishing, 1966

Thomas L: Notes of a biology-watcher: The technology of medicine. N Engl J Med 285:1366, 1971

V
SUMMARY, CONCLUSIONS, AND RECOMMENDATIONS

23

Summary, conclusions, and recommendations

John P. Bunker
Benjamin A. Barnes
Frederick Mosteller
John P. Gilbert
Bucknam McPeek
Richard Jay Zeckhauser

At the outset of this book, the authors posed the question, "How can we get the most from the resources we allocate to surgery?" We have examined attributes of a surgical procedure: the medical benefits it provides, the risks to life and health, and the resources it uses. Thus we want to achieve large benefits with small risks for modest cost. An economist might rephrase our original question as "How can we achieve the greatest net medical benefits for a given amount of resources?" Appraising this requires us to appreciate the tradeoffs among the different possible benefits, risks, and costs.

To illustrate the techniques, this volume emphasizes surgical procedures whose risks and costs almost outweighed their benefits because these problems are particularly difficult to study, and they force us to display the methods in detail. We selected for study elective inguinal herniorrhaphy in patients over the age of 65; elective hysterectomy for the relief of moderate or transient symptoms in the absence of demonstrable uterine pathology; elective cholecystectomy for asymptomatic or minimally symptomatic gallstones; and appendectomy for minimal and equivocal symptoms. We further selected coronary artery bypass graft for symptomatic coronary artery disease, the treatment of end-stage renal disease, and a variety of conditions requiring intensive care as examples of surgical care entailing very large costs.

Outcomes of Surgery

The authors used available data to carry out their cost-benefit analyses. These data were largely limited to costs of medical care (both direct and indirect), mortality, and morbidity. Data on costs were often adequate. Information on mortality, however, is limited, for the most part, to knowing whether death and the operation under study occur during a single hospital admission. Death may, and quite often does, occur following discharge, either at home, or on readmission to the same or to a different hospital. Current, routine data do not identify such deaths with the earlier operation. Morbidity as a consequence of treatment is even less well documented; and when the data are available they suffer from incompleteness and inadequate follow-up.

Mortality and morbidity data are essential for an adequate data base to assess the risks and benefits of operations intended to correct an acute, life-threatening condition, such as appendicitis. For many operations, however, the effect on life expectancy may be small, and other issues, such as quality of life, costs, and morbidity become the dominant considerations. Thus, for example, a good risk 49-year-old man is estimated to gain 16 days of life expectancy by undergoing cholecystectomy for minimally symptomatic gallstones, whereas a poor risk 60-year-old woman is estimated to lose 14 days for the same condition. Under these circumstances, we need to know how much the patient was relieved of the symptoms, and how successfully the patient was restored to function. That is, we need to judge the operation in terms of its effect on the quality, as well as on the quantity, of life.

When postoperative survival is the rule, physicians direct the therapeutic effort in the first instance to improvement of the quality of life by the relief of symptoms, disability, discomfort, or dysfunction. Under these circumstances, failure to survive therapeutic efforts intended to improve the quality of life is clearly sufficient evidence of therapeutic failure, but survival alone can hardly be proof of success. Clearly, we need more information about overall outcomes of surgical care, and in particular the long-run effects of surgery on the quality of life.

Professional Uncertainty

Many of the examples of established surgical procedures and specific circumstances treated here were deliberately selected because of uncertainty and disagreement within the medical profession. It is understandable that we find the effects of competing strategies of management—surgical or nonsurgical—on life expectancy to be small, thus helping to explain the existence of uncertainty and the large variations in the rates at which these operations are performed. For example, mortality rates associated with appendectomy appear to be minimally affected by wide variations in appendectomy rates; and this suggests, perhaps surprisingly, that large geographic variations in appendectomy rates (and consequently large variations in the percentage of normal appendices removed) may be consistent with good medical practice, at least as measured by mortality rates, provided that we ignore the cost of hospitalization and morbidity associated with removing normal appendices.

We can only speculate as to whether the large observed geographic variations in other operations (e.g., tonsillectomy, hysterectomy, cholecystectomy, herniorrhaphy) are also consistent with the best health care, since the necessary outcome data are not available. In the absence of such data, it seems plausible that variations are tolerated in part as the result of a relatively flat mortality function. Indeed, it may be, as in the appendectomy example, that flat mortality functions make it possible for us to select alternative therapies in a complicated clinical situation reasonably well in medicine. In those cases where nature requires us to have everything pinpointed perfectly in terms of accurate diagnosis and a specific operation for success, it may be much more difficult to discover and execute a good strategy, costs aside. Thus, some problems may have narrow margins for good practice.

Costs and Resource Allocation

Whether or not these large variations in procedure rates can occur with little or no effect on life expectancy, it is clear that such variations do entail substantially different associated costs in dollars and morbidity. Thus, nationwide policies of appendectomy for narrow indications or for broad indications differ only slightly in the number of expected lives saved or lost, but the substantial difference in morbidity and hospitalization costs is estimated to amount to several million days of patient hospitalization per year. Similar arguments can be made about other operations where the indications are marginal.

Public and professional attitudes toward costs of medical care, to the extent that costs have been considered at all, have frequently taken the view that a human life is priceless, and that no cost can or should be spared in the effort to save life. Whether or not such a position was appropriate in the past, we are now capable of developing lifesaving methods well beyond our capacity to pay for them. Coronary artery bypass surgery or renal transplantation may be treatments for our society as a whole that cost more than we are able or willing to pay. The intensive care unit exemplifies our ultimate skill in prolonging life, sometimes at extraordinary cost. Thus, new medical triumphs create new moral and economic issues.

Society decides, and must decide, what resources to make available for medical care. In the past, for that four-fifths of the total national expenditure for health care which falls outside the federal budget, these decisions have been varied and largely local: the result of professional pressures, public enthusiasms, and economic considerations. In the future, it will be more and more imperative that national priorities be set to assure that allocation of public resources to medical care will be viewed as equitable and appropriate to the public need.

The public or its representatives must determine how much and what types of life-prolonging care will be available for critically ill patients, such as those suffering from end-stage renal disease or from heart disease which might benefit by valve replacement or coronary artery bypass surgery. And if we are willing to provide treatment in a modern intensive care unit for the young patient who has taken an overdose of a barbiturate, but who is in otherwise good health, at costs which may be as low as $100 for each year of life expectancy, should the same treatment be provided for the middle-aged alcoholic suffering from liver and kidney failure? For this unfortunate patient, costs of care are estimated to exceed a rate of $100,000 for a year of additional life and with the usual prospect of additional large expenses in the treatment of subsequent similar episodes of acute illness.

Surgical Innovation

Several authors' efforts were directed initially to assess the current status of a number of established operations and the conditions for which they are performed in order to become familiar with the balance between costs and benefits for each procedure. An equally important task was to determine how these and other surgical therapies were introduced and evaluated—that is, to study the process of surgical innovation.

At the beginning of the twentieth century, pioneering surgeons devised operations primarily on the basis of intuition and insight and assessed them by trial and error. This era produced many brilliant surgical advances as well as a number of operations which were discarded sometimes only after many years of application and after a large cost in dollars, morbidity, and even mortality. In this respect, surgery shared with other branches of medicine at the time a process of groping for effective therapies, a process that did not have the help of extensive knowledge in the basic biological sciences or the understanding of sophisticated experimental designs to permit logical inductions from multivariate clinical circumstances.

Clinical Trials

The randomized controlled trial was not developed until a third of the century had passed, and its application to clinical research in surgery has remained limited to relatively few instances. The reason is not that surgeons have been slow to accept new patterns of thought, but rather the very real conceptual, practical, ethical, and economic difficulties of carrying out in adequate numbers and sizes experiments involving complex surgical procedures in human beings.

However formidable these difficulties, we have learned from our review of surgical experiments in humans that the costs in dollars and in lives of a poor experiment, or of no experiment, are often much greater than those of a well-designed and executed clinical trial. This is dramatically exemplified by the enthusiastic and widespread adoption of gastric freezing for the treatment of duodenal ulcer and of internal mammary artery ligation for relief of angina pectoris. These procedures were promptly discarded following the demonstration of their lack of effect when subjected to randomized clinical trial.

It is not possible or necessary to conduct a randomized clinical trail to evaluate all new operations—and certainly not all old ones. Where the positive effects of a treatment appear to be very large, it would almost certainly be considered unethical to withhold from control patients the treatment which is thought to be superior. When a strong competitor appears, a trial may be justified. Ordinarily, two competitive treatments are compared, rather than a treatment with no treatment. (One investigation mentioned here, though, compared two standard treatments with no treatment, and no treatment was found to be superior.) Where the effect of a treatment or the difference between two treatments is modest, however, a properly controlled comparison is almost certainly necessary to detect the difference and to establish the more advantageous therapy. For some problems, such as the treatment of breast cancer, however, the issue is not just that clinical data are inadequate, but rather that the fundamental biological questions upon which to base rational therapy remain to be answered.

Ethical Considerations

The ethical issue has created much of the controversy about the proper evaluation of surgical, as well as medical, therapy. It is argued, on the one hand, that the patient should not be deprived of the innovation by being in a comparative clinical trial; and, on the other hand, it is argued that, if a treatment is unproven, the patient should not be put at risk with an unproven treatment in a clinical trial. In both arguments, often put simultaneously, the patient is somehow viewed as the loser.

Although these arguments might be turned around, we suggest rather that a different view is in order. From our review of clinical trials in surgery, it is apparent that the patient often does about equally well with alternate treatments, and that large differences between treatments are the exception rather than the rule. The fact that the differences are numerically small does not mean that they are unimportant, only that they are hard to measure. For example, a 5% reduction in deaths is important, clearly, but it does not follow that such an improvement is easy to measure. The great gain comes, of course, when we consistently select for the future those new therapies that come out ahead of the old therapies and drop those that lose.

In reviewing the ethical considerations associated with controlled trials, the authors noted that such considerations were given limited discussion in uncontrolled observational studies, though sometimes these studies seemed to have the same sorts of issues of informed consent and ethical practice as the controlled studies. Perhaps the ethical considerations were given appropriate thought and care but not reported as often. No doubt future papers will have discussion of such matters more frequently. Although some controversy surrounds the randomized clinical trial in current discussions, the fundamental issues have little to do with the technique of randomization, rather they deal with when and under what precautions suitable controlled investigations are to be carried out. These investigations need objectivity, blindness, statistical power, and careful control so that firm inferences can be drawn. Otherwise society may not receive the benefits from innovations.

RECOMMENDATIONS

We make four recommendations dealing with I) the need for further studies of surgical treatments, II) improving and extending our technical ability to do such studies, III) the teaching of economic, social, and epidemiological principles of medical care, and IV) improving the public's understanding of medical outcomes and costs through better presentations.

I. *Studies of surgical treatment.* We no longer have the ability to pay for all the medical care we may be technically able to provide, and so, as a society we increasingly encounter and must face hard decisions on resource allocation. Such allocation, if done rationally, requires at a minimum cost-risk-benefit analyses of the sort described in this book for consideration with other factors. Both decisions on resource allocation and policies about medical treatment are being made in 1977 without the kinds of quantitative analyses we can do using our current skills and resources. Although this omission flows partly from inadequate knowledge of the methods, it flows also from lack of facts, as we have seen repeatedly in this book. When the authors pose a solid question, the analysis brings out the need for specific kinds of information, some of which has not been gathered or is so uncertain that the outcome of the analysis is also left uncertain. And so we know that a variety of studies of surgical facts is needed. More randomized trials are needed and in some instances more observational studies.

In attempting to take fullest advantage of opportunities offered by observational studies, we should note the special opportunities of "natural experiments" such as described in Chapter 7. If, for example, as observed in Vermont for geographically identifiable subpopulations, the frequency of various surgical operations varies markedly both qualitatively and quantitatively, a study of the outcomes and costs of such natural variations in therapy should teach us a good deal concerning their relative effectiveness.

Thus surgery still needs a good deal more of the kind of information that fairly standard scientific approaches to clinical evaluation can give. These can be combined with cost-benefit analyses.

Recommendation I:

Appropriate studies of the effectiveness of surgical treatment should be carried out for selected conditions, particularly those where uncertainty leads to professional disagreement.

II. *Improving techniques for evaluation.* At the same time that studies using currently available methods must go forward, we have seen the need to improve our *ability to conduct* these urgently needed studies. A major problem is our presently inadequate information system. Separate records are kept for each patient by each physician or institution caring for him. In 1977 it is possible to identify outcome as related to an operation or other treatment only if the treatment and the observed outcome occur during a single continuous hospitalization. Even under these circumstances the standard medical record is not designed for easy information retrieval or the pooling of information across patients to study populations. It is frequently nearly impossible to document the treatment and health status found at previous examinations, especially if a different hospital or physician were responsible. Existing data cannot determine long-term outcomes or the end-result of surgery. Thus we are unable to find out, except for selected conditions such as malignant tumors and end-stage renal disease, how many patients survive one or more years after a particular operation. We cannot determine how many patients have been relieved of the condition leading to the operation, or how many have fully recovered from the effects of anesthesia and surgery and been able to return to full, pre-illness activity.

We are now able to perform useful cost-risk-benefit analyses, but present techniques need to be improved; for example, we are probably not sufficiently aware of second order effects or unanticipated consequences of proposed new policies. Perhaps we can learn to anticipate such "unanticipated consequences." Careful work still remains to be done on methodology of experimental design. It is not sufficiently widely recognized how long it takes to design an informative clinical trial or how difficult it is to execute the design once it has been chosen. We do not yet know enough about randomized trials and their consequences, their weaknesses, strengths, and costs compared with their alternatives. We still are not sure enough of when we should trust an observational study. We do not know how to combine epidemiology and observational and experimental information. We have not dealt with the ethical issues surrounding human experimentation and are still shouting at one another from fixed positions. We have not reviewed the complexities of our ethical problems in enough detail or sophistication.

Recommendation II:

Our grasp of the components of cost-benefit analysis and their interrelations, the values of the various data gathering techniques, and our understanding of the ethics of data gathering must be improved by theoretical and empirical work and by continued discussions in the public forums.

III. *Improving medical capabilities for evaluation.* In addition to assessing the efficacy of many existing treatments, we need to develop a policy for the introduction of new medical and surgical technology. Thus among the studies encouraged in Recommendation II, we would include further historical studies of past successes and failures. We call particular attention to two recently published studies. One, the "Study on Surgical Services for the United States" (Orloff et al., 1976), includes a survey of the major surgical advances of the past quarter-century and the research on which these advances were based. The second, entitled "Scientific Basis for the Support of Biomedical Science" (Comroe and Dripps, 1976), examines in detail the research basis for recent advances in the surgical and medical treatment of cardiovascular and pulmonary diseases. Studying only successes or failures can have weaknesses that a balanced approach may avoid.

Even when the technology and data may be available, the current methods need to be more widely understood in the medical research and medical policy communities as well as among medical students and their teachers. Naturally, we cannot expect all to be experts. But physicians themselves must be better educated in the analytic techniques necessary for them to make a more informed discrimination among therapeutic programs or techniques, and they must be educated in the economic, social, and epidemiological principles of medical care which will allow them to participate as leaders of society in advising on or helping to make priority decisions.

Recommendation III:

These principles of cost-benefit evaluation should be included as an integral part of the medical school curriculum; and their application to the assessment of the efficacy of medical care should be incorporated into clinical practice and continuing medical education.

We note in particular that medical students at the beginning of their clinical training may feel little pressure to know much about the design of clinical trials or of policy analysis. Later, when working in the hospital and trying to read and appraise results presented in research papers or in participating in research, knowledge of these matters absorb the young physician's attention. Thus, we stress continuing education.

IV. *Improving public understanding.* In addition to educating itself, the medical community has an obligation to inform the public. Here we would note a distinction made by the sociologist Paul Lazarsfeld between advising and deciding. After data are gathered by good methods and carefully analyzed, the scientist or physician needs to advise the client, here the community, about the findings. The community takes this advice and tempers it with political, legal, social, and moral considerations and then decides. We should improve our advice so that it will be useful in the decision process.

Recommendation IV:

Information on outcomes as well as costs of medical care should be routinely formulated in a manner suitable for presentation to the public.

References

Orloff, MJ et al: Contributions of Surgical Research to Health Care, 1945–1970. Report of the Research Subcommittee of the Study on Surgical Services for the United States. 1976, American College of Surgeons and American Surgical Association

Comroe JH Jr, Dripps RD: Scientific basis for support of biomedical science. Science 192:105, 1976

Index